An Atlas of Amplitude-Integrated EEGs in the Newborn

This new edition updates the definitive clinical atlas textbook on interpreting continuous amplitude-integrated electroencephalography monitoring in neonatal units. It presents a comprehensive instructive overview linking tracings, scans, neuroimaging, real-time tracing clips, and detailed clinical scenarios and is an invaluable guide to all those needing to learn how to use aEEG for the best and safest results. An online quiz is available to enhance training and performance.

This third edition of the aEEG atlas summarizes the experience and evidence of more than 40 years of aEEG monitoring in the newborn and also addresses the development and future of brain monitoring.

Access the Online Question & Answer material at: https://routledgelearning.com/anatlasofamplitude/

Access the Videos at: https://routledgelearning.com/anatlasofamplitude/videos

An Atlas of Amplitude-Integrated EEGs in the Newborn

Third Edition

Edited by
Lena Hellström-Westas MD, PhD
Senior Professor of Perinatal Medicine, Department of Women's and Children's Health
Uppsala University, Sweden

Linda S de Vries MD, PhD
Emeritus Professor in Neonatal Neurology at Utrecht and
Leiden University Medical Center, The Netherlands

Sampsa Vanhatalo MD, PhD
Professor, Departments of Physiology and Clinical Neurophysiology
Children's Hospital, Helsinki University Hospital and University of Helsinki, Finland

With contributions from
Sonia L Bonifacio MD
Medical Director, NeuroNICU, Clinical Professor of Pediatrics
Stanford Medicine Children's Health, California, USA

Mohamed El-Dib MD
Director, Neonatal Neurocritical Care, Brigham and Women's Hospital, Associate Professor of Pediatrics, Harvard Medical School, Boston, Massachusetts, USA

Kathi Salley Randall RN, MSN, CNS, NNP-BC
Synapse Care Solutions, Las Vegas, Nevada, USA

And a Foreword from
Geraldine Boylan PhD, MRIA
Professor of Neonatal Physiology, Department of Paediatrics & Child Health, and Director,
INFANT Research Centre, University College Cork, Ireland

CRC Press
Taylor & Francis Group
Boca Raton London New York

CRC Press is an imprint of the
Taylor & Francis Group, an **informa** business

Third edition published 2025
by CRC Press
2385 NW Executive Center Drive, Suite 320, Boca Raton FL 33431

and by CRC Press
4 Park Square, Milton Park, Abingdon, Oxon, OX14 4RN

CRC Press is an imprint of Taylor & Francis Group, LLC

ISBN: 978-1-032-25850-8 (hbk)
ISBN: 978-1-003-28622-6 (ebk)

DOI: 10.1201/b22858

Typeset in Warnock Pro
by Apex CoVantage, LLC

Access the Online Question & Answer material at: https://routledgelearning.com/anatlasofamplitude/
Access the Videos at: https://routledgelearning.com/anatlasofamplitude/videos

CONTENTS

FOREWORD

It is an honour and a genuine pleasure to introduce the third edition of *An Atlas of Amplitude-Integrated EEGs in the Newborn*. This latest edition, meticulously compiled by three leading authorities in the fields of neonatology, neurology, and neurophysiology—Lena Hellström-Westas, Linda S de Vries, and Sampsa Vanhatalo—marks a significant leap forward in our collective understanding of neonatal brain monitoring and its clinical applications.

Over the years, I have had the distinct privilege of collaborating closely with these three experts. Their unwavering dedication to advancing neonatal care, combined with their pioneering research and clinical expertise, has been a constant source of inspiration. Their collaborative efforts in creating this atlas reflect a deep commitment to improving outcomes for the most vulnerable patients—our newborns.

Since the publication of the second edition, the field of neonatal neurology has continued to evolve at a remarkable pace. The integration of amplitude-integrated EEG (aEEG) into neonatal care has expanded, and its importance in early diagnosis and intervention is now widely recognized. This third edition comes at a crucial time when the demand for accurate, real-time brain monitoring has never been greater. The authors have incorporated the latest advancements in technology, research, and clinical practice to provide a resource that is both comprehensive and practical.

The technological advancements in EEG and aEEG devices, as well as the development of more sophisticated algorithms for signal interpretation, are thoroughly covered. This edition also introduces excellent case studies and extensive illustrations, which greatly enhance the utility of the atlas for clinicians at all levels. The detailed illustrations of normal and pathological aEEG patterns are particularly valuable for those new to the field, offering clear guidance on how to interpret these signals. For seasoned practitioners, these enhancements provide new insights and approaches that can be directly applied in clinical practice.

This edition also expands on the clinical applications of aEEG beyond the traditional focus on hypoxic-ischaemic encephalopathy (HIE) and seizures. The authors explore the use of aEEG in monitoring infants with various metabolic, genetic, and infectious causes of encephalopathy, providing a broader perspective on the utility of brain monitoring in different clinical scenarios. The inclusion of chapters on EEG trends and computational measures reflects the growing role of advanced data analysis in enhancing our understanding of neonatal brain function.

The final chapters of this atlas emphasize the integration of EEG into a broader neurocritical care framework. The authors advocate for a multidisciplinary approach to neonatal care, where continuous brain monitoring plays a central role in decision-making. This holistic perspective is crucial as we continue to strive for better outcomes in neonatal intensive care units (NICUs) around the world.

What makes this third edition particularly valuable are the carefully compiled figures, case studies, and quiz included. These real-life examples not only illustrate the concepts discussed but also provide practical insights into the challenges and nuances of neonatal aEEG interpretation. For clinicians, these visual aids are indispensable tools for honing skills and improving confidence in using aEEG as a diagnostic tool.

In conclusion, the third edition of *An Atlas of Amplitude-Integrated EEGs in the Newborn* is an essential resource for anyone involved in neonatal care. The authors have succeeded in creating a comprehensive, up-to-date, and user-friendly guide that will undoubtedly serve as a cornerstone reference in the field. It is a testament to their expertise and dedication, and I am confident that this atlas will continue to shape the future of neonatal neurocritical care for years to come.

Geraldine Boylan PhD, MRIA
Professor of Neonatal Physiology
Department of Paediatrics & Child Health
Director, INFANT Research Centre
University College Cork, Ireland

aEEG ATLAS: LIST OF ABBREVIATIONS

ASM	anti-seizure medication
ABR	Auditory brainstem response
BSID-III	Bayley Scales of Infant Development, III ed.
BSN	Brain State of the Newborn
CC	Corpus cllosum
EEG	Electroencephalogram
aEEG	amplitude-integrated EEG
aEEG/EEG	aEEG monitoring with continuous display of single- or multichannel EEG
(a)EEG	aEEG and EEG—irrespective of how you display them
cEEG	continuous EEG
CNV	Continuous normal voltage
DNV/DC	Discontinuous normal voltage/discontinuous
BS (+/–)	Burst-suppression (dense/sparse burst appearance)
CLV	Continuous low voltage
FT/ I	Flat/inactive

CFM	Cerebral Function Monitor
CNS	Central nervous system
CT	Computed Tomography
GMFCS	Gross Motor Function Classification System
Hz	Hertz
IBI	interburst interval
ISI	Inter-SAT intervals in seconds
IVH	intraventricular haemorrhage
NIRS	Near-Infrared Spectrosocopy
PVL	Periventricular leukomalacia
SWC	Sleep-Wake Cycling
SAT	Spontaneous Activity Transient
SB	Seizure Burden
SDA	Seizure Detection Algorithm
rSO2	Regional cerebral oxygen saturation
cUS	Cranial ultrasound

1 MONITORING THE NEWBORN BRAIN

Lena Hellström-Westas, Sampsa Vanhatalo and Linda S de Vries

Brain monitoring with amplitude-integrated EEG (aEEG) has since the early 1990s become an important integrated part of neonatal intensive care for continuous evaluation of brain function in high-risk infants. The present practice emerged from a combination of several independent advances over more than two decades: First, there was the development of EEG compression for clinical use of brain monitoring in the intensive care. Second, the aEEG trends became part of the digitally recorded and displayed EEG devices. Third, the rapid advances in the neonatal intensive care units established the need for a continuous surveillance of brain function. This chapter will briefly outline this remarkable history, highlighting steps that led to our current routine of aEEG monitoring showcased from different perspectives in this book.

1.1 History of aEEG

In the late 1960s, the early pioneers of long-term EEG monitoring recorded the signals on paper. They realized that visual assessment of the conventional EEG is not feasible over longer time periods; however, they also understood that the clinically important information is essentially preserved even after reducing much of the complexity in the raw EEG signals. This foundational idea led to the development of Cerebral Function Monitor (CFM), the predecessor of the current aEEG monitors. It was built and tested at the London Hospital by a clinician-engineering team of Dr Pamela F Prior, Mr Douglas E Maynard and Dr Donald F Scott. The early CFM monitors used a hotwire pen on heat-sensitive paper to draw the CFM trend on the paper slip without showing the raw EEG signals (see Figure 1.1A–D), and its primary purpose was to monitor the recovery of brain function after cardiac arrest, and status epilepticus, in adults. A British obstetrician, Dr David A Viniker, showed that CFM recordings could be used also with newborn infants, or even with fetuses during delivery. In the late 1970s, Prof Ingmar Rosén, a neurophysiologist in Lund, Sweden, visited Dr Prior and brought back a CFM device to monitor brain function in rats during experimental hypoglycemia; however, he also started a collaboration with a neonatologist, Prof Nils Svenningsen, to record newborn infants admitted for intensive care. Professor Gorm Greisen in Copenhagen later coined the term "amplitude integrated EEG" (aEEG) in order to more accurately reflect its technical underpinnings and to make it more accessible to the neurophysiological community.

In the 1980s and early 1990s, there was a parallel, increasing interest in studying physiology and pathophysiology in the perinatal brain. A large number of scientific studies were published on neonatal brain function using CFM or EEG devices in several institutions across Europe, US, Japan and New Zealand. They were often combined with other complementary methods of newborn brain assessment, such as measures of brain blood flow and metabolism, or neuroimaging, and a variety of multimodal approaches became incorporated into clinical and research practice.

During the 1990s, the scientific interest increased further for investigating potential interventions and treatments of perinatal brain injury. Several studies demonstrated the high predictive value of the aEEG trends in asphyxiated newborns during the first hours after birth and in very preterm infants with intraventricular hemorrhages. There were also several studies making direct comparison between aEEG trends and reviews of the raw EEG signal, which helped in gaining wider acceptance of the aEEG and in translating the scientific literature across these monitoring modalities.

However, the increasing clinical research interest in monitoring faced a severe challenge when the production and further development of CFM monitors was halted due to limited commercial interests. The situation improved dramatically when Mr Edward (Ted) Weiler (Olympic Medical) developed the first generation of digital CFM monitors that could essentially replace the analog (pen and paper) versions of the CFM known to the pioneering generation. At the same time, digital aEEG monitoring was also made possible in Lund by a young engineer, Mr Lars-Johan Ahnlide, who programmed the computation of an aEEG trend on a laptop computer connected to an EEG amplifier, which became implemented in the Nervus EEG device. These advances changed the availability of aEEG trends dramatically, coinciding perfectly with a wide-scale need as the first clinical studies on hypothermia treatment of asphyxiated infants were initiated. Many other digital EEG systems with an aEEG trend display were soon developed in different countries (e.g. New Zealand, Japan, Italy, the Netherlands, Ireland and Iceland). Currently, aEEG trend is a standard trend option in the digital EEG systems and routinely used by clinicians.

During the first decades of CFM/aEEG practice, it was common to find hesitance and reluctance from neurophysiologists and neurologists trained for a visual EEG review. This was understandable because the early analog CFM devices showed the trend and it was not possible to compare it with the raw EEG signals. However, a large number of studies have now carefully characterized the correspondence between the aEEG trends and the raw EEG signals; moreover, the current aEEG devices always show also the raw EEG signals that need to be used for confirming the aEEG trend interpretation. These advances have brought transparency and understanding, lifting the unneeded conflict between the two initial modalities, and the aEEG trends are now seen as a key aid in assessing long-term neonatal brain monitoring.

1.2 Underpinnings of the CFM/aEEG Success

All the neurophysiologically innovative part was already done in the first analog CFM devices, which drew the trends onto heat-sensitive paper slips, in parallel with the recorded impedance as a measure of electrode contact. Later introduction of the digital aEEG monitors were only about replacing the original analog signal processing by a digital computation, in addition to also showing the full raw EEG signal for comparison purposes. However, it is important to recognize that the different digital aEEG trends are slightly different from each other, which may challenge their direct numerical comparison.

DOI: 10.1201/b22858-1

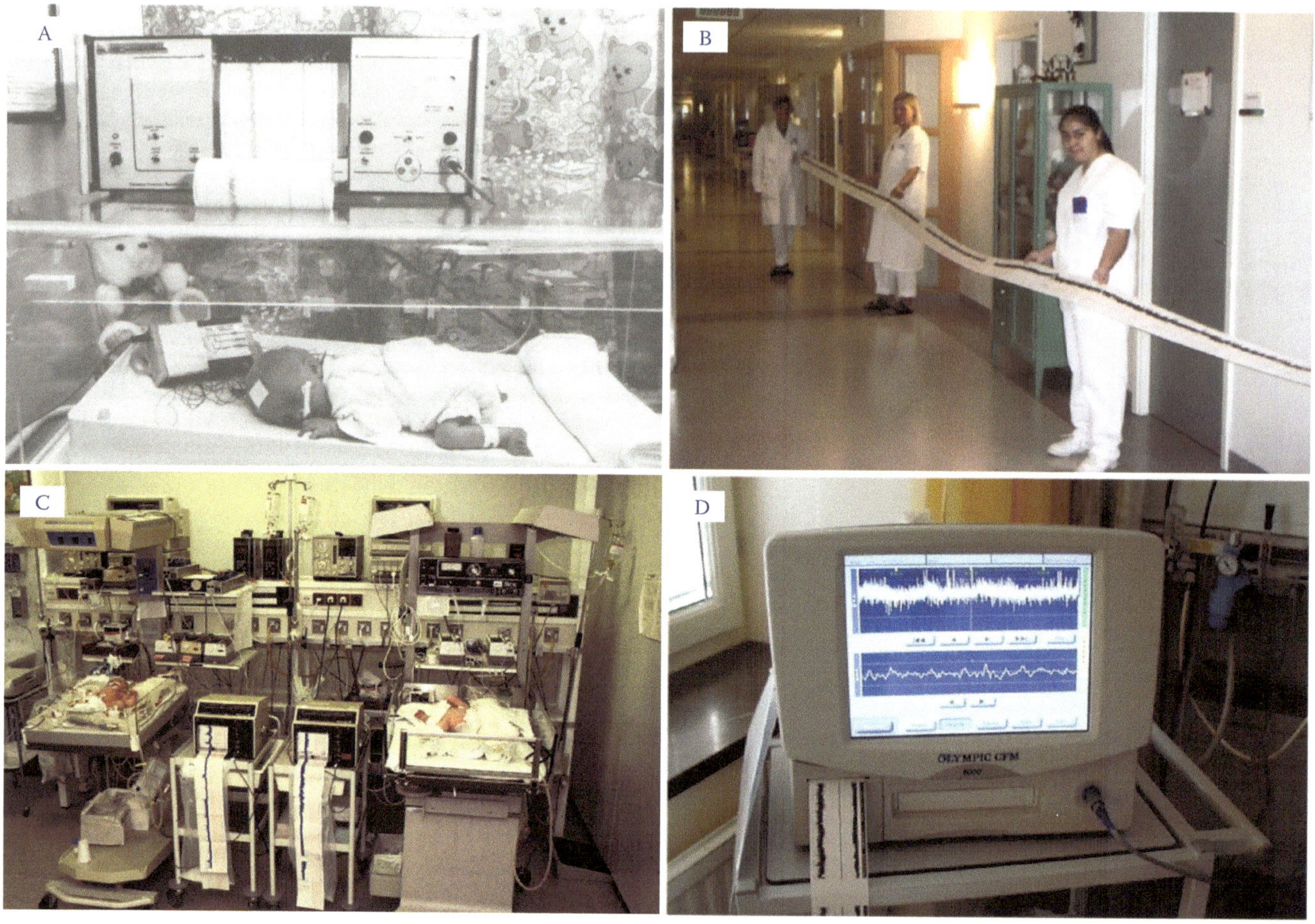

FIGURE 1.1 Early decades of history of CFM/aEEG monitors. **Figure A**, from 1990, shows an early Lectromed™ CFM on top of an incubator. The aEEG recording was continuously written out on heat-sensitive paper with a speed of 6 cm/hour. In parallel, impedance was also recorded. The raw EEG could not be inspected. **Figure B** shows an overview of the aEEG trend in a more than one-week duration, CFM recording. **Figure C** shows clinical monitoring with two CFM 4640 monitors, an updated version of the Lectromed™ CFM, and **Figure D** shows the Olympic™ CFM, a digital device, which recorded and displayed the raw EEG.

The original medtech innovation in the CFM trend was in combining four mutually linked aims into the analog circuits of the first CFM devices: First, the EEG data needed to be time-compressed to give a good overview of trends in brain function over several hours and to allow printing each hour of data to only a few centimeters of paper slip. Second, such time-compression required a strong reduction of the signal characteristics in a way that preserves and emphasizes the clinically important information (for the purpose of monitoring brain recovery and status epilepticus). Third, the EEG artefacts that typically destroy the signal in such clinical contexts (50/60 Hz, muscle activity, respiration, movements) needed to be removed or ignored in some way. Fourth, an analog circuit, the only option by that time, had to be able to perform all these operations.

In the following, these aims are explained in more detail (see also Figure 2.1).

Reduction of EEG signal and artefacts by filtering. The most significant component in aEEG computation is applying an "asymmetric bandpass filter". It keeps information between 2 Hz and 15 Hz so that all information is preserved around 10 Hz while the signal is increasingly attenuated below and above the 2–15 Hz range. This leads to an efficient removal of most NICU-relevant artefacts, both the low-frequency respiration and movement and the high-frequency muscle and 50/60 Hz artefacts. At the same time, the emphasis around the 10 Hz gives prominence to signal components that differentiate between the most important physiological and pathological brain states, such as EEG background, epileptic seizure or sleep state (see Figure 2.1). Unfortunately, such filtering cannot fully remove the interference of many common artefacts (e.g. ECG, high-frequency ventilation, nursing, gasping, movements, muscle activity, other medical devices), and sometimes (e.g. ECG or high-frequency ventilation) the filtering may even emphasize the artefact more than the brain activity (see Chapter 3). Some clinically important low-frequency activity, such as slow seizures, may be also removed by this filtering.

Emphasizing important features by rescaling the amplitudes. After filtering out the unneeded and/or interfering signal components (see previous section), the next step in the aEEG processing is measuring the signal magnitude and emphasizing the smallest signals. The signal magnitude is obtained by "rectification", followed by computing the "signal envelope" (or its height) and its average over the given time window (typically 10 seconds). Then the smallest signals are emphasized by plotting the signal magnitudes to a semi-logarithmic scale, where values are shown in a linear scale between 0 μV and 10 μV and in a logarithmic scale between 10 μV and 100 μV. Consequently, changes in the smallest signals (0–10 μV) become robustly visible, supporting the cornerstones in most clinical aEEG review rules (see Chapter 2).

Time-compression. Time-compression was initially done by slowing down the running speed of the CFM paper slip. The current digital aEEG devices offer more variable and adjustable ways to compute and display the aEEG trends. The user can readily change the number of hours visualized in one page, and some devices may even allow adjusting the time window under each dot in the aEEG trend. Notably, the time resolution in aEEG trends is nowadays defined by both the time window used for aEEG computation (the theoretically available resolution) and the length of the aEEG trend visualized in the screen (perceptual resolution, depending on the number of pixels available in the monitor).

1.3 Absolute Measures vs. Pattern Recognition in the aEEG Interpretation

All aEEG monitoring in the NICU aims to support the infant's clinical care, which requires understanding of the aEEG characteristics that correlate to physiological and pathological mechanisms. In this context, it is important to recognize that there is no clear evidence, neither theoretical nor practical, to claim the best and most optimal ways to use the aEEG trends. It is clear that a heavily time-compressed display improves review of long-term changes (e.g. background recovery after birth asphyxia), but it comes at the cost of losing temporal details (e.g. brief seizures). The initial output from the CFM devices was 6 cm/hour, and it was found to be a good compromise by most clinicians. See Figures 1.3 and 1.4 later. Current digital devices offer wider flexibility (see earlier), which may be helpful in many instances, but it also requires deeper understanding of the way aEEG trends are computed and how they reflect the original EEG characteristics. For everyday monitoring in the NICU, it is usually wise to use a "standardized" time-scale which allows the staff to faster learn and recognize the most common aEEG patterns.

Over recent decades, it has been common to apply fixed numerical thresholds for the aEEG interpretation (e.g. lower and upper border amplitudes) to allow an apparent harmonization across infants and sites. However, it has also become clear that a myriad of common artefacts (e.g. ECG, tiny electrical interference) may severely confound the aEEG amplitudes and even lead to diagnostic errors. Therefore, more recent practice and literature have emphasized the importance of aEEG pattern recognition, which looks at the overall pattern, or shape, of the aEEG trends. For instance, an inactive or burst-suppression background can be easily recognized even if a coincident artefact (e.g. ECG) brings the aEEG amplitudes to the formally "normal" level. Thus, reviewing aEEG by pattern recognition approach can effectively mitigate even severe confounding by trivial artefacts.

Recent introduction of additional trends and machine learning–based analytic tools (e.g. seizure detection algorithms, background measures and sleep state classifiers) may provide significant complementary tools for the EEG-based monitoring (see Chapter 8). Although new EEG trends and seizure-detection alarms can be very useful, another important option in some monitoring systems is the availability of remote access to the recording and evaluation of the aEEG/EEG by specialists.

1.4 Comparability between aEEG Devices

Clinical experience suggests that the commercial aEEG devices are sufficiently comparable. This has prompted technical comparisons of the commercial aEEG devices, showing that the signal filtering is very similar but not identical (see Figure 1.2). While the overall "asymmetric" shape of the band-pass filters is apparently comparable, there are small differences in the signal attenuation at both ends of the frequency spectrum. There may be other differences in the handling of the raw EEG signal and in the final aEEG output, but many manufacturers adjust the output to be as comparable as possible with the original analog aEEG devices.

Other differences in the visual aEEG trend can be created manually by different time windows, amplitude scaling and variations in color schemes. In spite of such differences, studies investigating aEEG trends in newborns report remarkably comparable results also with different monitors. The complementary information from the raw EEG should be acknowledged

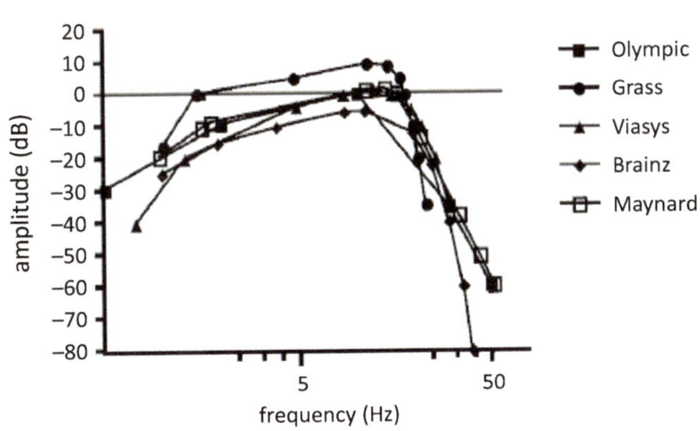

FIGURE 1.2A This figure shows a comparison of aEEG filter shapes in different aEEG monitors and also includes the original analog CFM monitor ("Maynard"). The graph shows the attenuation of the amplitude (dB) on the y-axis in relation to the different EEG frequencies (x-axis). Much of the EEG activity below 2 Hz and above 15 Hz is attenuated. Note that all filters have a comparable shape with the highest peak near 10 Hz. (From *Quigg and Leiner 2009, with permission.*)

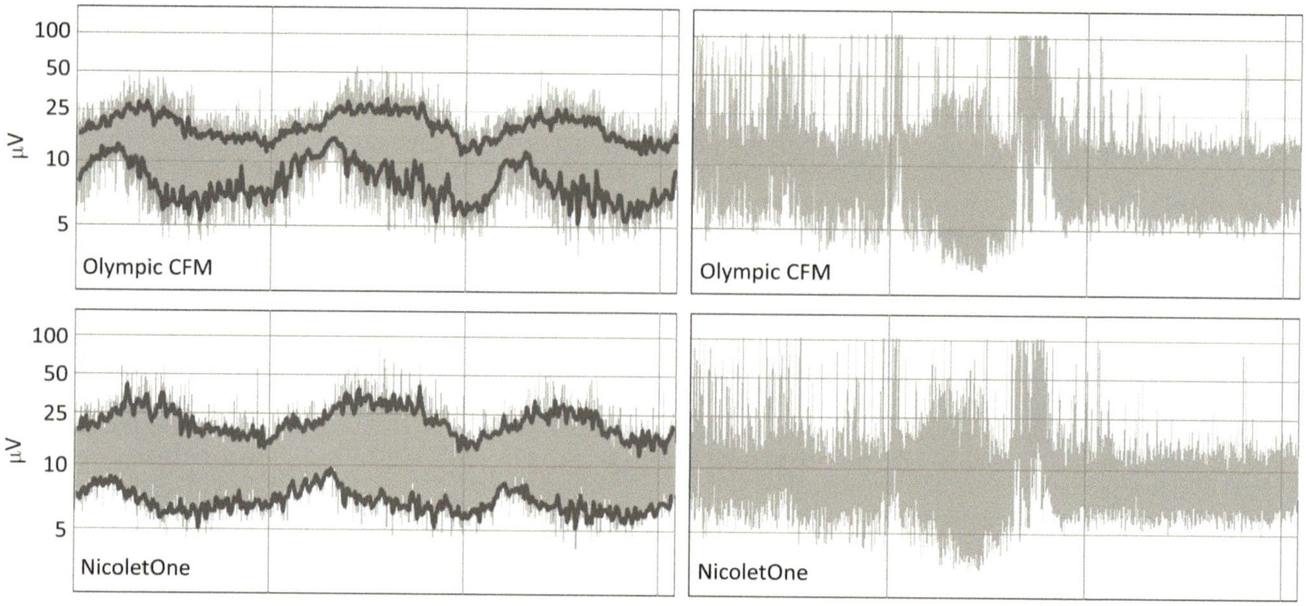

FIGURE 1.2B Another comparison also showed very similar filter shapes to the original CFM (Maynard) and also similar lower and upper border in several NICU monitors. The figure shows the aEEG output from a recording of a stable newborn infant and demonstrates the almost identical pattern from two commonly used aEEG monitors. When comparing multiple tracings, from neurologically stable infants, the mean difference in the lower and upper border amplitudes between the displayed two monitors were 1.55 μV and 2.12 μV, respectively. (Modified figure from *Werther et al. 2017, with permission.*)

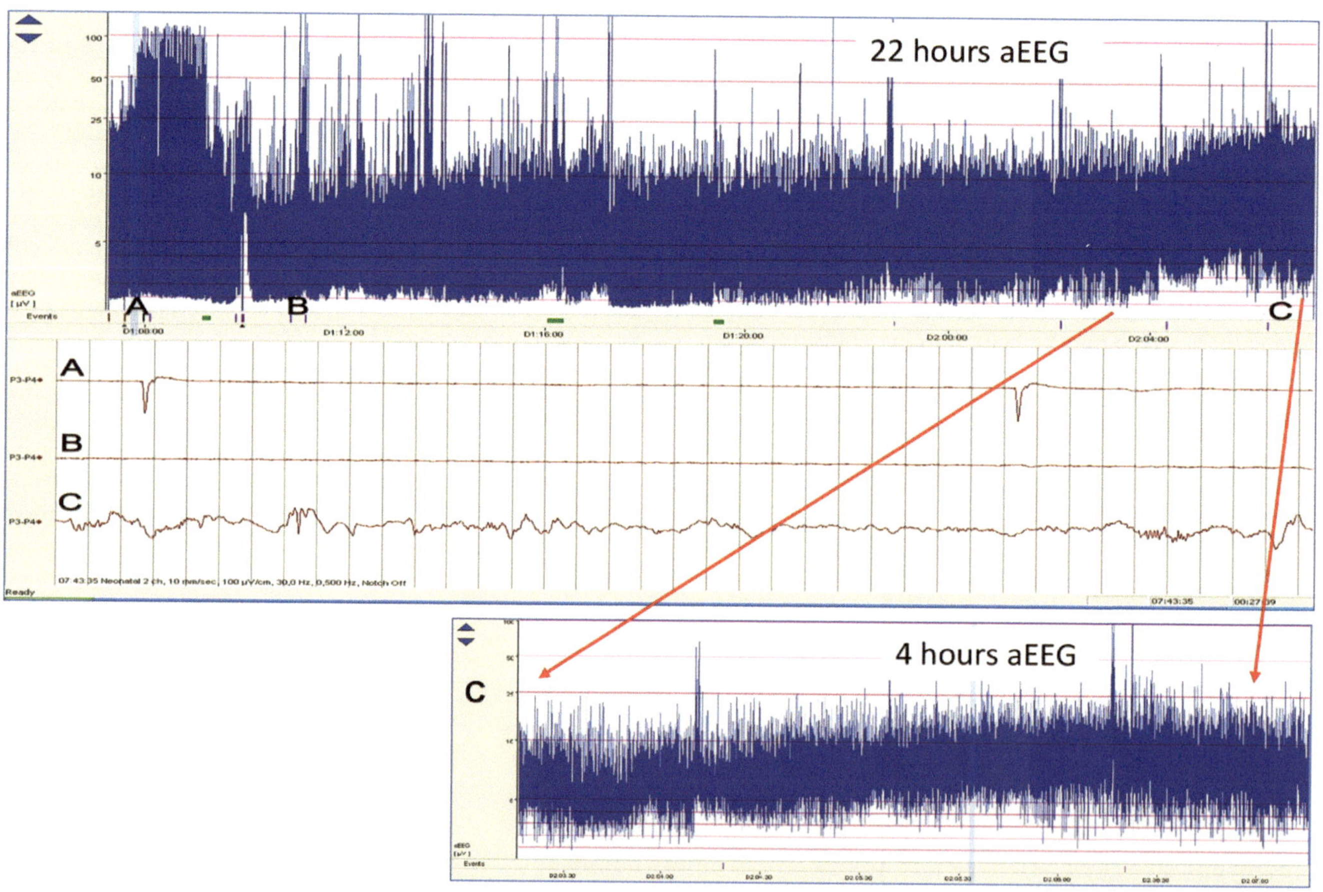

FIGURE 1.3 During clinical monitoring, the most common display is 4 to 6 hours of the aEEG output on the screen. By using a relatively standardized output, patterns of activity can be easier recognized and learned by the staff. Sometimes other timelines can be used in order to evaluate long-term trends in brain activity, as in the example earlier showing brain recovery during the first 24 hours (22 hours of aEEG) in a severely asphyxiated infant. Trace *A* shows the initially flat EEG with occasional gasping creating the suppression-burst-like aEEG pattern, trace *B* shows a flat EEG after initiation of hypothermia treatment and a loading dose of phenobarbital for a clinically suspected seizure, and trace *C* shows recovery of a continuous activity around 22–24 hours postnatal age, better seen in the 4-hour aEEG than in the very compressed 22-hour aEEG.

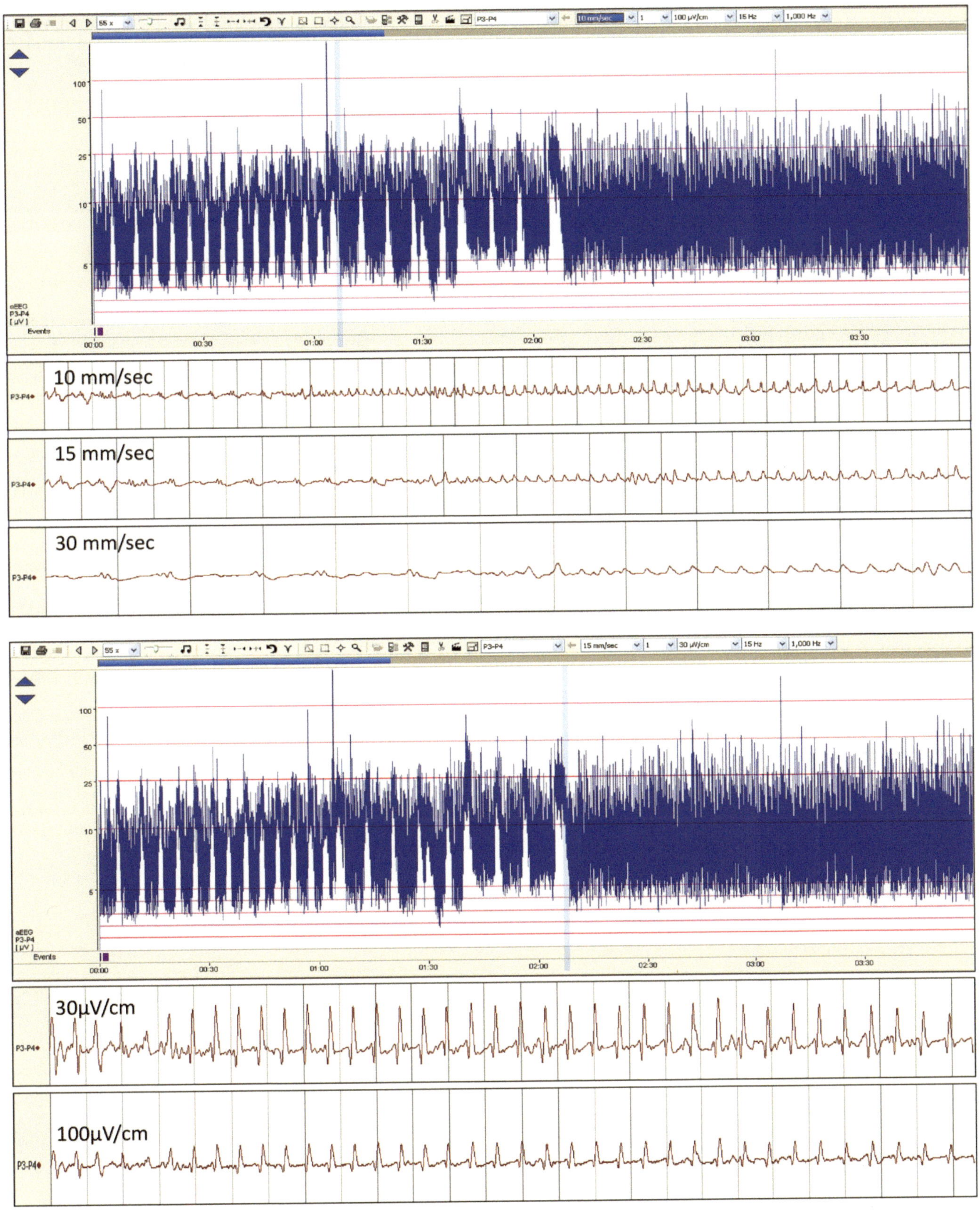

FIGURE 1.4 The NICU staff needs to be aware of the scaling of both the aEEG trend and of the EEG. The two examples come from the same recording demonstrating status epilepticus (in this case, 22 seizures during the first 2 hours) and, after that, a slightly discontinuous pattern (lower border below 5 µV). Example *A* shows how the EEG of the 14th seizure appears in different time-scales, and example *B* shows the EEG of the 22nd seizure with different amplitude scaling.

since it may help to distinguish artefacts from seizures and vice versa. It is necessary for the NICU staff in a hospital to learn and to recognize the most common aEEG patterns, and for this reason also, it is wise to use a "standardized" time-scale for everyday monitoring. The book contains examples from different monitors.

Acknowledgements

In this third edition of the aEEG atlas, we are summarizing the experience and evidence of more than 40 years of aEEG monitoring, but we are also addressing the development and future of brain monitoring. Additional EEG-derived trends, such as IBI and BSN (Chapter 8), may prove to be useful future adjunct trends to the aEEG. High-performing seizure-detection alarms will probably be standard in most monitors. However, for optimal management of at-risk newborns, a high level of knowledge at the bedside is of utmost importance but also close collaboration between neonatology, neurology and neurophysiology.

We are happy that Mohamed A El-Dib, Sonia Bonifacio and Kathi Salley Randall agreed to share their expertise and co-author some of the chapters, including creating questions for a quiz and some cases. Much of this work could not have been done without the enthusiastic support of all the nurses and EEG technicians in the different centers.

We are also extremely grateful to all contributors of figures, illustrations and cases for the atlas: Lina Chalak, Gabriel Variane, Marianne Thoresen, Elisabeth Norman, Maria-Luisa Tataranno, Lauren Weeke, Elisabeth Book, Douglas Hägerström, Sylke Steggerda, Ana Alarcon and Mar Velilla, Nathan Stevenson and Saeed Montazeri.

Finally, we want to express our admiration for the early pioneers of aEEG monitoring, the creators of the CFM and a concept that still holds true. We are especially grateful to Ingmar Rosén, neurophysiologist and co-author of the two first editions of this aEEG atlas, who promoted the use of CFM in newborns. There are many investigators around the world, not mentioned here but many of them are mentioned in the reference lists, that have made significant and important contributions to the CFM/aEEG development which has further promoted its use in the NICUs and also promoted brain care in high-risk newborns.

References

Ando Y, Hashimoto K, Yoshida K, et al. Cerebral function monitor (CFM) in neonates and prognosis (in Japanese). *No To Hattatsu*. 1988;20(2):151–157.

Archbald F, Verma UL, Tejani NA, Handwerker SM. Cerebral function monitor in the neonate. II: Birth asphyxia. *Dev Med Child Neurol.* 1984;26(2):162–168.

Bjerre I, Hellström-Westas L, Rosén I, Svenningsen N. Monitoring of cerebral function after severe asphyxia in infancy. *Arch Dis Child.* 1983;58(12):997–1002.

Bridgers SL, Ment LR, Ebersole JS, Ehrenkranz RA. Cassette electroencephalographic recording of neonates with apneic episodes. *Pediatr Neurol.* 1985;1(4):219–222.

Connell J, Oozeer R, Regev R, et al. Continuous four-channel EEG monitoring in the evaluation of echodense ultrasound lesions and cystic leucomalacia. *Arch Dis Child.* 1987;62(10):1019–1024.

Greisen G, Hellström-Vestas L, Lou H, et al. Sleep-waking shifts and cerebral blood flow in stable preterm infants. *Pediatr Res.* 1985;19(11):1156–1119.

https://collection.sciencemuseumgroup.org.uk/objects/co440044/cfam-i-cerebral-function-analyser-monitor-welwyn-garden-city-england-1977-cerebral-function-monitor

https://collection.sciencemuseumgroup.org.uk/objects/co8778064/the-london-hospital-survival-predictor-london-england-1972-survival-predictor

Maynard D, Prior PF, Scott DF. A continuous monitoring device for cerebral activity. *Electroencephalogr Clin Neurophysiol.* 1969;27(7):672–673.

Quigg M, Leiner D. Engineering aspects of the quantified amplitude-integrated electroencephalogram in neonatal cerebral monitoring. *J Clin Neurophysiol.* 2009;26(3):145–149.

Verma UL, Archbald F, Tejani NA, Handwerker SM. Cerebral function monitor in the neonate. I: Normal patterns. *Dev Med Child Neurol.* 1984;26(2):154–161.

Viniker DA, Maynard DE, Scott DF. Cerebral function monitor studies in neonates. *Clin Electroencephalogr.* 1984;15(4):185–192.

Werther T, Olischar M, Naulaers G, et al. Are all amplitude-integrated electroencephalogram systems equal? *Neonatology.* 2017;112(4):394–401.

2 BRAIN ACTIVITY AND GENERATION OF EEG SIGNAL

Sampsa Vanhatalo

SUMMARY

- Newborn EEG measures joint activity in large groups of cortical neurons.
- Visual review is based on pattern recognition of EEG waveforms and aEEG trends that are correlated to the patient's clinical course.
- The aEEG trends enable visual assessment of long-term changes in the spontaneous cortical activity (background activity).
- Visual review of aEEG/EEG is always subjective, and the exact details of interpretations need to be considered with care.

Brain functions are generated by networks of neuronal activity in widely distributed brain structures. Each trace (signal) in the newborn EEG recording comes from a relatively small cortical area under the given recording electrode. Newborn brain monitoring with aEEG trends from a limited number of electrodes assumes that the brain activity of interest covers wide cortical areas (e.g. epileptic seizures) or it is global (vigilance state or background activity). In the following, we will use abbreviation (a)EEG when referring to both the raw EEG signal and the aEEG trend.

2.1 Anatomy of the EEG Signal

Scalp-recorded EEG signals are generated by concerted activity of pyramidal neurons in the cerebral cortex. Activity in other cortical neurons or in subcortical neuronal structures is crucial for supporting synchronized activity in the pyramidal neurons. However, they do not directly contribute to the electric potentials measured by the EEG. Despite the selective signal generation at the cellular level, the raw EEG signals and the aEEG trends provide a unique non-invasive window to a wide range of whole brain functions, including subcortical mechanisms. For instance, vigilance (sleep) states are coordinated by extensive subcortical networks, but they also affect the cortical activity; thus, the aEEG can be an effective bedside readout of the fluctuations in sleep states, known as sleep-wake cycling (SWC).

2.2 Spatial View of the EEG Signal

Though the EEG signal is generated by only a thin cell layer in the cerebral cortex, it requires simultaneous neuronal activity over several square centimeters in the cortex. The actual spatial accuracy of the EEG signal is defined by two factors: the extent of the underlying cortical activity (e.g. extent of seizure discharge) and signal smearing (volume conduction) as it passes from the cortex through the skull and scalp to the EEG electrodes. The actual size of cortical activity underlying different EEG waveforms is unknown. Recent studies have indicated that the newborn EEG can be very focal as compared to older children or adults. In other words, each electrode only "sees" cortical activity within a couple centimeters around it. Such high spatial specificity is seen with many EEG signal waveforms. The common clinical experience is that epileptic seizures are surprisingly well detected even with sparse electrode configurations. This indicates that most newborn seizures extend over larger cortical areas, and they are sufficiently covered by the four-electrode configuration with frontal and parietal electrodes (Chapter 3).

2.3 General Aspects of Visual EEG Interpretation

The conventional visual EEG interpretation identifies particular waveforms ('graphoelements'), signal amplitudes, and fluctuating patterns ("oscillatory activity", measured by frequencies). The clinical relevance of the visually identified EEG waveforms is determined by their association with clinical situations. Such visual review struggles with assessing long-term changes. The clinical success with aEEG trends is essentially due to its ability to compress and visualize long-term changes in the power of band-limited EEG signal (see Chapter 1 and Figure 2.1).

2.4 Key Concepts in the Visual Review of EEG Signals and aEEG Trends

Visual EEG review assesses waveform patterns and their temporal behaviour: Overall signal amplitude, presence of visually identifiable rhythms (also called oscillations or frequencies), discrete waveforms with known clinical correlates, continuity of the rhythmic activity, differences between brain areas, presence of different vigilance (or sleep) states, as well as possible abnormal waveforms, such as seizure discharges. The spontaneous, ongoing activity is commonly called *background activity*, or background pattern. It describes the general type of brain activity during a time period ranging from minutes to hours. While these EEG concepts are lexically comparable between neonates and older subjects, most of the actual newborn EEG phenomenology is unique to this age window. The newborn EEG also matures on a weekly basis through the prematurity until some weeks after term age (see Chapter 7). Therefore, the newborn EEG needs to be considered in an age-specific manner and using nomenclature that is specific to the neonatal recordings.

DOI: 10.1201/b22858-2

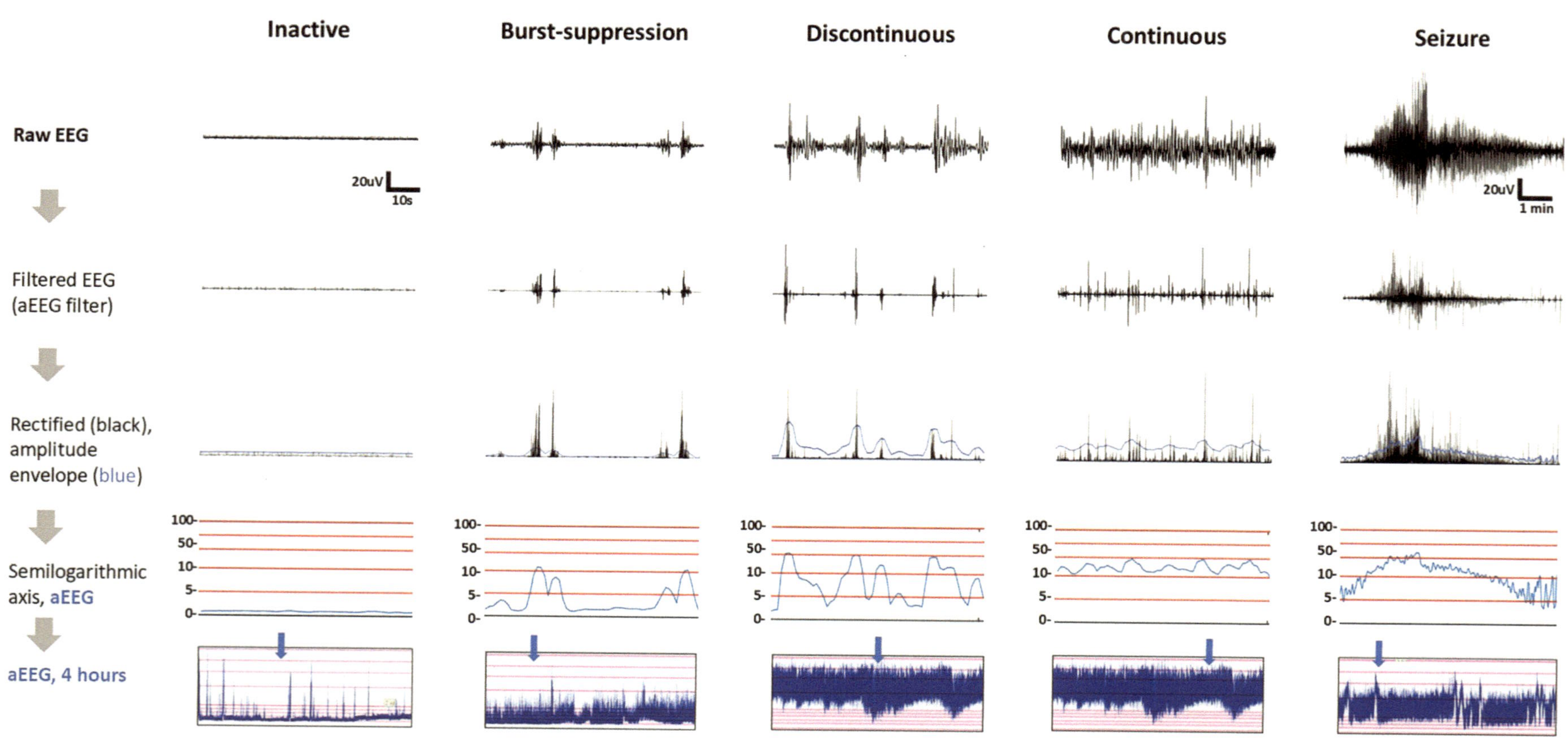

FIGURE 2.1 Computational process to generate aEEG trends from the raw EEG signals. Each of the five columns visualize transformation of one EEG signal type from the raw EEG signal to the corresponding aEEG trends. First, the raw EEG signal is bandpass filtered at mid-frequencies to remove the slowest and fastest activities. Second, the amplitude of the signal is estimated with amplitude envelope. Third, the amplitude is changed to a "semi-logarithmic" scale, which amplifies the difference between lowest (< 10 μV) and higher amplitudes. Fourth, these amplitudes are compressed to a typical 4 hours per window to yield the familiar appearance of aEEG trends. The duration of the raw EEG signals is 1 minute, except for the seizure example that shows 6 minutes to include the whole duration of this seizure. All aEEG trends show the same duration of 4 hours.

2.5 A Systematic Approach to Reviewing the aEEG Trend

During aEEG monitoring of a high-risk newborn, the clinical situation determines which aspects of compromised brain function should be evaluated in particular. The clinical expectations of each review instance should guide the aEEG assessment, including several aEEG characteristics: the type of background activity (continuous/discontinuous), presence of variability/cyclicity, suspected or clear seizures, clinical notes (medications, care procedures, observations), and whether the trends suggest recovery or deterioration. Potential artefacts (e.g. related electrode contacts, ECG, or high-frequency ventilation) must be noted and not let them confound the aEEG assessment. Any notable hemispheric difference needs checking technical reasons (electrode contacts, interelectrode distances, signal quality, other artefacts) that may be seen better in the raw EEG signal.

Bedside assessment of the aEEG trend:

- Lower border: Is it above or below 5 µV? What is the overall background pattern? Does it show variability over time or fluctuation compatible with SWC? Are there major changes in the aEEG trend, such as recovery or deterioration?
- Does the aEEG pattern match the clinical situation and the raw EEG signal? If no, check for artefacts (poor electrodes, high-frequency ventilation, care procedures/patting/sucking, unusual seizure patterns).
- Check clinical notes and observations—anything that needs closer look on aEEG/EEG.
- Are there suspected seizures? If so, inspect the raw EEG signal for verification.
- How does the raw EEG signal look like? Check 10–20 second epochs of raw EEG intermittently during the whole recording.
- Suspected findings or suspected seizures? Consult a senior or other experienced staff whether full montage EEG should be requested.
- Report observations and evaluation to bedside staff.

2.6 Review after Monitoring

- Assess aEEG background and major changes during the whole length of the recording. Evaluate the aEEG in the clinical context.
- Verify all aEEG observations by comparing with intermittent inspection of raw EEG throughout the recording (poor electrodes, artefacts, seizures).
- Conclude and write a note, according to local recommendations.

2.7 Rationale of the aEEG Trend

There are three key aims of the aEEG trend: First, to facilitate recognition of the overall cortical state, or 'background activity' (inactive, burst-suppression, and continuous activity). Second, to expedite recognition of seizure activity. Third, to visualize very long-term (hourly) changes between brain states, such as sleep-wake cycling or cortical recovery from injury. Figure 2.1 visualizes the rationale in computing the aEEG trends from different, clinically important EEG types. The apparent simplicity of aEEG trends has expanded its use as a surrogate index (i.e. use without physiological or technical rationale) in a large range of clinical and scientific contexts. It is essential to note, however, that aEEG is only a time-compressed display of band-limited EEG power with no clinical interpretation *per se*. The particular sensitivity of the aEEG trend to many artefacts (e.g. ECG, movement or mechanical ventilation) pose major challenges to the bedside aEEG interpretation, prompting development of other computational means in analyzing EEG signals (see Chapter 8).

2.8 Background Classifications

The concept "background activity" in the EEG signal and aEEG trend refers to the spontaneous, ongoing cortical activity. The clinical importance of evaluation of the aEEG background pattern comes from its close correlation to the overall brain health in high-risk or neurologically compromised infants (see Chapter 5). While discrete background categories are practical in the clinical use, the true cortical activity represents a continuous spectrum of brain states. It is important to be familiar with the key background categories that are recognized in the visual reading of EEG or aEEG. A number of classification schemes have been published to describe the same overall background types. For clarity, here we present classification schemes that are mostly comparable between reviews of the aEEG trends and the raw EEG signal.

In the healthy infant at term age or any time thereafter, the background activity exhibits continuous signal fluctuations at a wide range of frequencies. The vigilance state-related changes in background activity can be observed as sleep-wake cycling in the aEEG trend. Quiet sleep periods last usually up to 10–30 minutes, and they are characterized by a more discontinuous trace (*tracé alternant*). The more continuous periods in the aEEG represent wakefulness and active sleep, which may be difficult to distinguish without direct clinical observation of the infant. Vigilance state changes are seen as brief transitional periods. The key background categories (see later) can be also recognized in the preterm EEG; however, the highly discontinuous nature of the extremely preterm EEG challenges the background-based analysis as such (see also Chapter 7). See further Figure 2.2 and Table 2.1.

2.9 Continuous Background

Continuity is a commonly used concept in the EEG assessment. The cortical activity is considered continuous when the overall EEG amplitudes and frequency content is relatively constant. This is a purely visual perception, and it is best appreciated when reviewing the raw EEG activity. Assessing continuity is clinically important because the EEG activity may show lacking continuity in both physiological situations (early preterm EEG and quiet sleep in all newborn EEG) and in pathological situations (recovery from cerebral damage). Therefore, a separate recognition of continuity has context-dependent clinical implications. In the aEEG trends, continuity is assessed indirectly from the aEEG lower border (see e.g. Chapter 7).

2.10 Discontinuous Background

The electrocortical background activity can also be mainly discontinuous, i.e. be dominated by intermittent activity characterized by alternating periods of high- and low-amplitude activity, similar to the quiet sleep periods in the healthy term or near-term baby. Discontinuous activity can be seen in several circumstances: in the sedated or encephalopathic full-term

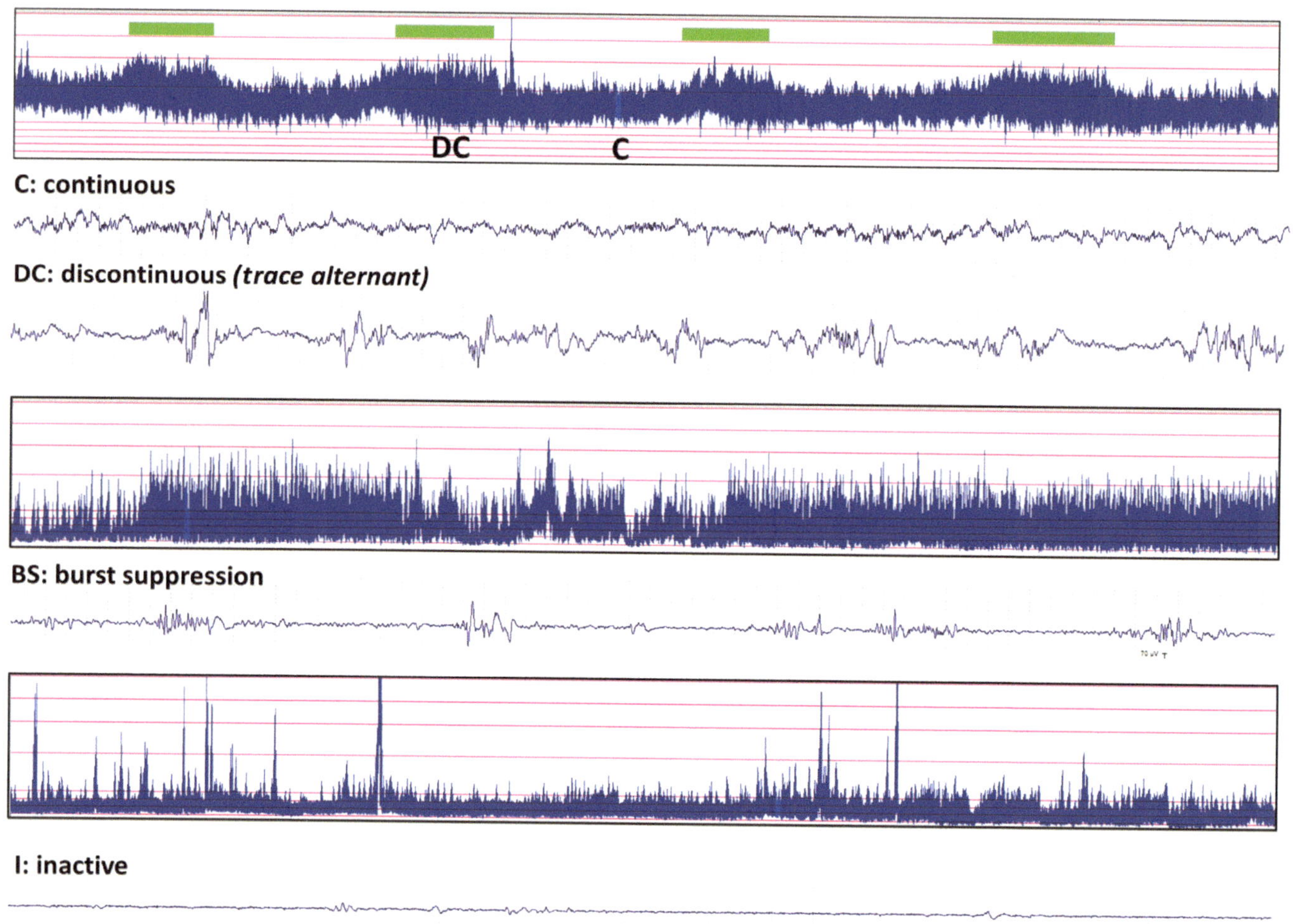

FIGURE 2.2 Comparison of the key types of background activity as seen in aEEG and EEG. Durations of the shown EEG signals are 60 seconds, and the aEEG trends are 4 hours.

TABLE 2.1: Comparison between EEG and aEEG Background Classifications

aEEG Review	EEG Review	Notes
CNV + SWC (Continuous Normal Voltage with SWC)	Continuous, fully normal appearing EEG with a clearly rhythmic sleep-wake cycling lasting over 6 hours	Clear periodicity in SWC
CNV + SWC	Continuous EEG with an observable sleep-wake cycling	No clear periodicity in SWC
CNV – SWC (Continuous Normal Voltage without SWC)	Continuous EEG without sleep-wake cycling	
DNV (Discontinuous Normal Voltage)	Clearly discontinuous EEG that is more reactive (i.e. temporally changing) than BS but also longer lasting than the typical quiet sleep epochs during later phase in recovery	
BS (Burst-Suppression)	Burst-suppression: Background activity < 10 μV, IBI duration between 10–60 s, no sleep-wake cycle	Frequency of bursts may be recognized as an additional descriptor
CLV (Continuous Low Voltage)	In the EEG review, this can be classified as inactive or burst-suppression	Very low amplitudes
I (Inactive)	Inactive: Background activity < 10 μV (or IBI duration > 60 s)	Very low amplitudes

Note: See also Figure 2.3 for illustrations of aEEG categories.

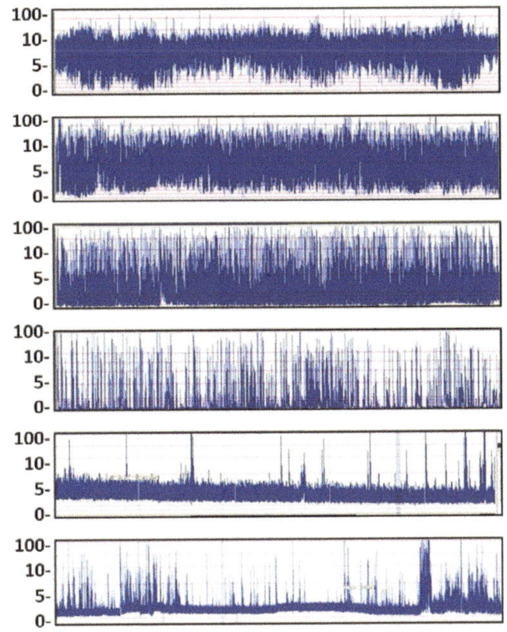

FIGURE 2.3 The commonly recognized aEEG background classes (see also Table 2.1).

infant, but also as normal activity in the very preterm infants. The more immature and younger the baby is, the longer the periods are with the attenuated activity. With increasing maturation, the pattern becomes more continuous.

2.11 Pathological Activities in the aEEG

There are three pathological forms of EEG activity that are essential to recognize to understand the clinical rationale in using the aEEG trend (see also Figures 2.2 and 2.3).

Burst-suppression background activity refers to a state where cortical activity is robustly intermittent, with prominent bursts separated by an inactive trace. Burst-suppression may graphologically resemble the physiological discontinuous activity (*tracé discontinu*) in the early preterm infants; however, physiological *tracé discontinu* is age-specific and changes with vigilance states or sensory stimulation. Burst-suppression is seen when the cortical activity recovers from an initially inactive state (e.g. severe asphyxia). Burst-suppression may persist in infants with severe prognosis, or it may be caused iatrogenically by heavy dosing of sedative medication. Notably, the traditional EEG terminology is based on brief EEG recordings with burst-suppression lasting throughout the recording, whereas long-term brain monitoring has made it clear that burst-suppression evolves over time and exhibits a range of variants. For instance, infants affected by HIE may exhibit long (hours or even days) times when the EEG is no more than the typical unreactive burst-suppression or an actual continuous EEG is neither a clear burst-suppression nor a clearly continuous EEG pattern, reflecting slower cerebral recovery. Such partly continuous/discontinuous background patterns lack accurate EEG definitions, and they may be easier to recognize as an evolving and recovering pattern in the aEEG trends as compared to the conventional EEG reading.

Inactive background activity refers to a state where cortical activity is absent or so low that nothing cortically generated can be recognized from either the EEG signal or the aEEG trend. This is characteristic in the acute phase after severe brain injury or ischemia or after high doses of sedative drugs.

Seizures are recognized by their stereotyped and evolving pattern that persists for several seconds (see Chapter 4). Briefer episodes are called single seizures, and frequently recurring seizures or continuously ongoing seizures are called status epilepticus, although there are no strict and objective criteria for diagnosing status epilepticus in newborn infants. Seizures can emerge from virtually any background activity, but they are more prevalent on depressed background activity. Seizures can be differentiated from many seizure-like EEG waveforms, such as respiration and pulse artefacts, by observing a clear "seizure triad": sudden onset, repetitive/rhythmic pattern, and evolution. See Chapter 4 for more details. It is essential to learn distinguish the seizures from other seizure-like events, such as respiration, care, or pulse artefacts.

In the aEEG signal, seizures typically appear as a transient elevation of the aEEG lower border, which is due to the increased middle-frequency components in the seizure waveforms. Of note, aEEG has some significant caveats that prompt a systematic comparison of the aEEG trend and the raw EEG signal to confirm the interpretation: Some seizures may only show smooth low-frequency waveform that can be difficult to identify in the aEEG, and many aEEG elevations are often caused by artefacts, such as muscle activity, movements, or care procedures. Consequently, the aEEG trend alone is an effective aid for rapid bedside scanning of seizures, but suspected events should always be confirmed by inspecting the corresponding raw EEG signal.

2.12 Early Maturation of EEG and aEEG activity

Preterm cortical activity, and the corresponding EEG signal, shows weekly developmental changes (for more details, see Chapter 7). In the visual EEG review, most developmental changes are observed in the background patterns and their relationship to sleep states, as well as in the occurrence of individual "immature" EEG waveforms. An experienced EEG reviewer may assess the age of infant (or EEG maturity) with an accuracy of a few weeks, while computational EEG measures of functional brain age may show even higher accuracies. Abnormal waveforms and delayed maturation of the EEG background may suggest a significant white matter brain injury in preterm infants. The developmental changes in the background activity in different sleep state are also seen in the aEEG trends. The most salient developmental aEEG changes include an increase in the lower border of aEEG (reflecting increased continuity) and the gradually emerging separation of sleep states with later organization as periodic sleep-wake cycling (SWC). Delayed maturation ('dysmaturation') of the aEEG activity may be seen in serial recordings in preterm infants with brain injury but can be very difficult to diagnose such maturation delays in single aEEG recordings. See Chapter 7 for an example of using aEEG review in estimating maturation.

The hallmark of the early (preterm) brain activity is intermittent bursting in all neuronal ensembles throughout the nervous system, including cortical neurons. Experimental studies have shown that these bursts belong to a large family of intermittent activities in the early neuronal networks. In the EEG tradition, they have been called by different graphological names (e.g. delta brush, or temporal theta) or by using category terms like burst or spontaneous activity transient (SAT). The bursting activity is developmentally important for guiding neuronal wiring and for supporting neuronal survival by the time of intensive neuronal network organization. In the youngest viable preterm infants, the bursts may be separated by up to tens of seconds of relative silence (a.k.a. interburst intervals), which becomes progressively shorter towards term age. In addition to the intermittent bursting, there is also a developmentally evolving rhythmic activity in the newborn EEG, with a handful of other visually identifiable EEG waveforms, such as local transients; however, they are not covered here due to their relative unimportance to the appearance of the aEEG trends.

For simplicity and for the sake of aEEG interpretation, it is practical to view a normal newborn EEG as a combination of early bursting and a superimposed continuous activity. Thereby, vigilance states are readily identified as markedly intermittent activities during quiet sleep, *tracé discontinu* in the young infants and *tracé alternant* in the older infants, while active sleep and wake are characterized by a more continuous activity with less prominent bursting. These two vigilance states are readily identified in the aEEG trend (see Figure 2.1).

2.13 Reliability in the Visual Review of aEEG Trends and Raw EEG Signals

When reviewing the EEG signals or aEEG trends, it is important to recognize the unavoidable uncertainty in visual interpretations, despite their apparently clear verbal descriptions. Several interrater agreement studies have shown that even trained experts may have substantial disagreements about aEEG and EEG assessments. The interrater agreement is lowest for the detailed characteristics, such as very brief seizures or borderline findings, while the experts may have modest to good agreement about more global and coarse features, such as the overall aEEG and EEG background over long time epochs. Therefore, very detailed aEEG or EEG review is bound to be inaccurate, and the clinical practice should emphasize broader interpretations, such as measuring the background over longer time periods or the overall seizure burden rather than the exact seizure counts.

References

Backman S, Rosén I, Blennow M, et al. Swedish consensus reached on recording, interpretation and reporting of neonatal continuous simplified electroencephalography that is supported by amplitude-integrated trend analysis. *Acta Paediatr.* 2018;107:1702–1709.

Bourgoin P, Barrault V, Loron G, et al. Interrater agreement between critical care providers for background classification and seizure detection after implementation of amplitude-integrated electroencephalography in neonates, infants, and children. *J Clin Neurophysiol.* 2020;37:259–262.

Burdjalov VF, Baumgart S, Spitzer AR. Cerebral function monitoring: A new scoring system for the evaluation of brain maturation in neonates. *Pediatrics.* 2003;112:855–861.

Durrani NUR, Dinan MH. Amplitude-integrated electroencephalography: A primer for neonatologists and practitioners in the NICU. *Neoreviews.* 2022;23:e96–e107.

Griesmaier E, Enot DP, Bachmann M, et al. Systematic characterization of amplitude-integrated EEG signals for monitoring the preterm brain. *Pediatr Res.* 2013;73:226–235.

Hellström-Westas L, Rosén I, de Vries LS, et al. Amplitude-integrated EEG classification and interpretation in preterm and term infants. *Neoreviews.* 2006;7:e76–e87.

Kidokoro H, Inder T, Okumura A, et al. What does cyclicity on amplitude-integrated EEG mean? *J Perinatol.* 2012;32:565–569.

Luhmann HJ, Kanold PO, Molnar Z, et al. Early brain activity: Translations between bedside and laboratory. *Progress in Neurobiology.* 2022;213:102268.

Massey SL, Shou H, Clancy R, et al. Interrater and intrarater agreement in neonatal electroencephalogram background scoring. *J Clin Neurophysiol.* 2019;36:1–8.

Odabaee M, Freeman W, Colditz P, et al. Spatial patterning of the neonatal EEG suggests a need for a high number of electrodes. *NeuroImage.* 2013;68:229–235.

Stevenson NJ, Lauronen L, Vanhatalo S. The effect of reducing EEG electrode number on the visual interpretation of the human expert for neonatal seizure detection. *Clin Neurophys.* 2018;129:265–270.

Stevenson NJ, Palmu K, Wikström S, et al. Measuring brain activity cycling (BAC) in long term EEG monitoring of preterm babies. *Physiol Meas.* 2014;35:1493–1508.

Stevenson NJ, Clancy RR, Vanhatalo S, et al. Interobserver agreement for neonatal seizure detection using multichannel EEG. *Ann Clin Transnl Neurol.* 2015;2:1002–1011.

Stevenson NJ, Tataranno M-L, Kaminska A, et al. Reliability and accuracy of EEG-based age estimates in the preterm infant: Comparison of conventional EEG, amplitude-integrated EEG and an age prediction algorithm. *Ann Clin Transl Neurol.* 2020;7:1564–1573.

Vanhatalo S, Kaila K. Development of neonatal EEG activity: From phenomenology to physiology. *Seminars in Fetal and Neonatal Medicine.* 2006;11:471–478.

Walsh BH, Murra DM, Boylan GB. The use of conventional EEG for the assessment of hypoxic ischaemic encephalopathy in the newborn: A review. *Clin Neurophysiol.* 2011;122:1284–1294.

3 ELECTRODE APPLICATION, RECORDING CAVEATS AND ARTEFACTS

Kathi Salley Randall and Sampsa Vanhatalo

SUMMARY

- The aEEG trend and its underlying raw EEG signal are very sensitive to interference from various technical and biological artefacts, such as other electronic equipment, any movement of the infant, muscle activity and ECG.
- A good electrode contact is required for good signals. The electrode impedance is useful for monitoring the electrode contact; however, the bedside staff must also recognize loose electrodes as a source of artefacts.
- Frequent clinical notes about care procedures and medication are needed to facilitate later interpretation.
- Electrodes should not be applied over fontanelles, sutures, cephalic hematoma or other skull abnormalities.
- The electrodes should not be in direct contact with bedding or other devices.
- The raw EEG signal and the synchronized video recording are often invaluable for supporting the aEEG interpretation.

A successful brain monitoring session requires recording of high-quality signals that are essentially free from artefacts. In practice, the quality of brain monitoring relies on securely and accurately placed scalp electrodes, continuous inspection of signal quality and removal of any sources of artefacts. There are a large variety of both technical and biological factors that can cause artefacts and distort the EEG recording in the NICU. An interference in the raw EEG signals is always a potential problem for the aEEG trends as well. In this chapter, we present the essential principles of how to achieve a quality EEG or aEEG recording using scalp electrodes, as well as the potential effects of common artefacts on the aEEG trend.

3.1 Number of Electrodes

Historically, aEEG devices required at least three electrodes attached to the infant scalp, two measuring electrodes placed typically over central or parietal regions and one ground electrode. A minimum of two measuring electrodes are required because the EEG signal is generated from the difference in electrical potentials (voltage) between two scalp locations.

Nowadays the most common neonatal montage for aEEG consists of four measuring electrodes and one ground electrode. Two electrodes are placed over the left and right parietal lobes, and two electrodes are placed over the frontal lobes (or central sulcus), respectively. The ground electrode is commonly placed somewhat away from the recording electrodes, such as on the infant's forehead, neck or trunk, but it can also be attached elsewhere on the body. Some monitors require an additional "reference" electrode, which is typically placed near the scalp midline, to be easy to maintain and to reduce interference with care or other medical devices (Figure 3.1).

The aEEG trend can be computed from any pair of measuring electrodes (commonly referred to as "channels") available on the bedside monitor; notably, the most critical consideration for any electrode placement is the signal quality that determines whether the aEEG trends can be computed reliably enough for clinical interpretation and decision-making. Additional electrodes (EEG and polygraphic channels) can be applied on the scalp with most monitors. However, this comes at a cost of more maintenance during monitoring, thereby offsetting the benefits and ease of use of aEEG at the bedside—for instance, the common four-electrode neonatal aEEG montage shown in Figure 3.2 allows assessment of the left and right cerebral hemispheres separately, as well as a combined "cross-cerebral" view.

3.2 Alternatives for the Electrode Attachment

There are multiple alternatives for the recording electrodes and their attachment on infant's scalp. It is important to note that the aEEG trend is computed from the recorded EEG signal, so the aEEG trend will be affected by the quality of the EEG signal, not by the type of electrode. Therefore, the type of electrodes and their methods for attachment can be chosen according to the clinical and practical needs and preferences.

Three issues are important for obtaining a reliable aEEG:

- First, the recorded EEG signal must remain free of artefact ("clean") throughout the long duration of infant's brain monitoring. The electrode wires need to be placed away from other electrical devices and wires (such as IV pumps, ventilatory tubing and electric wires) to minimize their interference with the EEG signal.
- Second, the electrodes must be placed correctly on the infant's scalp to maintain appropriate interelectrode distances, at least 2–3 cm (too closely attached electrodes decrease the signal amplitude).
- Third, the electrode attachment needs to be mechanically stable to ensure a good contact with the scalp for long periods (days to weeks). This may be achieved by using medical tape, a head wrap or net, or their combination.

The recording electrodes can be non-invasive (using a variety of electrode materials for EEG recording, such as disc electrodes or adhesive electrodes) or invasive (small subdermal needles). The preferred option is non-invasive electrodes. However, the choice for electrode types is decided locally, defining an optimal balance between minimal invasiveness, staff safety and resources available for maintaining good-quality recordings. It is always helpful to request on-site training from the local EEG technicians when starting aEEG monitoring with new types of electrodes.

DOI: 10.1201/b22858-3

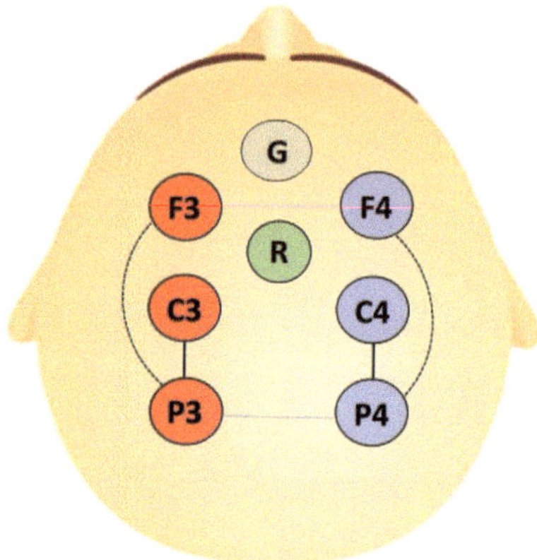

FIGURE 3.1 The preferred electrode placement for aEEG monitoring, according to the international 10–20 standard, consisting of two parietal electrodes (P3, P4) and two frontal electrodes (F3, F4). Some hospitals may use a less optimal central location (C3, C4). The four EEG signals are derived from the two intra-hemispheric (black) and two cross-cerebral (grey) electrode pairs. Ground (G) and reference (R) electrodes are usually placed near midline at a convenient location.

3.3 Non-Invasive Electrodes

The aEEG/EEG is usually recorded with electrodes attached on the scalp surface using reusable metal discs or cups, electrode caps or disposable peel-and-stick adhesive electrodes. All these electrode types require attention to the electrode-skin attachment on the scalp:

- Long-term mechanical stability during movement and caregiving activities can be increased with additional adhesive gel or a head wrap of different kinds.
- Second, the skin is an electrically active organ that interferes with the cortical EEG signals. This interference can be reduced by rubbing (exfoliating creme) the epithelium. The electrode impedance goes down with skin rubbing, but it is not sufficient to ensure quality signal.

In the very preterm infants, hydrogel electrodes are preferred. Their skin impedance is typically very low, and electrodes can be easily applied after very gentle rubbing. In more mature infants, rubbing the epithelial surface and securing the electrodes may need some more training to achieve a good-quality signal. Attachment of electrode cups or plates needs adhesive pastes, glue or a textile, such as a head wrap or netting bandage or their combination.

Many aEEG monitors can display the "electrode impedance" to measure electrical resistance between recording sites. This can be helpful for adjusting skin preparation; however, it provides only a partial assessment needed for setting up a noise-free recording.

In the typical situation, electrical contact at the epithelial surface improves over time, while a large range of other biological and technical artefacts may increase during the intensive care stay and impact the quality of the aEEG recording. These specific artefacts and targeted actions are described below in the section on artefacts.

Regardless of the type of non-invasive electrodes, it is essential that the bedside NICU staff is trained to inspect the quality of the raw EEG signal at least hourly to ensure that aEEG trends remain reliable. The staff should also be trained to maintain and troubleshoot the most common problems that may compromise signal quality.

When choosing the types of non-invasive electrodes, it is essential to consider practical aspects, such as availability of supplies and staff training needed for the solution. Maintaining sufficient signal quality over long-term in the NICU environment is often the greatest challenge that ultimately determines the method of choice in each case.

3.4 Invasive Electrodes

In some NICUs, aEEG recording in term or near-term infants is mostly performed using sterile stainless steel subdermal needle electrodes that are inserted superficially under the skin and fixed with tapes and dressings. Recordings with these electrodes are not contaminated by the skin-borne artefacts, and they yield a maintenance-free recording for extended periods of time.

However, this procedure does require skin breaking and theoretically places the infant at risk for infection at the insertion site. Insertion of sterile needle electrodes causes pain and should be done after skin disinfection. The other important consideration is staff safety, as needle-stick hazards are possible, or the exposed needles may even damage infant's bedding or other medical devices.

It is important to note that the entire shaft of the needle electrodes is conductive, and therefore, the placement and orientation of the needle is as important as the site of insertion (or skin penetration). Give special attention to the interelectrode distance and needle orientation, as they can substantially impact the area of the cortical activity that is monitored. Note that the interelectrode distance may vary even three times if needles are pointing towards vs. away from each other (Figure 3.3). Consequently, the aEEG trend can be substantially affected by the needle orientation alone. The needle orientation is most important in smaller infants (see also Chapter 7).

When inserting the needle electrodes, it is important to always follow the same protocol in your NICU. A few best practices to keep in mind are the following:

- Start needle insertion a few millimeters above the desired scalp location, and avoid pointing the needle tip towards the other needles.
- Keep all electrodes in the same (parallel if possible) orientation with the electrode wires to help orienting during maintenance.
- Ensure that the distances between the recording electrodes are symmetric.

In summary, the advantages of needle electrodes are easy maintenance over long periods of time, while the two disadvantages are invasiveness due to skin breaking and potential for needle hazards; in addition, the needles can be painful, especially when the needles are pulled by changing the wire positions during any care procedures.

3.5 Training for aEEG Recording

Practical skills for performing a good-quality aEEG/EEG monitoring session are best taught and learned at the bedside with the guidance and example of more experienced personnel. Published literature and other teaching material for extending

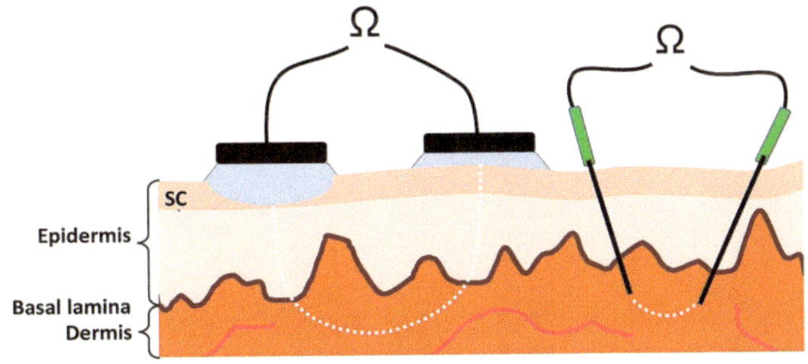

FIGURE 3.2 Principles of the electrode-skin contact in the non-invasive (left side) and invasive (right side) electrodes. The white stippled line depicts the body part of the "recording circuit" that makes up the aEEG and EEG signal, and the "electrode impedance". For the case of non-invasive electrodes, the impedance is the sum of all tissues as the current passes through the epidermis to basal lamina to dermis and back again to the other electrode. There are two important tissue layers causing high impedance: the dry epithelium of stratum corneum (SC) and the tight layer of basal lamina. Skin rubbing before non-invasive electrode application aims to reduce thickness of SC layer. For the case of invasive (needle) electrodes, the impedance measurements are very low because the electrical connection happens only within the highly conductive dermis layer.

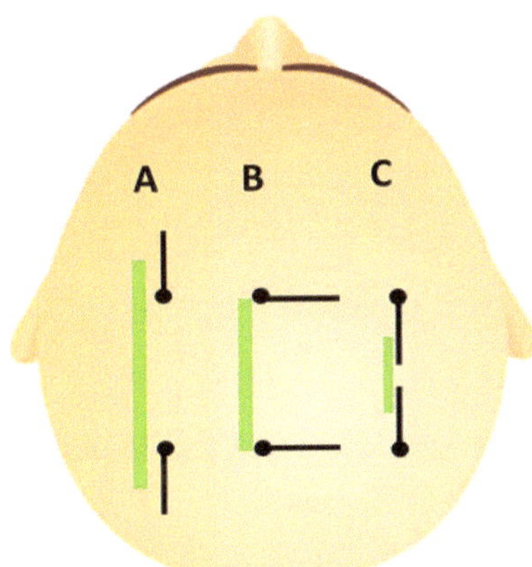

FIGURE 3.3 Needle orientation may cause as much as a threefold difference in the effective measuring distance (green bars) between two needle electrodes, even if the skin penetration sites (black dots) are fixed.

the skills (for instance, see the link to multimedia material in the references) are also useful to learn the best practice. Some hospitals may use lab training sessions with dolls to practice electrode application; however, simulations cannot be used as replacement for hands-on training at the bedside.

3.6 Pitfalls and Caveats, Artefacts

3.6.1 Impedance vs. Electrode Contact vs. Signal Quality

It is important to remember that the artefacts must be eliminated at bedside, i.e. during the recording. Therefore, it is essential that the bedside staff is trained and able to do the following:

i) recognize an artefact,
ii) identify the cause of artefacts in the present situation, and
iii) choose appropriate action to eliminate it.

Electrode-skin contact is routinely assessed by measuring impedance, which is essentially a measure of electrical contact over the whole recording circuit that goes from the amplifier via electrode to the skin and back to the amplifier through another electrode (Figure 3.2). As the epithelial cells create the biggest obstacle (or resistance) for the electrical contact, the skin preparation procedure involves mechanical removal of the vernix and oils and outermost epithelial layers. It is important to note, however, that a good-quality EEG signal also needs mechanically stable attachment of the electrode on the scalp. A "loose electrode" may show good impedance levels while it remains very sensitive to even tiny movements, such as respiration, pulse or moving of electrode wires. Moreover, many NICU-related electrical artefacts may jump directly into the EEG wires by magnetic induction if the electrodes are located too near to other NICU devices (incubator, pumps, monitors). It is important to note that such artefacts are not eliminated by rubbing the skin for lower impedance. However, repositioning the electrodes wires will readily reduce these artefacts.

3.6.2. Artefacts

EEG signals and aEEG trends are easily confounded by several sources of biological and technical artefacts that may lead to misinterpretation of an infant's condition (see Table 3.1 and the Appendix). There are only two ways to avoid confusions created by artefacts: The best way is to minimize or eliminate the artefacts by the time of recording, which requires continuous surveillance and rapid bedside actions for better data quality when suspected artefacts are noted. It is equally important to carefully inspect the aEEG trend and its underlying raw EEG signals before making clinical judgements about the aEEG patterns. Notably, identifying the source of aEEG artefact is only possible by inspecting a synchronized video recording and the raw EEG signal. The most common appearance of an artefact in the aEEG trend is a raised lower aEEG border, which resembles the finding in very many clinical conditions (as described throughout this book). Artefacts can exhibit an abrupt increase caused by a temporary effect, such as care procedure, or the aEEG levels may be persistently elevated due to a long-standing cause, such as subtle head movements caused by high-frequency respiratory support or an intrusion of cardiac activity or arterial pulse into the signal. Both of these latter effects may have very low amplitude and may not be easy to recognize in the

TABLE 3.1: The Main Categories of EEG and aEEG Artefacts with Advice for Their Bedside Elimination

Artefact	Description	EEG Appearance	aEEG Appearance	Elimination
Mains noise (50 Hz or 60 Hz), technical	This is present in all modern environments. It may come to the aEEG/EEG signal through the infant's body or by induction ("jumping") from other wires, including bed and other metal structures.	A thick-looking trace that clears with applying the "notch filter" (obviously it only removes the noise from the view, not from the recorded signal!).	Only limited effect due to aEEG-specific filtering.	Check the electrode impedance; move other wires and tubes away from the EEG leads.
Other interference from electrical devices (technical)	May look much like the 50/60 Hz noise (see earlier), and it is identified by a regular waveform when "zoomed in" (higher amplitude and time-scale). These may consist of many different frequencies, depending on the interfering device.	A thick-looking trace, much like the 50/60 Hz noise. This is not affected by the "notch filter".	Depending on its frequencies, the effect on the aEEG trace may range from minimal to significant elevation of the baseline, even > 100 uV.	Try to identify the device causing the artefact, e.g. by shutting them off one by one. Remove that device away from the patient or the EEG device, if possible. Else, make a note of it for the reviewing clinician.
Cardiac activity from the heart (ECG) or pulse from the artery (biological)	ECG: The "ECG peaks" may project through the neck to the head, especially if the neck is thicker and electrode placement is lower. Pulse: Electrodes may move by arterial pulse below them. Appearance may be like ECG, but it is generated by movement rather than cardiac signal.	A little bump in the EEG signal that is very periodic and coincides with R-peaks in the ECG signal. If ECG is not recorded in the device, you may recognize its rate and the lack of evolution (i.e. not a seizure).	The aEEG level is constantly elevated.	Changing infant's position or electrode positions may reduce it substantially.
Muscle activity, biological (EMG)	Mixed and high-frequency activity that often contaminates signals to varying degrees. It is worst in frontal and temporal areas.	Rapid activity that is clearly a mixed frequency, and it fluctuates over time, making it different from the electrical interference.	Elevation of aEEG level during EMG activity. Needs to be confirmed from the raw EEG signal.	Calm the infant's. Check the electrode positions; moving frontal electrodes more posteriorly may reduce forehead EMG.
Movement, biological	This can be a very variable combination of skin-borne potential that changes when the epithelium is stretched (slow), or if there is an effect at the electrode/gel or gel/skin interphases (rapid).	Typically, slow and high-amplitude jumps/potentials; sometimes also fast jumps. These are always related to movement at the electrode-skin contact, which is not necessarily seen elsewhere in the infant. Note that movements can easily mimic many pathological activities, such as epileptic seizures; thus, identification of the cause from synchronized videos is often necessary.	Elevation of the aEEG level that coincides with movement-like artefacts in the raw EEG signal. Movement artefacts with only slow components may be fully ignored by aEEG trends.	Reduce movements of the infant and wires/electrodes as much as possible. If this does not help, check the electrode impedance to reduce epithelial potentials.
High-frequency ventilation, technical/biological	This results from the high-frequency movement of infant's head, causing a frequency-specific movement artefact (see earlier).	A persisting rhythm at about 10 Hz. This is often so low amplitude that it doesn't interfere with visual EEG review. It is typically more prominent on the side of the head lying against the pillow.	Due to its frequency, this causes a prominent increase in the aEEG baseline and may readily result in misinterpretations. This is typically more prominent on the side of the head lying against the pillow.	Infant's head and wires can be stabilized to remove at least some of the artefact.
Respiration, biological (including hiccups)	Respiration may cause very low-frequency (1–2 seconds per cycle; 0.5–1 Hz) movement of infant's head and wires, causing a frequency-specific movement artefact (see earlier). Sometimes the movement may be sharp, such as hiccups, causing sharper artefacts, respectively.	A slow fluctuation in the signal that persists longer than expected for cortical signals (i.e. not a seizure). Comparison to respiration confirms the finding.	aEEG trends are not affected if the respiration artefact is only a slow wave activity. However, sometimes respiration may also have sharper waveforms that causes elevation of the aEEG baseline.	Infant's head and wires can be stabilized to remove at least some of the artefact.
Care/handling (biological and/or technical)	Any care/handling-related movements may affect the electrode-skin attachment and the epithelial potential by mechanical stretching.	The waveforms can be almost anything, but they always relate to the care/handling. Oftentimes, the artefact can be only defined by comparing them to synchronized video recordings.	Elevation in the aEEG baseline when the artefact includes sharper waveforms.	Minimize handling when possible. Minimize moving electrode wires, and stabilize the electrode attachment on the skin to reduce electrode movements.

raw EEG signal, but they still give significant contribution to the aEEG levels (see Chapter 2 about aEEG computation).

Taken together, the artefacts mostly relate to a brief or sustained elevation of the lower border of the aEEG trend, which is also the key aEEG characteristic of seizures or background state, respectively. This may easily lead to significant misinterpretations and treatment decisions, so it is essential to confirm any significant aEEG interpretations from comparing it to corresponding EEG signals.

A multimedia presentation about common artefact mechanisms, their appearance in the EEG signal, as well as advice for their elimination is available as an interactive multimedia presentation (www.babacenter.fi/nemo/index.html).

Note: For examples of different artefact types, see the Appendix.

References

Bruns N, Blumenthal S, Meyer I, et al. Application of an amplitude-integrated EEG monitor (cerebral function monitor) to neonates. *J Vis Exp.* 2017;(127):55985.

Cordeiro M, Peinado H, Montes MT, et al. Evaluation of the suitability and clinical applicability of different electrodes for AEEG/CEEG monitoring in the extremely premature infant. *Anales de Pediatría (English Edition).* 2021;95(6):423–430.

El Ters NM, Mathur AM, Jain S, et al. Long term electroencephalography in preterm neonates: Safety and quality of electrode types. *Clin Neurophysiol.* 2018;129(7):1366–1371.

Foreman SW, Thorngate L, Burr RL, et al. Electrode challenges in amplitude-integrated electroencephalography (aeeg): Research application of a novel noninvasive measure of brain function in preterm infants. *Biol Res Nurs.* 2011;13(3):251–259.

Hellström-Westas L. Amplitude-integrated electroencephalography for seizure detection in newborn infants. *Semin Fetal Neonatal Med.* 2018;23(3):175–182.

Lloyd R, Goulding R, Filan P, et al. Overcoming the practical challenges of electroencephalography for very preterm infants in the neonatal intensive care unit. *Acta Paediatrica.* 2015;104(2):152–157.

Multimedia resource for demonstrating different electrode attachments and for trouble-shooting artefacts. https://www.babacenter.fi/nemo/index.html

Shah D, Mathur A. Amplitude-integrated EEG and the newborn infant. *Curr Pediatr Rev.* 2014;10(1):11–15.

Shah NA, Wusthoff CJ. How to use: Amplitude-integrated EEG (AEEG). *Arch Dis Child—Educ Pract Ed.* 2014;100(2):75–81.

Tsoi K, Yam KK, Cheung HM, et al. Improving consistency and accuracy of neonatal amplitude-integrated electroencephalography. *Am J Perinatol.* 2024;41(3):330–336.

APPENDIX: EXAMPLES OF ARTEFACTS

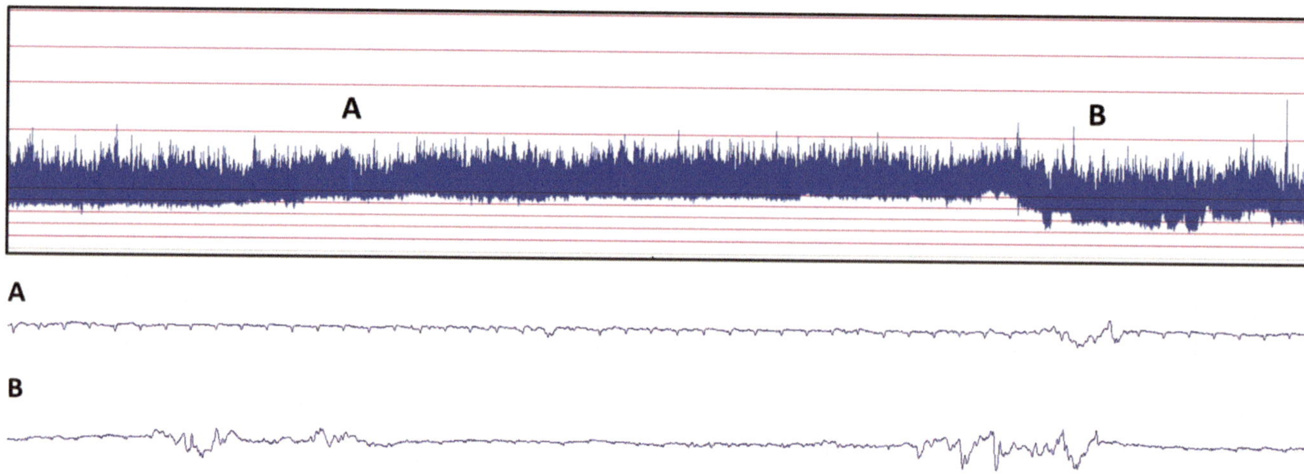

FIGURE 3.4 ECG.

An aEEG recording with a prominent ECG artefact raising the lower aEEG border (A), which comes down when infant's head is turned to another position (B). Note the sparse burst-suppression that is almost inactive first (A) and a more clear burst-suppression later (B). This aEEG pattern could be easily misinterpreted as normal voltage without reviewing the raw EEG signal.

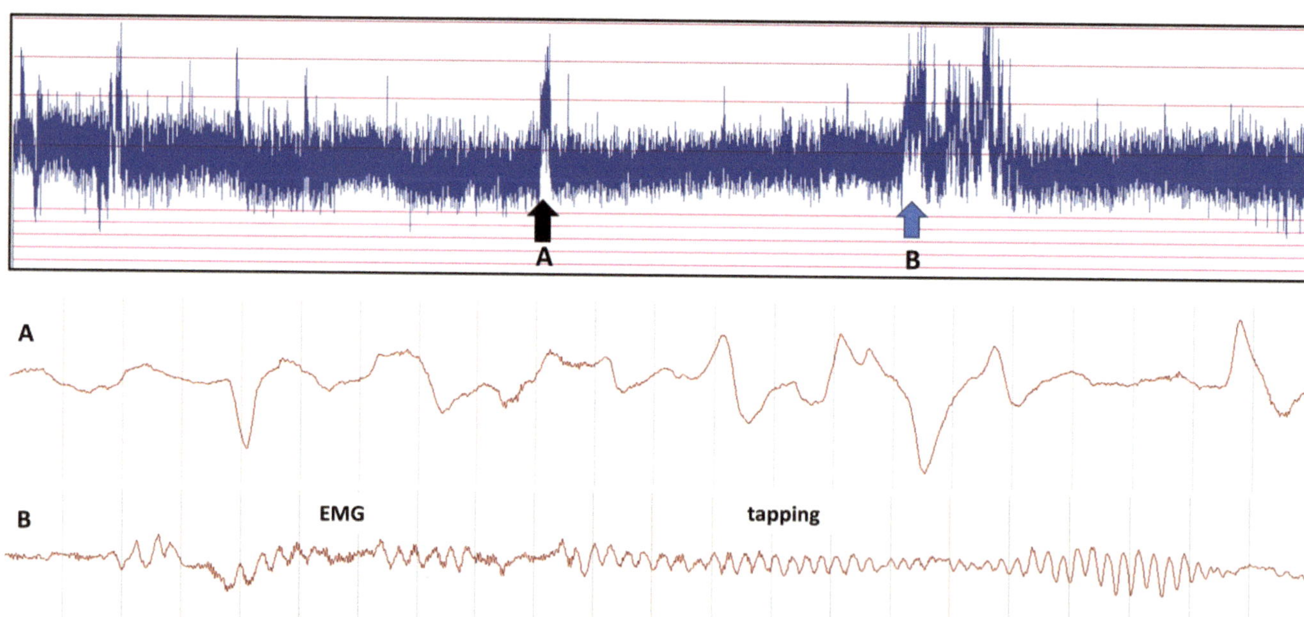

FIGURE 3.5 Muscle (EMG), tapping, movements.

This is an example of a combination of artefacts caused by movements, intermittent muscle (EMG) activity and tapping of infant during parental soothing. Note the irregular high-amplitude waveforms that are typical of spontaneous movements (A), higher-frequency activity typical of EMG (B) and tapping causing artefacts with often quite periodic fluctuation. Tapping is often difficult or impossible to confirm without reviewing a synchronized video that is available in the modern brain monitors; however, tapping may be suspected from the spindle-shape appearance of the characteristic frequency (3–5 Hz). In the aEEG signal, these both may cause raising of the lower border that may be misdiagnosed as a seizure. For properly excluding a seizure, it is often necessary to review the video from at least one of such episodes.

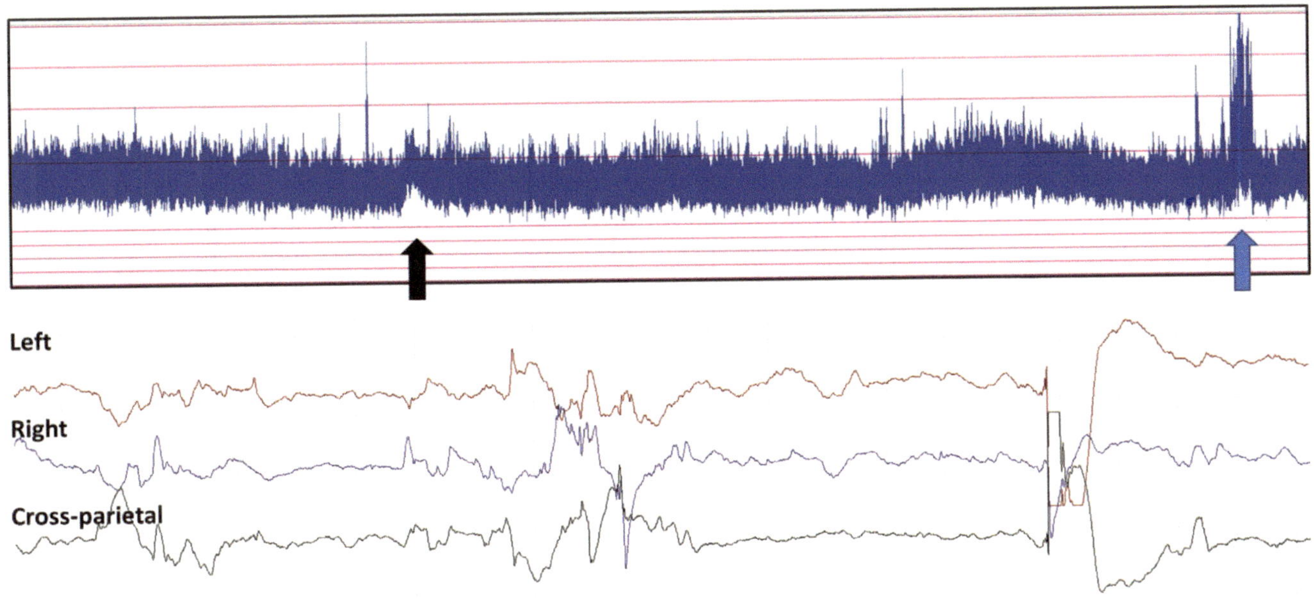

FIGURE 3.6 Movements and care procedures.

Body movements alone would typically cause slow artefacts that may have other superimposed components (left side of the EEG signals), while care procedures may cause almost any kind of movement-related artefacts. There are often very sharp and high-amplitude components in the EEG signal when the infant is moved during care (left side of the signal). In the aEEG trend, the smoother artefacts will appear as smaller raising of the aEEG lower border (black arrow), resembling very much a seizure event. The artefacts with sufficiently high sharper components will result in an aEEG trend with raised lower and higher aEEG borders (blue arrow), which are easier to distinguish as artefact from the aEEG.

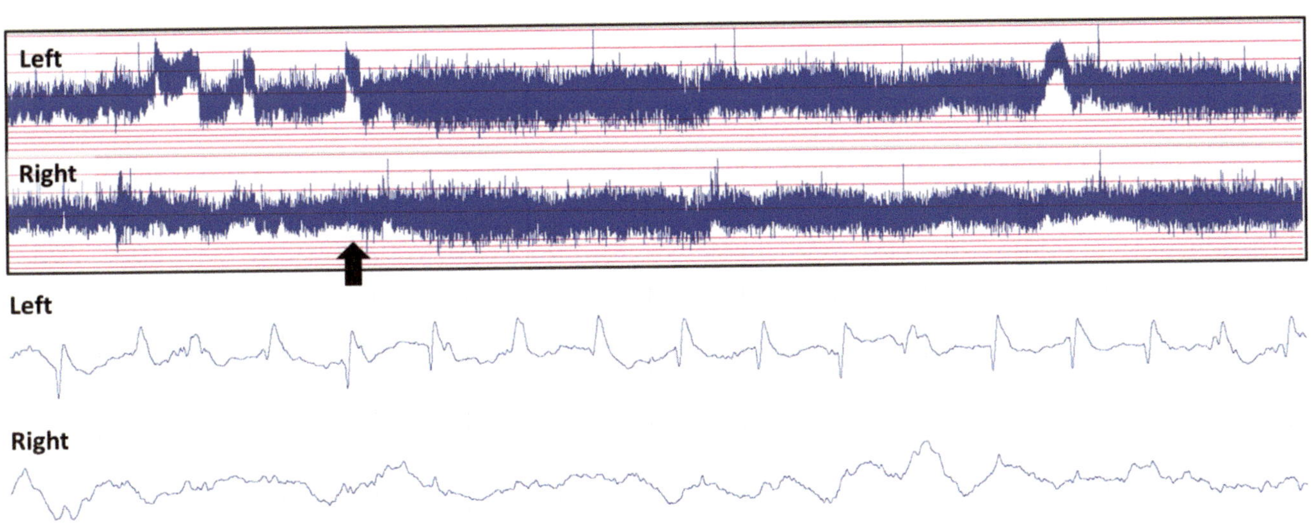

FIGURE 3.7 Movements and seizure.

The left-side EEG signal shows a clear seizure activity that also appears in the aEEG trend. The right-side EEG shows slow irregular fluctuations typical of milder movements; there are also little epileptic spikes visible in the EEG signal without correlates in the aEEG trends.

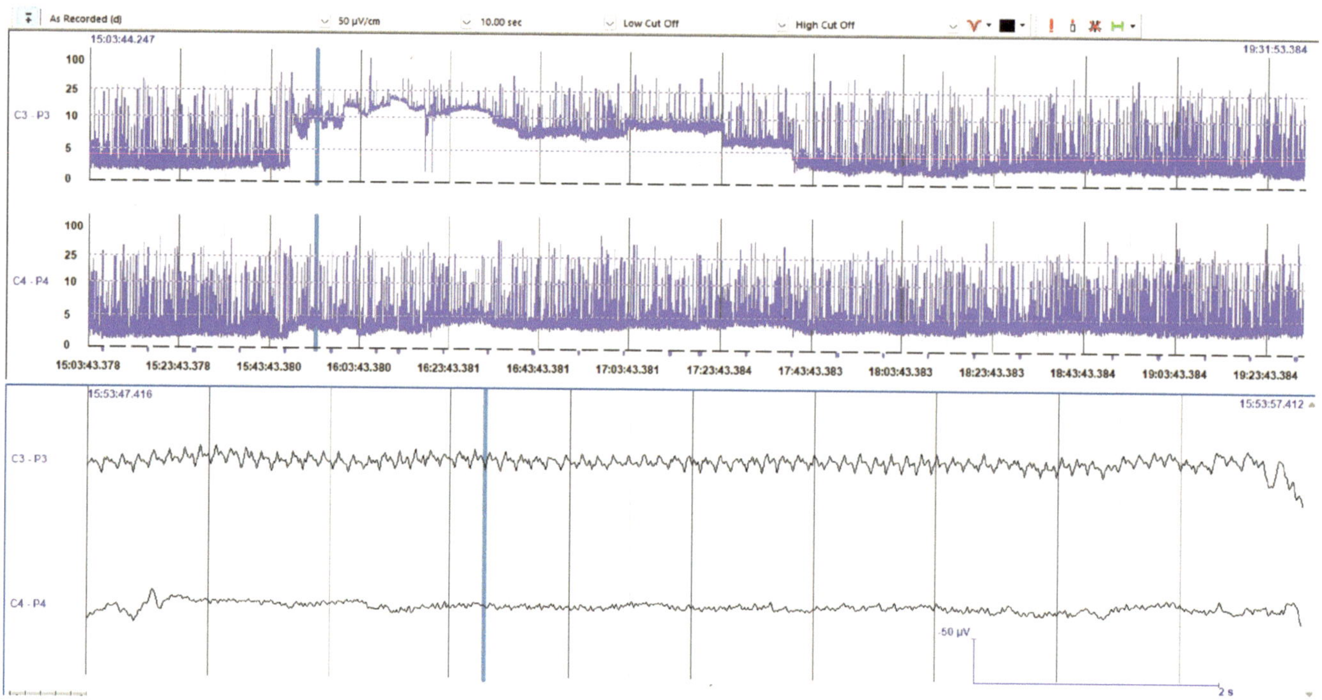

FIGURE 3.8 High-frequency ventilation (HFV).

Respiration causes slow fluctuation at respiration frequency, which is often best visible in the EEG channel that is between the infant and the pillow (here, right-side channel; compare to the left where respiration artefact is not visible). The appearance of respiration artefact in the aEEG trend is typically a raised lower border (arrow; indicates the time of EEG samples shown later), which may be easily mistaken for a seizure if synchronized video is not considered. Additional hints to distinguish respiration from seizures: respiration artefact is often very long-standing, with stable frequency (even hours), and it likely changes with the infant's position (as was the case with this example).

High-frequency ventilation produces a constant rapid movement of the head, leading to corresponding rhythm (~10 Hz) in the EEG signal. This leads to a substantial rise in the aEEG baseline that can be easily misinterpreted as an "aEEG seizure". The constant high frequency in the raw EEG signal confirms the observation. This artefact is typically asymmetric, higher in the electrodes between infant's head and the pillow.

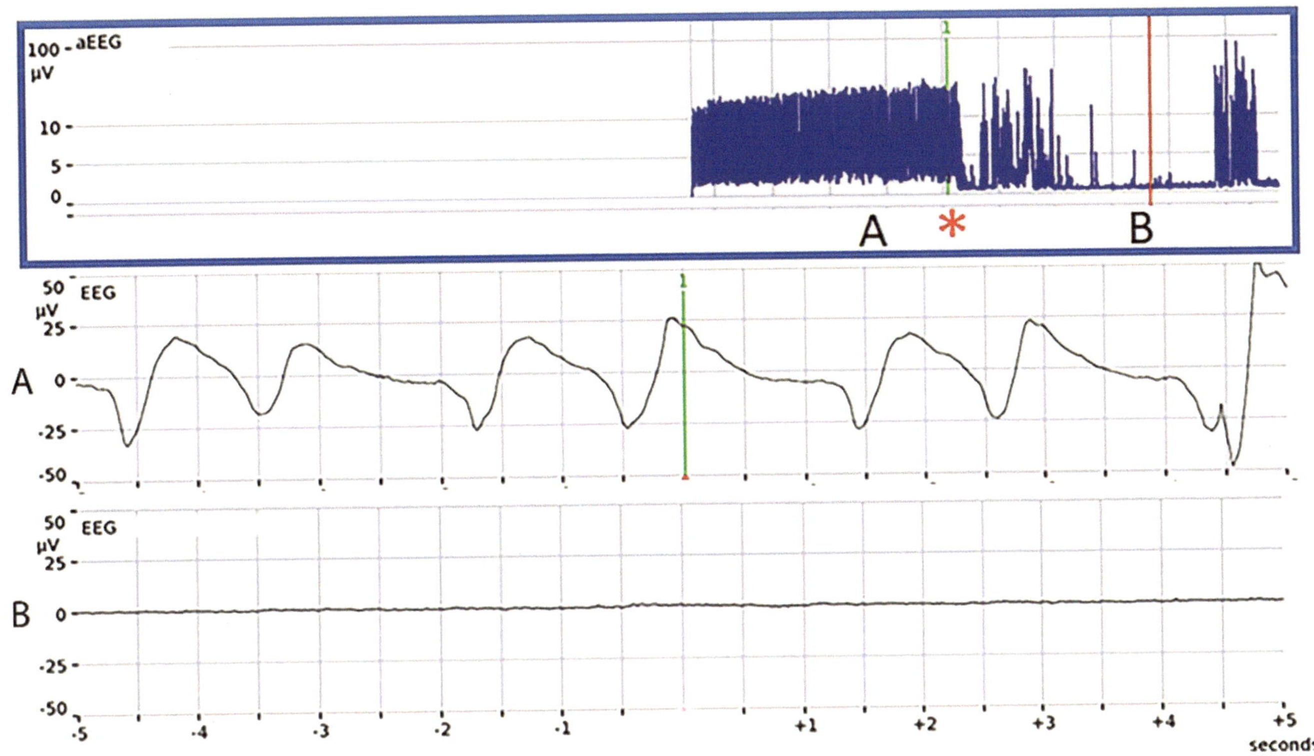

FIGURE 3.9 Gasping.

Artefacts due to gasping (or hiccup) are rare, but they should be considered when the aEEG exhibits a dense "BS pattern" in an infant who is gasping (see Video 3.1). When the infant is mechanically ventilated, a muscle relaxant can be administered to assess the background activity (administered at *). A muscle relaxant only affects the muscle activity but not the cortical activity.

4 SEIZURES

Mohamed El-Dib, Sampsa Vanhatalo and Lena Hellström-Westas

SUMMARY

- Clinical recognition of neonatal seizures is unreliable.
- High-risk neonates should preferably be monitored before seizures appear.
- Infants with unclear symptoms should be monitored with aEEG/EEG as soon as possible.
- A bilaterally recorded aEEG trend, with intermittent inspection of the raw EEG signal, is sufficient for long-term monitoring of seizure occurrences.
- It is essential for the bedside clinician using the aEEG/EEG to be familiar with the raw EEG readings to distinguish true seizure activity from various artefacts.
- Conventional EEG is needed to detect all individual seizures.

The aEEG has a unique role in the management of neonatal seizures. Monitoring the electrocortical activity is necessary for a reliable diagnosis of seizures and for evaluating the treatment response to antiseizure medications. Since early evaluation of seizures is crucial, aEEG monitoring should begin as soon as a risk of seizures is identified or when suspected seizures are observed. Irrespective of the number of EEG recording electrodes, having the aEEG display available for bedside staff is often helpful in expediting seizure identification and treatment.

4.1 Etiology and Diagnosis of Neonatal Seizures

Seizure semiology describes typical clinical symptoms during a seizure event, but in most infants with seizures, the clinical characteristics are nonspecific for etiology. However, some types of clinical seizures may be associated with a specific etiology, e.g. multifocal myoclonic seizures and tonic seizures in some neonatal epilepsies and unilateral focal clonic seizures in those with perinatal stroke. A common phenomenon in newborns is the transformation of clinically recognized seizures to electrographic only 'nonclinical' seizures after administration of antiseizure medications. This phenomenon has been described as 'uncoupling' or 'electroclinical dissociation'. Thus, continuing/ongoing nonclinical seizure activity after antiseizure medication can only be confirmed when using continuous monitoring with aEEG/EEG.

Continuous aEEG/EEG monitoring is recommended in infants, including preterm infants, with conditions associated with increased risk for seizures, including perinatal asphyxia, stroke, sepsis/meningitis, severe hypoglycemia, acute bilirubin encephalopathy, intracranial hemorrhages, intraventricular hemorrhages, and in infants undergoing major surgeries.

4.2 Postnatal Age at Seizure Onset

The majority of neonatal seizures develop during the first 3 days of life. In asphyxiated infants, seizures tend to develop 6–24 hours after birth and reach maximum intensity within the next 24 hours, followed by a spontaneous resolution within days. In perinatal stroke, seizures commonly occur during the first day following the stroke occurrence. Seizures related to metabolic diseases (see also Chapter 6) tend to develop on the second and third day, and seizures related to infections typically emerge later during the first week. In very preterm infants, seizures may occur within the first few days after birth, often in connection with the development of large intraventricular hemorrhages. Seizures in moderately preterm infants often arise somewhat later (10–12 days) since infections are a prevalent cause of seizures in this population. Taken together, the postnatal age at seizure onset is not specific for a certain etiology, and the investigations should be broad unless the underlying cause is known.

4.3 Electrographic Seizure Definition

Based on the International League Against Epilepsy (ILAE) definition 2021, a seizure in the newborn is defined as follows:

> "an electrographic event with a pattern characterized by sudden, repetitive, evolving stereotyped waveforms with a beginning and end. The duration is not defined but has to be sufficient to demonstrate evolution in frequency and morphology of the discharges and needs to be long enough to allow recognition of onset, evolution, and resolution of an abnormal discharge."

A very comparable definition was also proposed by the American Clinical Neurophysiology Society (ACNS) in 2013, with criteria also including a minimum duration of 10 seconds for the electrographic event. The ACNS definition has been used in several scientific publications, and the minimum duration is clinically helpful to ignore large numbers of otherwise ambiguous epochs.

The bedside clinician must be familiar with these seizure definitions when assessing rhythmic EEG activities for confirming observations in the aEEG trend. Since neonatal seizures may appear in various shapes, forms, and frequencies on the raw EEG signal, it is important to recognize the compulsory "seizure triad": 1) To be *sudden*, the seizure activity looks different from the earlier EEG activity in the given infant. 2) To be *repetitive* or *stereotyped*, the seizure activity needs to have a waveform that keeps repeating and that often (but not necessarily) has a sharper waveform. 3) To be *evolving*, there must be a clear change over time, typically within seconds or tens of seconds. This change is often a combination of frequency, waveform, and location. Indeed, lack of evolution is perhaps the

DOI: 10.1201/b22858-4

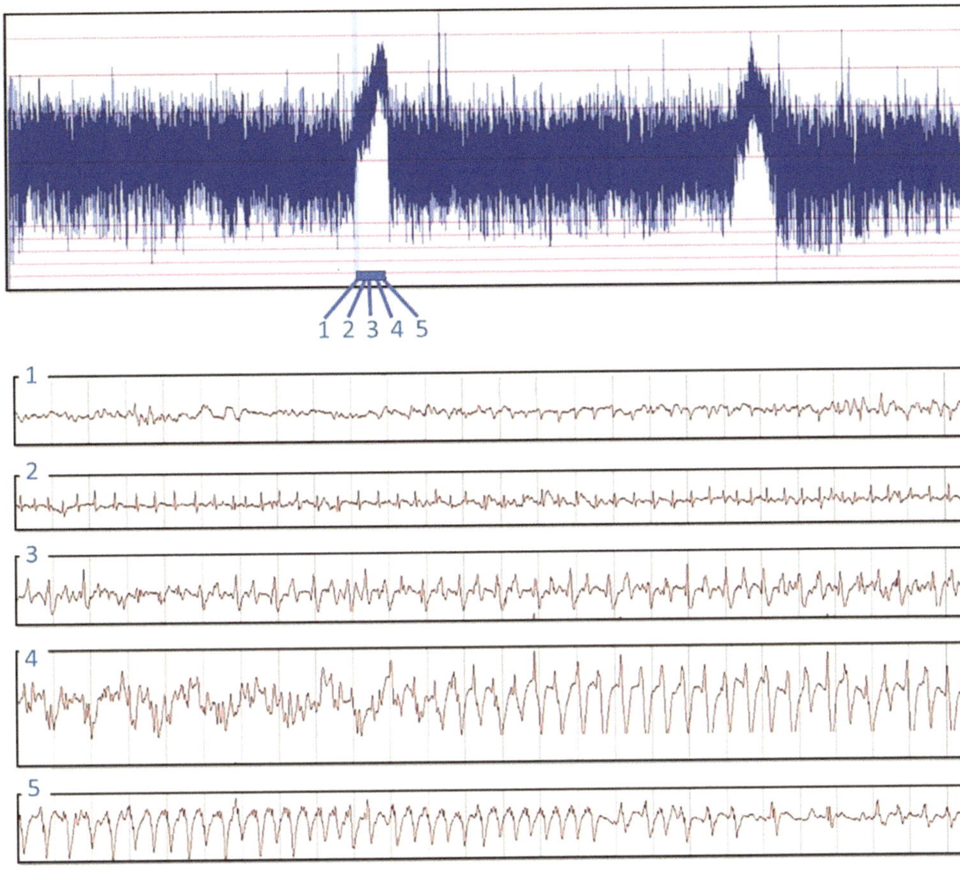

FIGURE 4.1 Four hours of aEEG with two seizures in a full-term baby after cardiac surgery. The aEEG pattern is mainly continuous with no sleep-wake cycling. The numbers 1–5 depict consecutive epochs of raw EEG signal as indicated in the aEEG trend later (5 times, 26 seconds), showing how the rhythmic sharp waves first increase in amplitude and frequency, reach a maximum, and subsequently decrease in amplitude and frequency. This is an example of the evolution that needs to be observed on the raw EEG signal when confirming seizures in the aEEG monitoring.

most common hint that the suspected waveform is not a seizure but may arise from other etiologies, e.g. respiration. Taken together, the clinician must inspect the full 'evolution' of the seizure, from beginning to end, before making firm interpretations. If available, it is helpful to review the synchronized video recording to exclude external interference, such as patting or nursing that may look very similar to actual seizure activity.

Most electrographic neonatal seizures observed on aEEG are characterized by a sudden transient rise in the lower margin, often accompanied by a smaller increase in the upper margin, which leads to a narrowing of the bandwidth. This happens because the peak-to-peak amplitude of a neonatal seizure is generally greater than the amplitude of the interictal background. (See further Figures 4.1–4.3 and Video 4.2.)

Especially in extremely preterm infants, unspecific rhythmic EEG activities that are not seizures may be misinterpreted as seizures in the aEEG. These activities lack the typical evolution of EEG seizures and may represent movement artefacts, nursing care, and patting and often disappear after repositioning. (See Figure 4.4.)

The appearance of seizures in the aEEG trend is rarely suggestive of the etiology, except for some rare conditions like SCN2A, KCNQ2, and KCNQ3-related epilepsy in neonates and EIEE (Early Infantile Epileptic Encephalopathy) (see Chapter 6) (Figure 4.5), and the immediate response to pyridoxine administration in infants with pyridoxine deficiency can be diagnostic (Figure 4.6).

4.4 Seizure Detection with aEEG

Seizures may occur as single events, they can recur for shorter periods or with relatively long intervals ('repetitive' or 'recurrent'), or they may re-occur or be continuous over a prolonged period (usually more than 30 minutes) which is then called status epilepticus. In the aEEG trend, repetitive seizures often create a 'sawtooth' appearance (see Figure 4.7). However, there are no universally adopted criteria for the term 'status epilepticus'. A traditional (by ACNS) definition of status epilepticus is based on total seizure duration being ≥ 50% of an arbitrarily defined one-hour epoch, while other definitions may be based on observing repetitive or continuous seizures for at least 30 minutes.

4.5 Seizure Types That May Go Unnoticed in the aEEG Trend

Brief seizures (< 30 seconds) may go unrecognized since the aEEG trend is compressed in time and a brief event will not create any notable changes. However, brief seizures may also

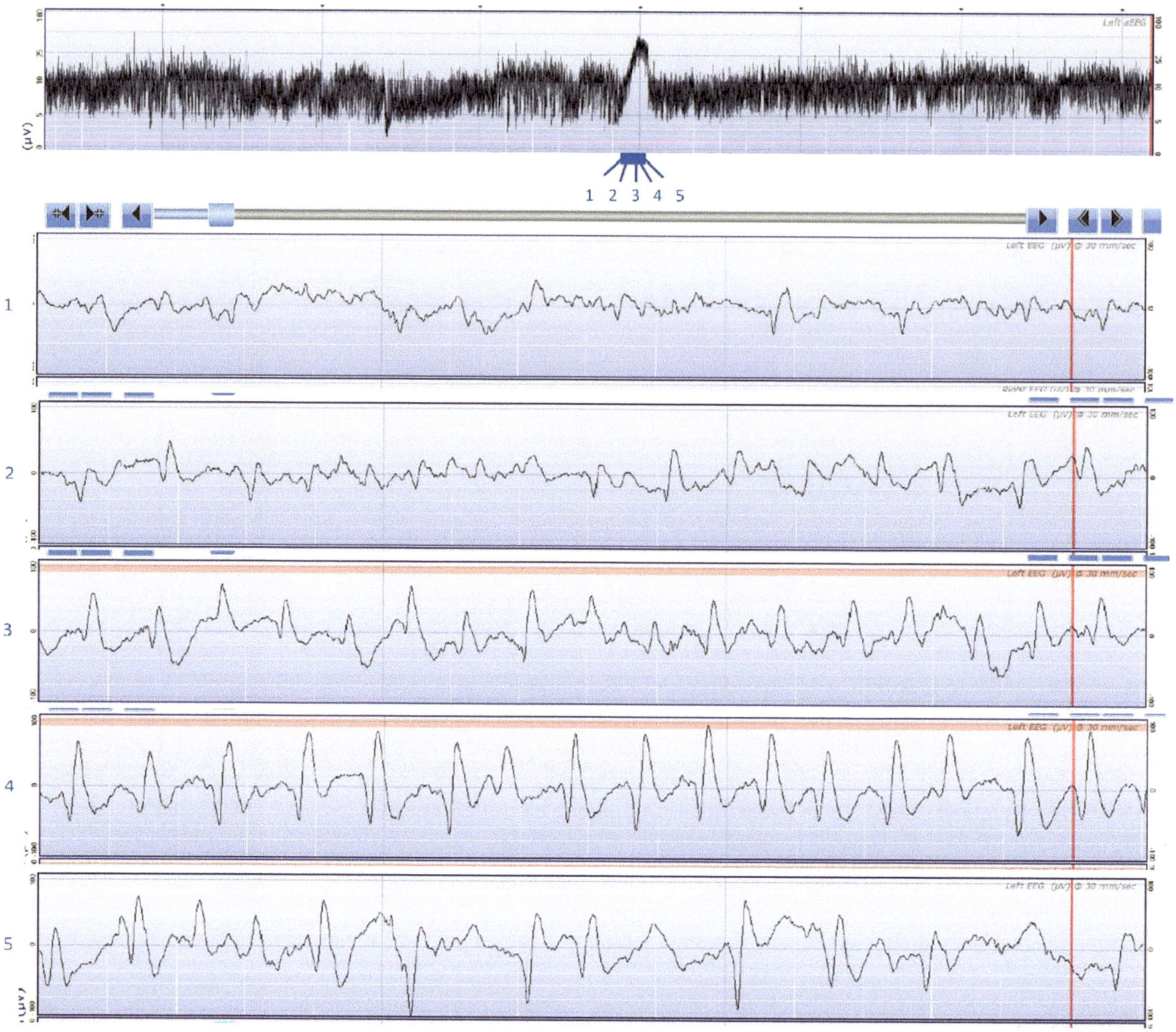

FIGURE 4.2 Another similar example of the evolution of the EEG waveforms *in a full-term baby with HIE*. The background activity is continuous, and a single seizure is present in the middle of the aEEG trace. Below the aEEG are raw EEG traces (each with a duration of 16 seconds) demonstrating the seizure pattern. Video 4.2 also demonstrates the evolution of EEG waveforms.

be challenging to diagnose on the raw EEG, and even very experienced EEG reviewers may show substantial interrater disagreement when seizures are shorter than 30 seconds. The safest approach for bedside aEEG monitoring is, therefore, to always inspect the raw EEG when suspected seizures appear on the aEEG trend.

Very long seizures are relatively rare but may be difficult to discern in the aEEG trend because the lower border is typically elevated throughout the whole seizure (see Figure 4.8). However, they are often easy to recognize in the raw EEG by visual review or by using automated seizure detections.

Seizures with slow EEG waveforms (< 2 Hz) will not show in the aEEG trend since almost all EEG activity below 2 Hz is filtered out by the specific aEEG filter settings (see Figure 2.1). Such seizures are sometimes seen in both preterm infants and in full-term infants after birth asphyxia. These seizure can be easier recognized with automated seizure detection.

Focal seizures may go unnoticed if they occur far from the recording electrodes. Obviously, a higher number of EEG recording electrodes can be more sensitive in capturing focal seizures and their full duration.

When reviewing a single-channel aEEG/EEG recording, the risk of not detecting seizures is increased especially when the seizure originates from cortical areas at a distance from the recording electrode locations. However, in a recent study, reviewing raw EEG signals from the four channels used in the recommended aEEG monitoring (see Chapter 3) yielded detection accuracy that compares well with the conventional neonatal montage (Figure 4.9). This is explained by the predominance of neonatal seizures in the central and parietal areas. Notably, placing the anterior electrodes on the frontal

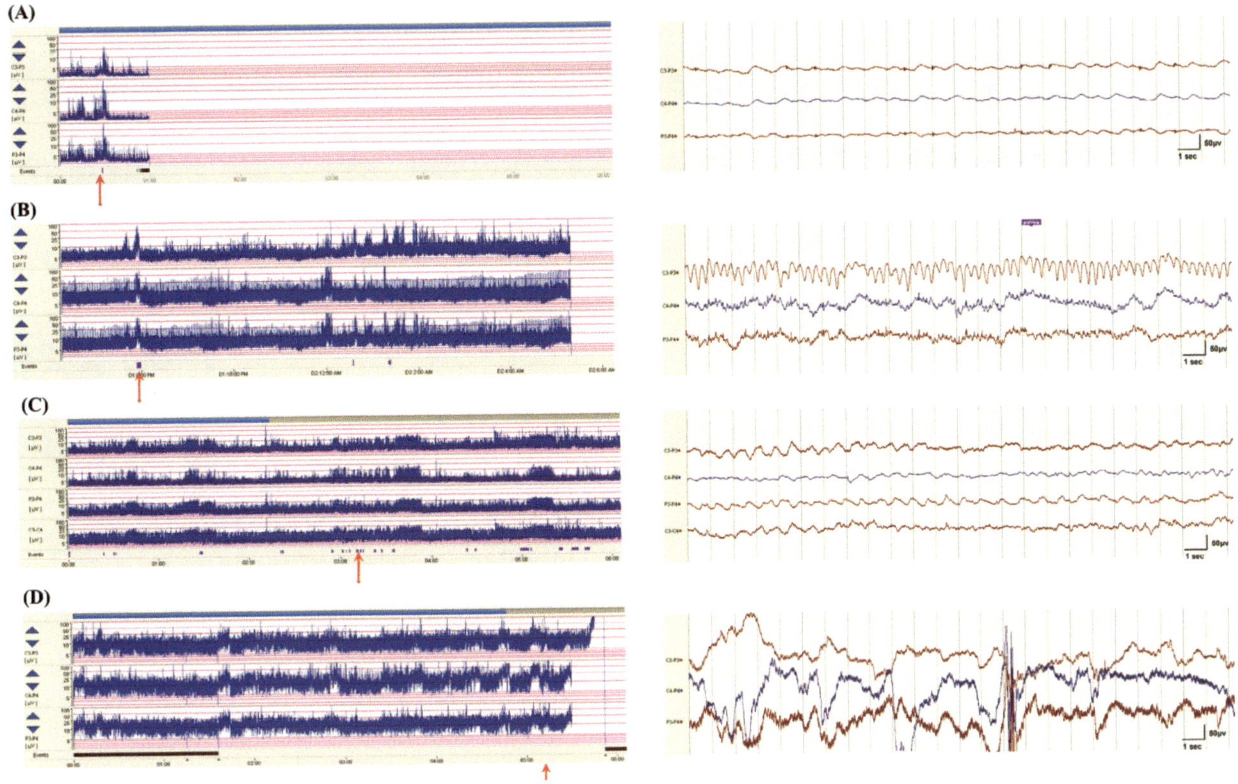

FIGURE 4.3 The examples later show seizure-like changes in the aEEG, while the EEG reveals that these are artefacts and not seizures (arrows indicate where the EEG was displayed): (A) ventilator artefact, (B) patting artefact, (C) chewing artefact, and (D) electrode artefact. (The aEEG is displayed at 6 cm/hour and the EEG at 15 mm/sec.) (From *El-Dib et al. 2009, with permission.*)

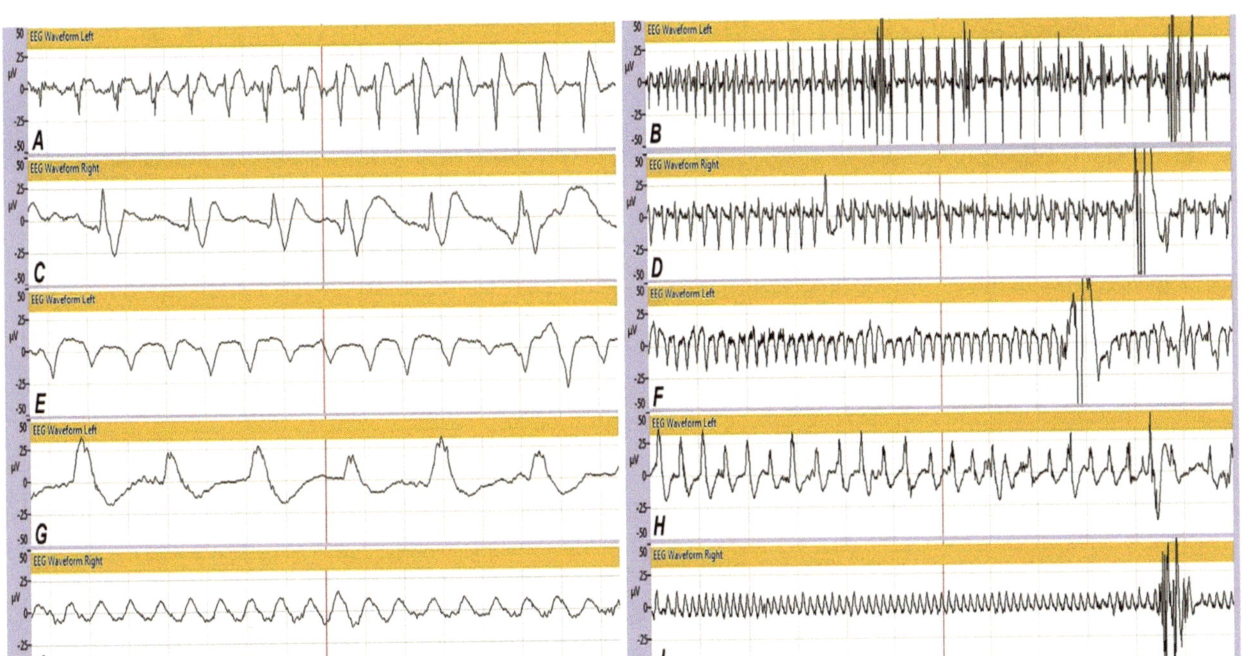

FIGURE 4.4 Examples of seizures and rhythmic activities mimicking seizures in extremely preterm infants. These paired examples of EEG traces come from five infants with rhythmic activities identified by a seizure detection algorithm. The displayed EEGs on the left side (A, C, E, G, I) show 15 seconds of EEG, and the corresponding trace of the same recording on the right side (B, D, F, G, J) shows a more compressed EEG with a duration of 1 minute. The upper two examples (A–B and C–D) show a seizure with typical characteristics, as described earlier. The three lower examples (E–F, G–H, and I–J), show artefacts that can be distinguished since they do not have the typical evolution of seizures. They also disappeared when the infants' head positions were changed. (From *Weeke et al. 2017, with permission.*)

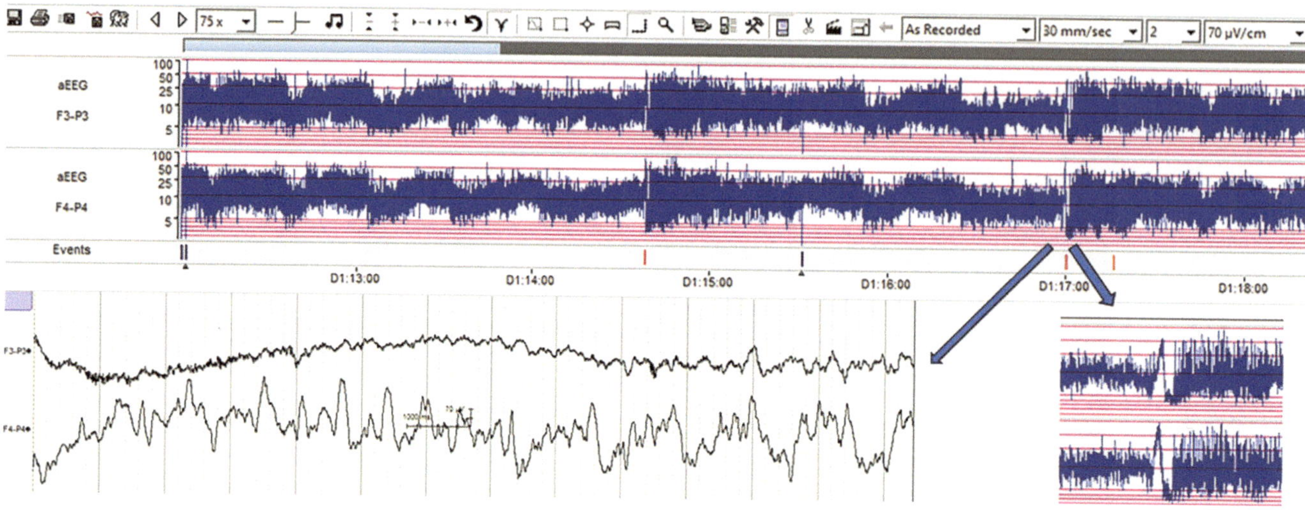

FIGURE 4.5 Distinct seizure morphology in an infant with KCNQ2 mutation. Top: Two seizures can be seen, with a brief interruption of the background pattern. In the less compressed aEEG trend (later), the seizure is easier to recognize and shows the typical brief uplift followed by a marked suppression can be recognized.

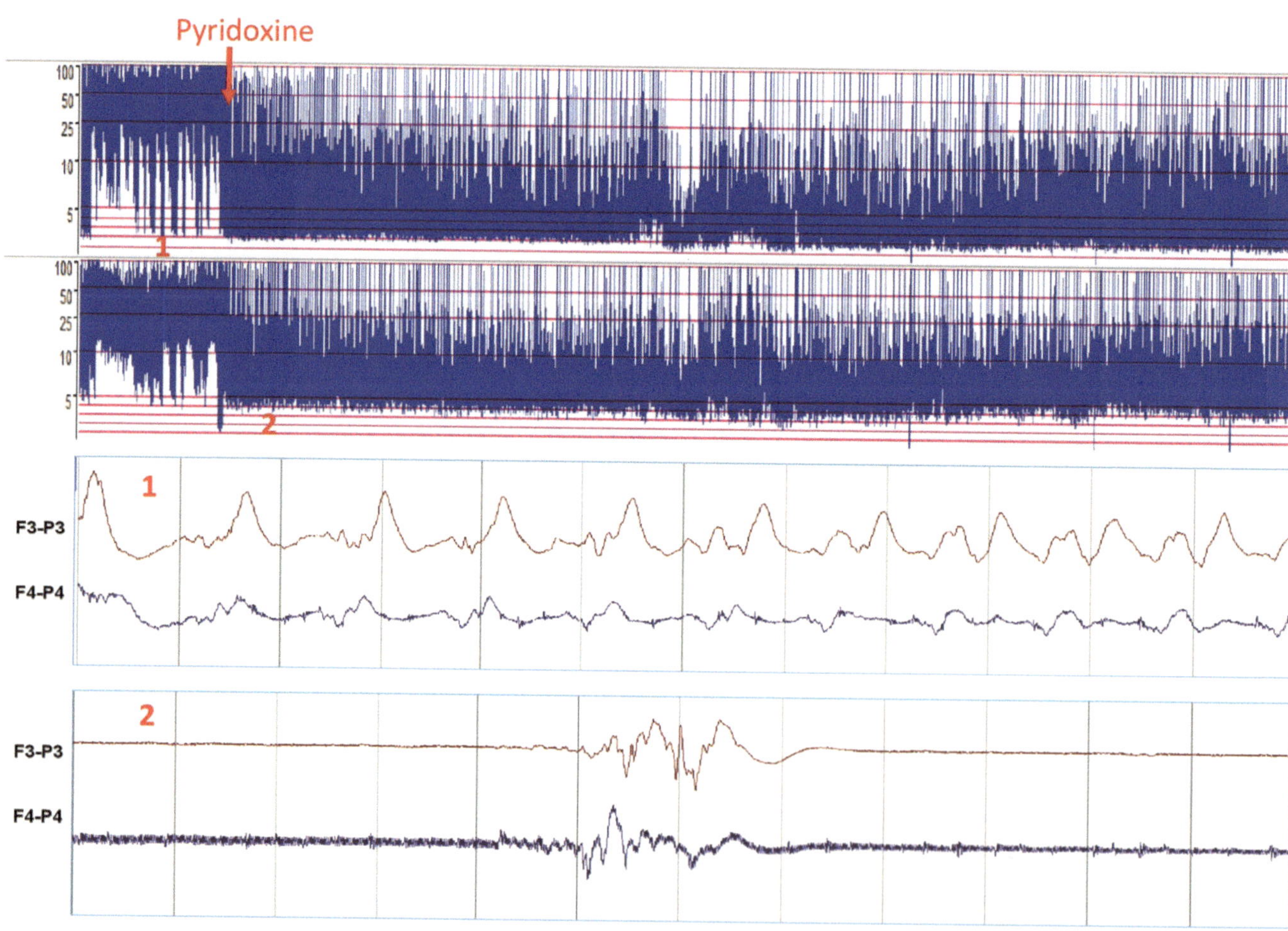

FIGURE 4.6 *aEEG in* pyridoxine deficiency. Late preterm infant presenting with ongoing seizures that were therapy-resistant. After administration of pyridoxine (arrow), the aEEG and EEG show immediate resolution of the seizure pattern and the background activity becomes severely discontinuous with a burst-suppression pattern. Similar, very rapidly occurring responses to pyridoxine have appeared in other infants with pyridoxine dependency after administration, and some infants become entirely flaccid and apneic. It is recommended that trained NICU staff and equipment for assisted ventilation are available when pyridoxine is tested in infants with seizures. (By courtesy of Elisabeth Book and Douglas Hägerström.)

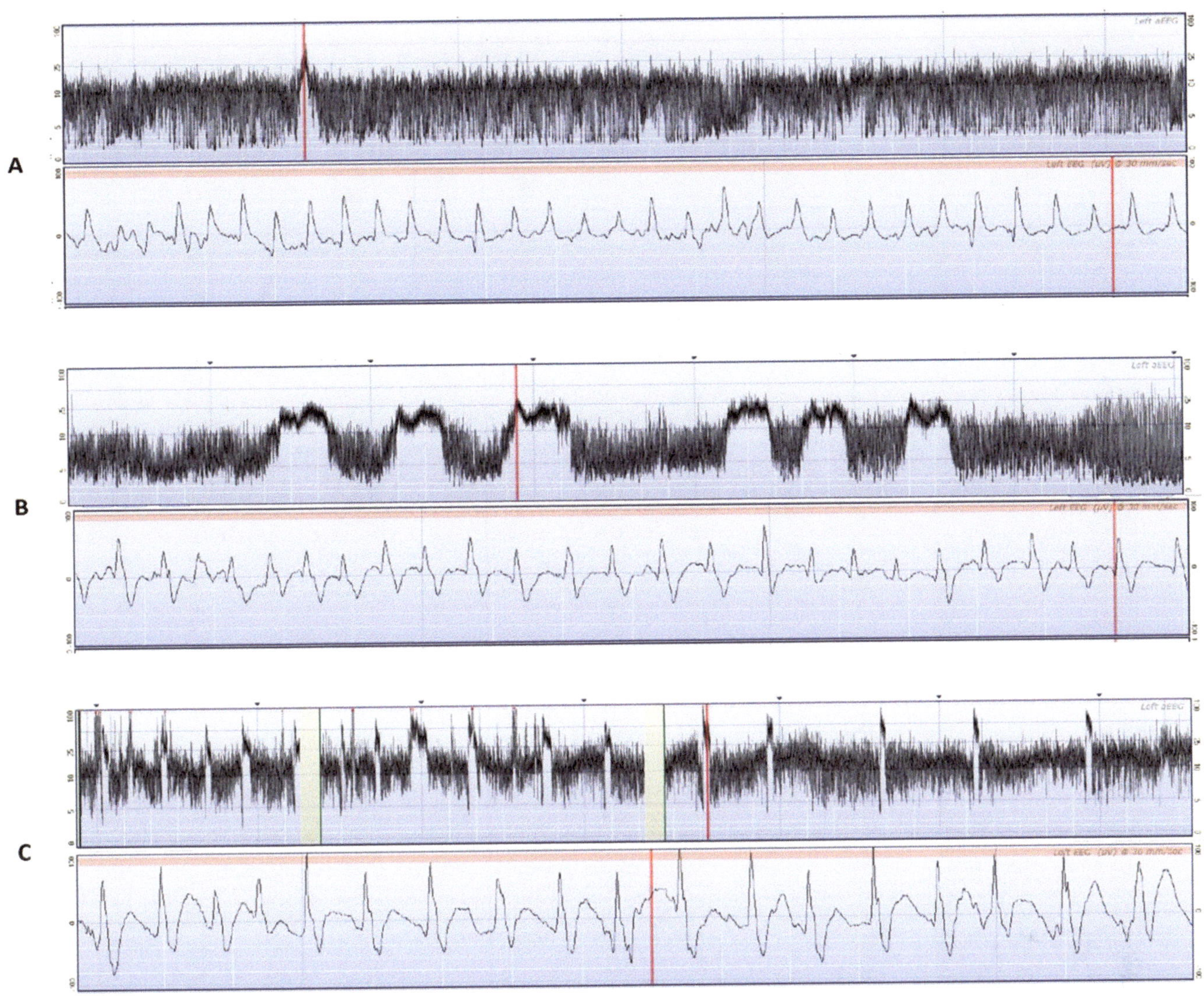

FIGURE 4.7 Different seizure occurrences in the aEEG trace (verified by the corresponding raw EEG): (A) single seizure, (B) repetitive prolonged seizures, and (C) repetitive seizures (short). Both (B) and (C) can fulfill the diagnosis of status epilepticus.

region instead of the central areas will significantly improve the cortical coverage. Irrespective of the electrode configuration used for the recording, better clinician skills and experience in both aEEG and raw EEG review will lead to improved seizure detection.

4.6 Seizure Burden (SB)

Seizure burden (SB) is a measure of the cumulative amount of seizures within a given time, such as the number of minutes with seizures in an hour (min/h; alternatively, the percentage of time). A commonly used definition of status epilepticus is the presence of seizures occurring ≥ 50% of an arbitrarily defined one-hour epoch. Recognizing such a high SB is easy with aEEG/EEG, but measuring lower SB requires detection of all seizure occurrences. The SB concept has several intuitive, (patho)physiological, and practical advantages: First, it reflects the total seizure load experienced by the brain during a given time. Second, it overcomes the uncertainty with detecting every brief seizure that may have a minimal cumulative effect on the SB, or the neonatal brain. Third, SB provides a more robust assessment than counting the number of individual seizures. Several publications have now demonstrated that a high total seizure burden in asphyxiated newborn infants is associated with poorer neurodevelopmental outcomes. A rough assessment of the SB can also be readily obtained from the aEEG trend. Notably, the seizure detection algorithm (SDA) outputs can be displayed directly as SB trends in some monitors (see Figure 8.4 *and* Chapter 8 more generally).

4.7 Role of Automated Seizure Detection

Automated seizure detection algorithms (SDAs) are increasingly implemented in commercial aEEG monitors to facilitate bedside review and evaluation of suspected seizures. SDAs rely on the raw EEG signal, and their output can be shown as an additional trend (Figure 4.10; *see also* Chapter 8). To reduce false detections, many SDAs focus on longer (> 30 seconds) seizures only. While the modern SDAs may even perform at the level of an expert EEG reviewer, it is important to note that the algorithms are not replacing the bedside clinician, but they can support in the clinical decision-making. In other words, the automated seizure detections need the clinicians'

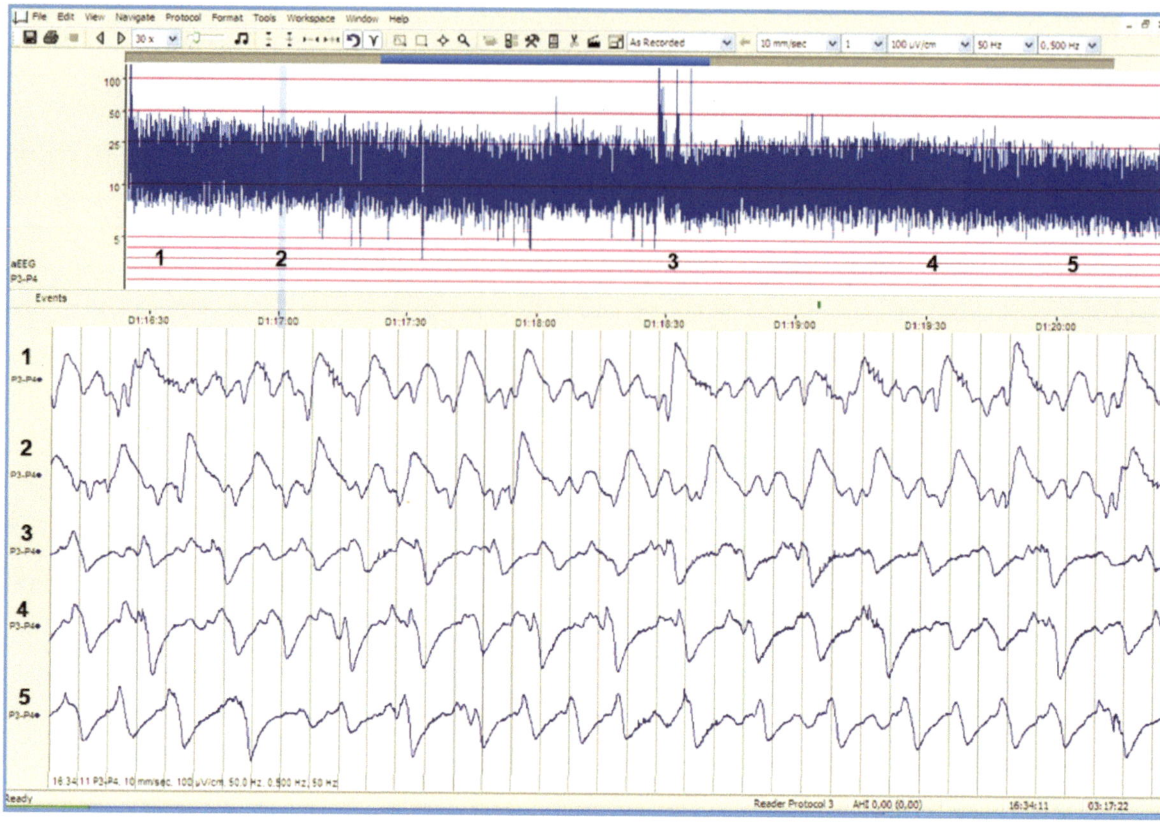

FIGURE 4.8 aEEG showing suspected continuous seizure activity over several hours. Since the seizure activity continues with only minor changes of waveforms, there are no waxing-waning patterns, and the aEEG pattern looks (falsely) continuous. This full-term baby was severely asphyxiated and undergoing therapeutic hypothermia.

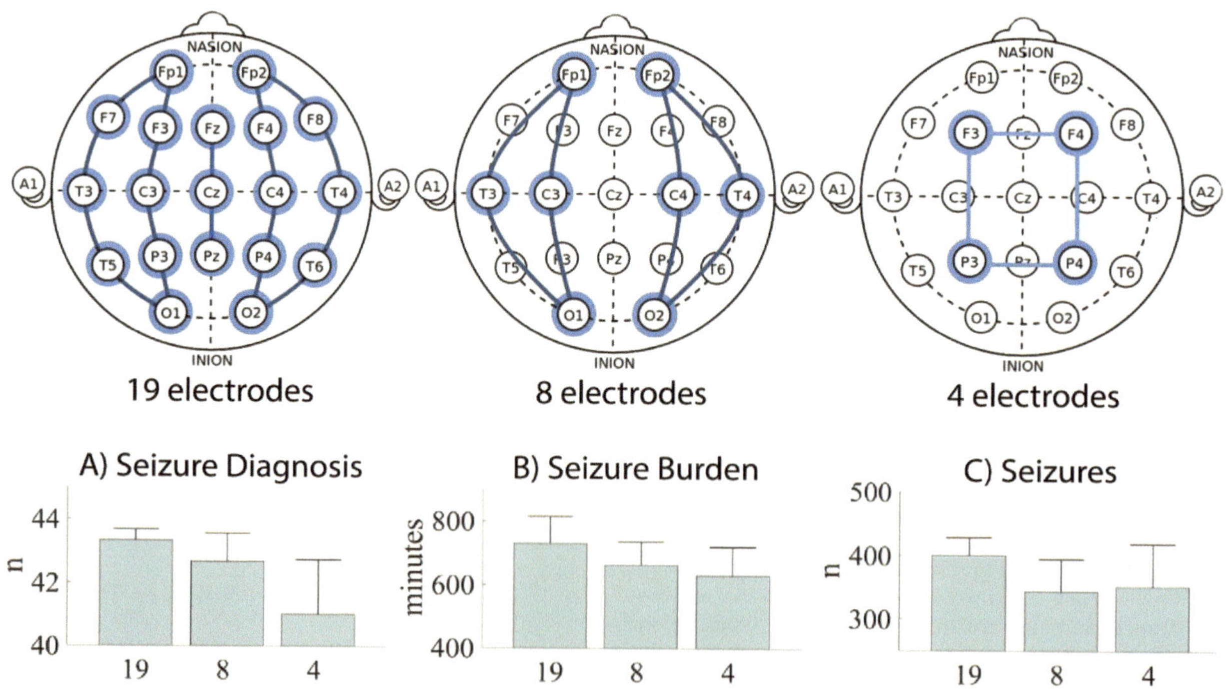

FIGURE 4.9 Comparison between different numbers of recording electrodes (19, 8, and 4 electrodes) in the visual detection of seizures. Upper panel illustrates the compared montages: The 19-electrode montage corresponds to the standard 10–20 system that was used as the ground truth in comparisons. The 8-electrode montage represents a conventional 'full neonatal montage', and the 4-electrode montage represents the current recommendation for 'aEEG monitoring'. The lower panel summarizes montage comparisons: (A) how many infants were identified as having seizures (seizure diagnosis), (B) how much seizure burden was detected, and (C) how many seizures were observed. When the seizure detections were compared across three blinded and very experienced EEG reviewers, the overall outcome was this: The 8- and 4-channel recordings did not differ significantly, while both of them showed poorer seizure detection as compared to the 10–20 standard montage with 19 electrodes. (From *Stevenson et al. 2018, with permission.*)

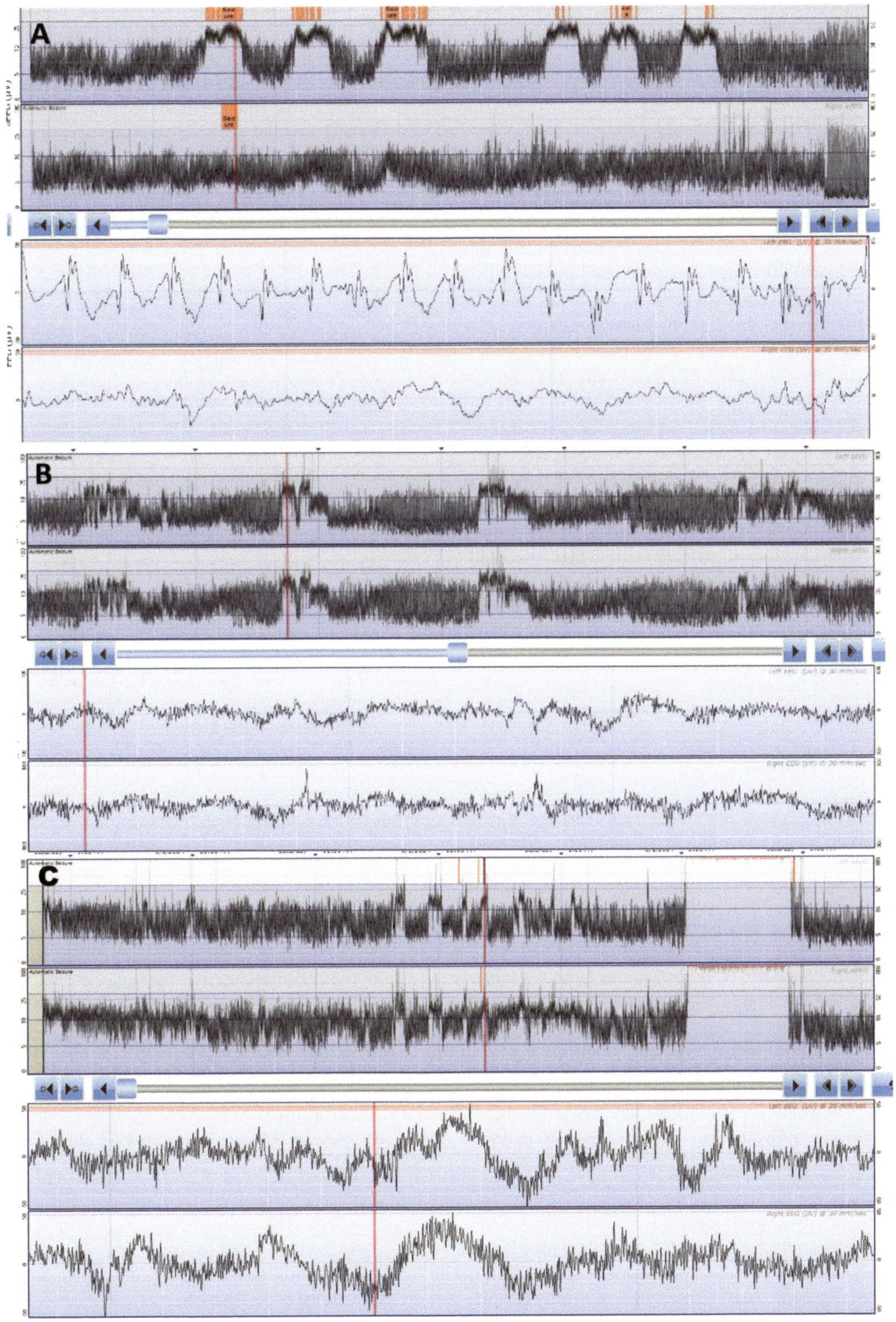

FIGURE 4.10 Examples of SDA in three infants: (A) with seizures correctly diagnosed by SDA, (B) without seizures, correctly excluded by SDA, and (C) without seizures but with three false short positive SDA alerts. Although the aEEG patterns appear suspicious for seizures in all three cases, the raw EEG pattern in (A) was correctly flagged as seizures by SDA (orange ribbon). A similar aEEG pattern in (B) was not flagged by SDA since it represented artefacts on the raw EEG. Finally, although baby (C) had no seizures, artefacts triggered three short SDA alerts. These cases demonstrate how SDA is helpful as a tool, but reviewing raw EEG continues to be the most reliable method.

confirmation, and at least an intermittent visual review of the raw EEG should be performed in the NICU. Future work is needed to show the added value of SDAs in different clinical situations, as well as to compare their performance with the agreement between human experts.

To summarize, the diagnosis of neonatal seizures requires confirmation from the raw EEG signals. High-risk neonates, with or without seizure suspicion, should be continuously monitored to allow timely detection of seizure onset. Seizure detection algorithms can assist in detecting seizures, but seizure diagnosis and treatment decisions need the bedside clinician with sufficient skills in raw EEG reading.

Bilaterally recorded aEEG/EEG from four electrodes over both hemispheres can pick up a majority of neonatal seizures. The evaluation requires that raw EEG is inspected. Single brief seizures may be challenging to diagnose in both aEEG and multichannel EEG recordings, and interobserver agreement is far from 100%, even between experienced interpreters. Detection of brief seizures is difficult for both human experts and SDAs. The most important is to routinely initiate monitoring of infants at high risk for seizures, or with suspected clinical seizures, and to regularly review the raw EEG. Studies evaluating 'neonatal neurocritical care' have demonstrated improvement in the accuracy of diagnosing seizures and more precise administration of antiseizure medications, see Chapter 9. Clinical cases with seizures in various conditions are presented in multiple cases in other chapters of this book.

References

Alharbi HM, Pinchefsky EF, Tran MA, et al. Seizure burden and neurologic outcomes after neonatal encephalopathy. *Neurology.* 2023;100(19):e1976–e1984.

Boylan GB, Stevenson NJ, Vanhatalo S. Monitoring neonatal seizures. *Semin Fetal Neonatal Med.* 2013;18(4):202–208.

El-Dib M, Chang T, Tsuchida TN, Clancy RR. Amplitude-integrated electroencephalography in neonates. *Pediatr Neurol.* 2009;41(5):315–326.

Glass HC, Shellhaas RA, Tsuchida TN, et al. Seizures in preterm neonates: A multicenter observational cohort study. *Pediatr Neurol.* 2017;72:19–24.

Hellström-Westas L. Comparison between tape-recorded and amplitude-integrated EEG monitoring in sick newborn infants. *Acta Paediatr.* 1992;81(10):812–819.

Hellström-Westas L, Blennow G, Rosen I. Amplitude-integrated encephalography in pyridoxine-dependent seizures and pyridoxine-responsive seizures. *Acta Paediatr.* 2002;91(8):977–980.

Janáčková S, Boyd S, Yozawitz E, et al. Electroencephalographic characteristics of epileptic seizures in preterm neonates. *Clin Neurophysiol.* 2016;127(8):2721–2727.

Kharoshankaya L, Stevenson NJ, Livingstone V, et al. Seizure burden and neurodevelopmental outcome in neonates with hypoxic-ischemic encephalopathy. *Dev Med Child Neurol.* 2016;58(12):1242–1248.

Lloyd RO, O'Toole JM, Pavlidis E, et al. Electrographic seizures during the early postnatal period in preterm infants. *J Pediatr.* 2017;187:18–25.e12.

Pavel AMJ, Rennie JM, de Vries LS, et al. A machine-learning algorithm for neonatal seizure recognition: A multicentre, randomised, controlled trial. *Lancet Child Adolesc Health.* 2020;4(10):740–749.

Pijpers JA, Au PYB, Weeke LC, et al. Early recognition of characteristic conventional and amplitude-integrated EEG patterns of seizures in SCN2A and KCNQ3-related epilepsy in neonates. *Seizure.* 2023;110:212–219.

Pisani F, Barilli AL, Sisti L, et al. Preterm infants with video-EEG confirmed seizures: Outcome at 30 months of age. *Brain Dev.* 2008;30(1):20–30.

Pressler RM, Abend NS, Auvin S, et al. Treatment of seizures in the neonate: Guidelines and consensus-based recommendations—special report from the ILAE task force on neonatal seizures. *Epilepsia.* 2023;64(10):2550–2570.

Pressler RM, Cilio MR, Mizrahi EM, et al. The ILAE classification of seizures and the epilepsies: Modification for seizures in the neonate. Position paper by the ILAE task force on neonatal seizures. *Epilepsia.* 2021;62(3):615–628.

Ronen GM, Penney S, Andrews W. The epidemiology of clinical neonatal seizures in Newfoundland: A population-based study. *J Pediatr.* 1999;134(1):71–75.

Shah DK, Mackay MT, Lavery S, et al. Accuracy of bedside electroencephalographic monitoring in comparison with simultaneous continuous conventional electroencephalography for seizure detection in term infants. *Pediatrics.* 2008;121(6):1146–1154.

Shellhaas RA, Chang T, Tsuchida T, et al. The American Clinical Neurophysiology Society's guideline on continuous electroencephalography monitoring in neonates. *J Clin Neurophysiol.* 2011;28(6):611–617.

Shellhaas RA, Clancy RR. Characterization of neonatal seizures by conventional EEG and single-channel EEG. *Clin Neurophysiol.* 2007;118(10):2156–2161.

Shellhaas RA, Soaita AI, Clancy RR. Sensitivity of amplitude-integrated electroencephalography for neonatal seizure detection. *Pediatrics.* 2007;120(4):770–777.

Stevenson NJ, Lauronen L, Vanhatalo S. The effect of reducing EEG electrode number on the visual interpretation of the human expert for neonatal seizure detection. *Clin Neurophysiol.* 2018;129(1):265–270.

Stevenson NJ, Tapani K, Vanhatalo S. Hybrid neonatal EEG seizure detection algorithms achieve the benchmark of visual interpretation of the human expert. *Annu Int Conf IEEE Eng Med Biol Soc.* 2019:5991–5994.

Tsuchida TN, Wusthoff CJ, Shellhaas RA, et al. American Clinical Neurophysiology Society standardized EEG terminology and categorization for the description of continuous EEG monitoring in neonates: Report of the American Clinical Neurophysiology Society critical care monitoring committee. *J Clin Neurophysiol.* 2013;30(2):161–173.

Vilan AJ, Mendes Ribeiro J, Striano P, et al. A distinctive ictal amplitude-integrated electroencephalography pattern in newborns with neonatal epilepsy associated with KCNQ2 mutations. *Neonatology.* 2017;112(4):387–393.

Weeke LC, van Ooijen IM, Groenendaal F, et al. Rhythmic EEG patterns in extremely preterm infants: Classification and association with brain injury and outcome. *Clin Neurophysiol.* 2017;128(12):2428–2435.

Zhang L, Zhou YX, Chang LW, Luo XP. Diagnostic value of amplitude-integrated electroencephalogram in neonatal seizures. *Neurosci Bull.* 2011;27(4):251–257.

5 NEONATAL ENCEPHALOPATHY IN THE FULL-TERM INFANT DUE TO HYPOXIA-ISCHEMIA AND FOCAL BRAIN LESIONS

Linda S de Vries and Lena Hellström-Westas

SUMMARY

- A continuous or a slightly discontinuous aEEG pattern within the first hours after birth in asphyxiated infants is associated with a favourable outcome.
- Hypothermia-treated infants with burst-suppression, or a more depressed aEEG background pattern, at 36–48 hrs of age have a high risk for adverse outcome.
- Hypothermia-treated infants with emerging sleep-wake cycling at 36–48 hrs of age have a good chance of recovery.
- As seizures can occur during and following rewarming, continue the aEEG recordings for at least 84 h.
- Sedative and anticonvulsive medications can depress the aEEG background activity and contribute to a more uncertain evaluation of brain activity.

The neonatal EEG is depressed during and immediately after an acute hypoxic-ischemic insult. The degree and duration of the EEG depression correlates with the severity of the brain injury. During recovery, the EEG subsequently contains information on the severity of the previous hypoxic-ischemic insult. In newborn infants, the electrocortical activity is a highly sensitive predictor of neurologic outcome when recorded early after a hypoxic-ischemic insult. In most full-term infants with NE (neonatal encephalopathy) and acute symptomatic seizures, the electrocortical background will normalize within 1–2 weeks, also in infants who start with severely abnormal electrocortical activity.

It is recommended to use aEEG as part of the initial evaluation in full-term infants with suspected hypoxic-ischemic encephalopathy (HIE). The electrocortical background activity identified with the aEEG trend should preferably be supported by simultaneous assessment of the underlying raw EEG signal. Assessment of cortical activity by EEG/aEEG may provide more reliable brain assessment than the clinical neurological status in the given critical care situation and may assist in decisions on whether to cool or not. Care should also be taken with only looking at the numerical aEEG amplitudes because various NICU-related technical artefacts may cause a persistent elevation of the aEEG lower border (see Chapter 3, Artefacts).

The main focus, when monitoring infants with neonatal encephalopathy, irrespective of the underlying cause (e.g. hypoxia-ischaemia, metabolic, infectious or other), is the electrocortical background activity, as reflected by the aEEG pattern. The aEEG trend shows the variability in brain activity over time, including recovery or deterioration, sleep-wake cycling and seizures.

Clinical evaluation of the aEEG trend is mainly based on pattern recognition, where the reviewer assesses the lower border, its fluctuation over time, as well as the overall pattern of the aEEG trend. In severely depressed aEEG tracings, the number of bursts over a certain time period (e.g. 1 hour) can be used as a semi-quantitative measure. When two bilateral leads are recorded, side differences caused by, for example, unilateral brain injury or technical artefacts can sometimes be detected. Evaluation of the aEEG trend is usually performed with pattern recognition, although amplitude-based assessment of the aEEG trend before hypothermia treatment has also been used in some studies. However, it is important to be cautious when using numerical amplitude cut-offs, as artefacts may affect and elevate the lower margin. It is also safer to perceive that the clinical information of the aEEG trend is embedded in the overall pattern rather than in any absolute aEEG value. Checking the raw EEG for artefacts can often be very helpful in infants with depressed brain activity.

5.1 Neonatal Encephalopathy (NE) Due to Hypoxia-Ischemia

5.1.1 aEEG Background Activity

Prior to the introduction of therapeutic hypothermia, several studies showed that crude outcome (good or poor) could be accurately predicted from the aEEG trend already during the first hours after birth. Table 5.1 shows the results of a systematic review investigating the predictive value of aEEG in asphyxiated term infants. The study included 12 studies of normothermic infants (most of the infants recorded before hypothermia treatment was introduced) and seven studies of hypothermia-treated infants and showed the high predictive value of the aEEG at different time points for predicting both good and poor outcomes. The two graphs in Figure 5.1 summarize the findings in one study, demonstrating results close to the meta-analysis. The graphs demonstrate clearly how the hypothermia intervention, which aims to improve outcome, changes the early predictive value of the aEEG.

A recent study (Meder et al. 2022) evaluated aEEG monitoring in hypothermia-treated infants for 84 hours, including the rewarming period, and created a score for the aEEG background pattern, including sleep-wake cycling. Longitudinal aEEG background analysis combined with sleep-wake cycling score had an excellent predictive value (AUC, 0.90; 95% CI, 0.85–0.95), better than single aEEG scores at any individual time point. The prediction tool can be accessed online: *https://suneonatalgroup.shinyapps.io/aeegpredictiontool/.*

5.1.2 Sleep-Wake Cycling (SWC)

The infant's ability to express different sleep states in a rhythmic manner (SWC) is considered to reflect restored functional integrity in wide subcortical brain networks. Therefore, SWC may provide a useful surrogate for assessing brain recovery wider than the cortical function. While sleep-wake cycling will develop eventually in almost all children who survive, and also in

DOI: 10.1201/b22858-5

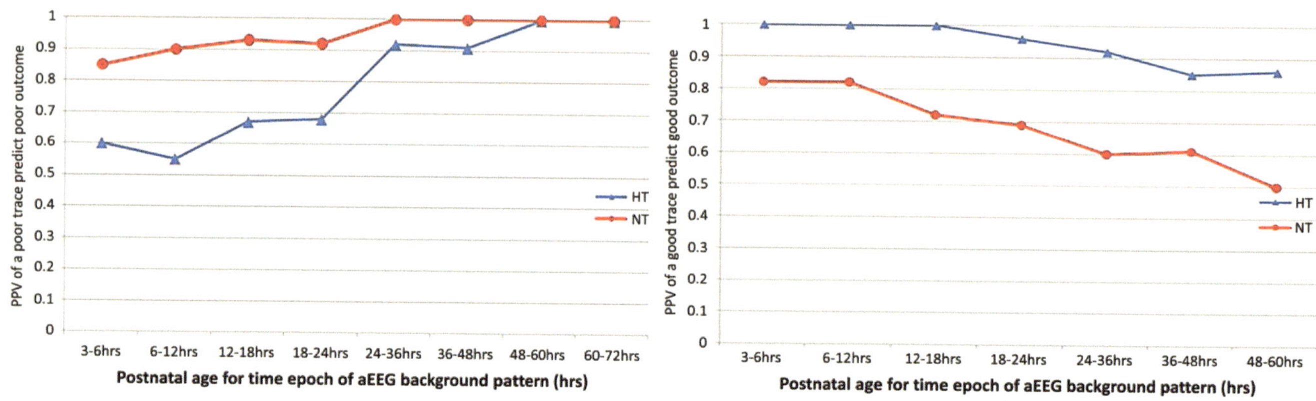

FIGURE 5.1 The graphs show the PPV for a poor trace to predict poor outcome (left) and the PPV for a good trace to predict good outcome (right) in non-cooled (red) and hypothermia-treated (blue) infants. In the left part, the change in PPV (due to the intervention, blue line) which is due to the hypothermia treatment and occurs during the first 36 hours is clearly seen. The very high PPV of a poor trace to predict poor outcome (red trace) is clear. On the right part of the figure, it is shown how a good pattern predicts good outcome. The PPV is decreasing over time, as a result of the recovery to a good pattern of infants with poor outcome. Also in this part, the difference in trajectories, due to the hypothermia intervention, is evident. (Left, from *Thoresen et al. 2010 with permission*; Right, courtesy of Marianne Thoresen.)

some of those who do not survive the neonatal period, the time of SWC onset is associated with the severity of HIE. Recovery of SWC before 36 hours was associated with better outcome in non-cooled infants, while therapeutic hypothermia seems to delay the development of SWC, which usually starts to appear around 48 hours. Presence of SWC by the time of rewarming is associated with good outcome, while never developing SWC during hypothermia treatment is predictive of poor outcome.

5.1.3 Reactivity to Care

The aEEG trend often responds to caregiving with a short transient rise in the aEEG background. It does likely reflect infant's arousal to higher vigilance state, and it is best seen when the aEEG is discontinuous without being too ill or heavily sedated. Reactivity is not usually clearly discernible in infants with a CNV aEEG background and can be even confused with an ictal discharge (see Figure 3.2). The raw EEG is needed to make this distinction.

5.1.4 aEEG, NIRS and Biomarkers

By combining aEEG monitoring with NIRS during hypothermia treatment, early PPV can be increased to values seen in normothermic infants with asphyxia. Several studies have also shown correlations between various biomarkers, e.g. neuron-specific enolase, and lactate dehydrogenase and outcome. However, these biomarkers have not been proven to be predictive early after birth, when decisions of hypothermia treatment need to be taken.

5.1.5 Preterm Infants with HIE

There is less evidence about the ability of the aEEG trend to predict outcome after hypoxic-ischemic events occurring in moderately-late preterm infants or later in the neonatal period or infancy. The available scarce data suggest that the same overall relationship holds true between the recovery of the aEEG background and the subsequent outcome.

5.1.6 Seizures in Infants with NE Following HI or Focal Brain Lesions

When the initial electrocortical background pattern is discontinuous in encephalopathic infants, the risk of developing seizures is increased. While initially suspected seizures are often clinical, they often become electrographic without clear clinical symptoms after administration of antiseizure medication. This phenomenon has been called "uncoupling" and stresses the importance of continuous aEEG or EEG monitoring in infants with suspected seizures. While the corresponding single- or two-channel EEG in the aEEG monitor may display more than 80% of seizures present in a conventional EEG, the sensitivity varies a lot in the literature and can be explained by the variable experience of the staff, the duration and the location of the seizures. When users are experienced and also look at the raw EEG and have access to a seizure-detection algorithm, the sensitivity of the aEEG/EEG is higher.

In infants with mild HIE or NE with normal EEG background activity, presence of electrographic seizures does not seem to be a strong predictor of outcome. However, the seizure burden, expressed as a high total seizure burden or a high maximum hourly seizure burden, are associated with adverse outcome. Following the introduction of hypothermia, seizures have become less common and are reported in 20–30% of the infants. Recurrence of seizures during or following rewarming are, however, not uncommon. Infants with a depressed aEEG/EEG background pattern were especially at risk to develop seizures during rewarming.

The incidence of status epilepticus, reported in aEEG and cEEG studies, varies around 15–20%, depending on whether the infant received hypothermia treatment. See further Table 5.2.

5.2 Neonatal Encephalopathy Due to Causes Other Than Hypoxia-Ischemia

Clinical seizures are usually the presenting symptom in infants with focal brain lesions, such as perinatal arterial ischemic stroke (PAIS) or cerebral parenchymal hemorrhage. The onset of seizures in infants with PAIS is more common beyond 12h in infants with HIE, and these infants are more likely to present with clinical hemiconvulsions. Bilateral aEEG monitoring may show depression of activity (including poorer sleep-wake cycling) and more seizures over the affected hemisphere.

TABLE 5.1: Predictive Values of Abnormal Background Patterns (BS, CLV, FT) from 6 to 72 Hours of Life to Predict Adverse 138 Outcomes (Death or Handicap)

aEEG-Death/Serious Disability		Normothermia	Hypothermia
6 h	Studies (n)	12 (671)	7 (360)
	AUC	0.87	0.94
	Sensitivity (95% CI)	0.84 (0.78 to −0.88)	0.95 (0.9 to 0.98)
	Specificity (95% CI)	0.79 (0.63 to 0.89)	0.61 (0.51 to 0.69)
	Positive LR (95% CI)	4.34 (2.31 to 7.73)	1.57 (1.37 to 1.85)
	Negative LR (95% CI)	0.2 (0.14 to 0.29)	0.12 (0.05 to 0.25)
24 h	Studies (n)	5 (267)	4 (141)
	AUC	0.95	0.86
	Sensitivity (95% CI)	0.84 (0.77 to 0.89)	0.89 (0.71 to 0.96)
	Specificity (95% CI)	0.96 (0.89 to 0.98)	0.65 (0.46 to 0.81)
	Positive LR (95% CI)	24.2 (7.48 to 59.3)	2.76 (1.48 to 5.27)
	Negative LR (95% CI)	0.16 (0.1 to 0.23)	0.19 (0.04 to 0.53)
36 h	Studies (n)	3 (76)	3 (126)
	AUC	0.95	0.93
	Sensitivity (95% CI)	0.79 (0.59 to 0.9)	0.89 (0.76 to 0.95)
	Specificity (95% CI)	0.95 (0.81 to 0.99)	0.84 (0.74 to 0.9)
	Positive LR (95% CI)	26.6 (4.43 to 94.9)	5.73 (3.35 to 9.43)
	Negative LR (95% CI)	0.23 (0.09 to 0.44)	0.14 (0.05 to 0.28)
48 h	Studies (n)	3 (77)	3 (123)
	AUC	0.95	0.85
	Sensitivity (95% CI)	0.76 (0.61 to 0.86)	0.79 (0.64 to 0.89)
	Specificity (95% CI)	0.95 (0.79 to 0.99)	0.93 (0.85 to 0.97)
	Positive LR (95% CI)	23.3 (3.55 to 85.7)	14.4 (5.51 to 32.5)
	Negative LR (95% CI)	0.26 (0.15 to 0.41)	0.22 (0.11 to 0.37)
72 h	Studies (n)	3 (64)	3 (119)
	AUC	0.82	0.91
	Sensitivity (95% CI)	0.73 (0.54 to 0.85)	0.61 (0.45 to 0.75)
	Specificity (95% CI)	0.89 (0.58 to 0.97)	0.97 (0.9 to 0.99)
	Positive LR (95% CI)	9.04 (1.69 to 31.6)	24.3 (5.89 to 71.3)
	Negative LR (95% CI)	0.32 (0.17 to 0.56)	0.39 (0.25 to 0.57)

Source: From Del Río et al. 2016.

AUC = Area under the curve; 95% CI = 95% Confidence Interval; LR = Likelihood ratio.

TABLE 5.2: Summary of Impact of Different aEEG Features for Prediction of Outcome in Hypothermia-Treated Asphyxiated Full-Term Infants

	Age				
	0–12 h	12–24 h	24–36 h	36–48 h	48–72 h
Background pattern	++	+	+	+++	++
Single seizures	–	–	–	–	–
Status epilepticus	++	++	++	++	++
Sleep-wake cycling	+	+	+	++	++
Reactivity to care	–	–	–	–	–

The EEG may also show specific unilateral bursts of theta activity with sharp waves or spikes intermixed. Apneas are often a presenting symptom in infants with a temporal lobe hemorrhage. Infants with cerebral parenchymal hemorrhages can develop seizures that are difficult to control.

Critically ill and unstable neonates may experience several events during intensive care that may negatively affect brain function, e.g. periods with low or unstable oxygenation and blood pressure. Such high-risk infants include babies with congenital heart defects and congenital diaphragmatic hernia, infants with persistent pulmonary hypertension of the newborn, infants developing a pneumothorax and infants with severe infections. With the aEEG, it is possible to follow the impact on the brain in such infants. Combining regional cerebral oxygen saturation (rSO_2), fractional cerebral tissue oxygen extraction (FTOE) measured by near-infrared spectroscopy (NIRS) and aEEG after perinatal asphyxia can be of additional value.

Critically ill infants may suffer severe hypoxic-ischemic or other insults before they are stabilized on *ECMO*. Cannulation and initiation of ECMO is not associated with acute aEEG changes, except that administered anaesthetic medications may transiently depress electrocortical activity. Comparable to infants with HIE, the depressed aEEG background activity is predictive of death or moderate to severe intracranial neuropathology (moderate to severe hydrocephalus, ischemia, infarction or hemorrhage documented on neuroimaging or autopsy), and electrographic seizures are not unusual. An abnormal aEEG background activity after 24 hours on ECMO is associated with unfavourable outcome with a high specificity.

Monitoring with aEEG in infants undergoing *neonatal heart surgery* has also been shown to be of value in several studies. Around 20% of infants have been reported to develop ictal discharges postoperatively. An abnormal BGP and ictal discharges are more frequent in neonates with new postoperative brain injury. Besides an abnormal postoperative background pattern, lack of SWC has also been reported to predict poorer intelligence quotient in early childhood.

References

Alharbi HM, Pinchefsky EF, Tran MA, et al. Seizure burden and neurologic outcomes after neonatal encephalopathy. *Neurol.* 2023;100(19):e1976–e1984.

Al Naqeeb N, Edwards AD, Cowan FM, Azzopardi D. Assessment of neonatal encephalopathy by amplitude-integrated electroencephalography. *Pediatrics.* 1999;103(6 Pt 1):1263–1271.

Arnaez J, Sanchez-Acosta CG, Fasce J, Garcia-Alix A. Usefulness of two-channel amplitude-integrated EEG recording in a neonatal setting. *J Matern Fetal Neonatal Med.* 2021;34(14):2248–2258.

Bjerre I, Hellström-Westas L, Rosén I, Svenningsen N. Monitoring of cerebral function after severe asphyxia in infancy. *Arch Dis Child.* 1983;58(12):997–1002.

Caramelo I, Coelho M, Rosado M, et al. Biomarkers of hypoxic-ischemic encephalopathy: A systematic review. *World J Pediatr.* 2023;19(6):505–548.

Chahine A, Chenouard A, Joram N, et al. Continuous amplitude-integrated electroencephalography during neonatal and pediatric extracorporeal membrane oxygenation. *J Clin Neurophysiol.* 2023;40(4):317–324.

Chalak LF, Pappas A, Tan S, et al.; Eunice Kennedy Shriver National Institute of Child Health and Human Development Neonatal Research Network. Association between increased seizures during rewarming after hypothermia for neonatal hypoxic ischemic encephalopathy and abnormal neurodevelopmental outcomes at 2-year follow-up: A nested multisite cohort study. *JAMA Neurol.* 2021;78(12):1484–1493.

Chandrasekaran M, Chaban B, Montaldo P, Thayyil S. Predictive value of amplitude-integrated EEG (aEEG) after rescue hypothermic neuroprotection for hypoxic ischemic encephalopathy: A meta-analysis. *J Perinatol.* 2017;37(6):684–689.

Claessens NHP, Noorlag L, Weeke LC, et al. Amplitude-integrated electroencephalography for early recognition of brain injury in neonates with critical congenital heart disease. *J Pediatr.* 2018;202:199–205.e1.

Del Río R, Ochoa C, Alarcon A, et al. Amplitude integrated electroencephalogram as a prognostic tool in neonates with hypoxic-ischemic encephalopathy: A systematic review. *PLoS One.* 2016;(11):e0165744.

El-Dib M, Abend NS, Austin T, et al.; Newborn Brain Society Guidelines and Publications Committee. Neuromonitoring in neonatal critical care part I: Neonatal encephalopathy and neonates with possible seizures. *Pediatr Res.* 2022;94(1):64–73.

Guidotti I, Lugli L, Guerra MP, et al. Hypothermia reduces seizure burden and improves neurological outcome in severe hypoxic-ischemic encephalopathy: An observational study. *Dev Med Child Neurol.* 2016;58(12):1235–1241.

Gunn JK, Beca J, Hunt RW, et al. Perioperative amplitude-integrated EEG and neurodevelopment in infants with congenital heart disease. *Intensive Care Med.* 2012;38(9):1539–1547.

Herzberg EM, Machie M, Glass HC, et al.; Neonatal Seizure Registry Study Group. Seizure severity and treatment response in newborn infants with seizures attributed to intracranial hemorrhage. *J Pediatr.* 2022;242:121–128.e1.

Hoogstraate SR, Lequin MH, Huysman MA, et al. Apnoea in relation to neonatal temporal lobe haemorrhage. *Eur J Paediatr Neurol.* 2009;13(4):356–361.

Jiang CM, Yang YH, Chen LQ, et al. Early amplitude-integrated EEG monitoring 6 h after birth predicts long-term neurodevelopment of asphyxiated late preterm infants. *Eur J Pediatr.* 2015;174(8):1043–1052.

Kharoshankaya L, Stevenson NJ, Livingstone V, et al. Seizure burden and neurodevelopmental outcome in neonates with hypoxic-ischemic encephalopathy. *Dev Med Child Neurol.* 2016;58(12):1242–1248.

Latal B, Wohlrab G, Brotschi B, et al. Postoperative amplitude-integrated electroencephalography predicts four-year neurodevelopmental outcome in children with complex congenital heart disease. *J Pediatr.* 2016;178:55–60.

Lemmers PM, Zwanenburg RJ, Benders MJ, et al. Cerebral oxygenation and brain activity after perinatal asphyxia: Does hypothermia change their prognostic value? *Pediatr Res.* 2013;74(2):180–185.

Low E, Boylan GB, Mathieson SR, et al. Cooling and seizure burden in term neonates: An observational study. *Arch Dis Child Fetal Neonatal Ed.* 2012;97(4):F267–F272.

Low E, Mathieson SR, Stevenson NJ, et al. Early postnatal EEG features of perinatal arterial ischaemic stroke with seizures. *PLoS One.* 2014;9(7):e100973.

Mebius MJ, Oostdijk NJE, Kuik SJ, et al. Amplitude-integrated electroencephalography during the first 72 h after birth in neonates diagnosed prenatally with congenital heart disease. *Pediatr Res.* 2018;83(4):798–803.

Meder U, Cseko AJ, Szakacs L, et al. Longitudinal analysis of amplitude-integrated electroencephalography for outcome prediction in hypoxic-ischemic encephalopathy. *J Pediatr.* 2022;246:19–25.e5.

Osredkar D, Toet MC, van Rooij LG, et al. Sleep-wake cycling on amplitude-integrated electroencephalography in term newborns with hypoxic-ischemic encephalopathy. *Pediatrics.* 2005;115(2):327–332.

Pappas A, Shankaran S, Stockmann PT, Bara R. Changes in amplitude-integrated electroencephalography in neonates treated with extracorporeal membrane oxygenation: A pilot study. *J Pediatr.* 2006;148(1):125–127.

Parmentier CEJ, Steggerda SJ, Weeke LC, et al. Outcome of non-cooled asphyxiated infants with under-recognised or delayed-onset encephalopathy. *Arch Dis Child Fetal Neonatal Ed.* 2022;107(4):364–370.

Sansevere AJ, Kapur K, Peters JM, et al. Seizure prediction models in the neonatal intensive care unit. *J Clin Neurophysiol.* 2019;36(3):186–194.

Sirsi D, Nadiminti L, Packard MA, et al. Apneic seizures: A sign of temporal lobe hemorrhage in full-term neonates. *Pediatr Neurol.* 2007;37(5):366–370.

Srinivasakumar P, Zempel J, Trivedi S, et al. Treating EEG seizures in hypoxic ischemic encephalopathy: A randomized controlled trial. *Pediatrics.* 2015;136(5):e1302–e1309.

Thoresen M, Hellström-Westas L, Liu X, de Vries LS. Effect of hypothermia on amplitude-integrated electroencephalogram in infants with asphyxia. *Pediatrics.* 2010;126(1):e131–e139.

van Rooij LG, Toet MC, van Huffelen AC, et al. Effect of treatment of subclinical neonatal seizures detected with aEEG: Randomized, controlled trial. *Pediatrics.* 2010;125(2):e358–e366.

Case 5.1 Full-Term Infant with Mild HIE and Slow Recovery

Term infant, born at 39 weeks' gestation, birthweight grams, born by ventouse extraction in a delivery complicated by cord prolapse. Apgar scores were 3, 5 and 5 at 1, 5 and 10 minutes, respectively. Slow recovery with insufflation breaths and Positive End Expiratory Pressure (PEEP). At 15 minutes, a capillary blood gas showed a pH of 6.95 and arterial lactate of 12.8 mmol/L. The Thompson score was 7, and the infant was admitted to the NICU.

The *aEEG* was started soon after admission (5 hrs of age) and showed a DNV pattern, and it was decided to start hypothermia (Figure 5.1A). The transient elevation of the lower margin at the end of the trace was due to care. The infant never developed seizures. At around 48 hrs, the background pattern was a mixture of DNV and CNV and imminent SWC was observed (Figure 5.1B). The background activity improved further to CNV, but SWC was not completely established when rewarming started (Figure 5.1C).

The *MRI* (Figure 5.1D) at 4 days did not show any abnormalities except for an increased signal intensity on the T2 (a) and diffusion restriction of the mammillary bodies. on DWI (b). Diffusion restriction was also seen in the corpus callosum (not shown). Outcome at 2 years was within the normal range.

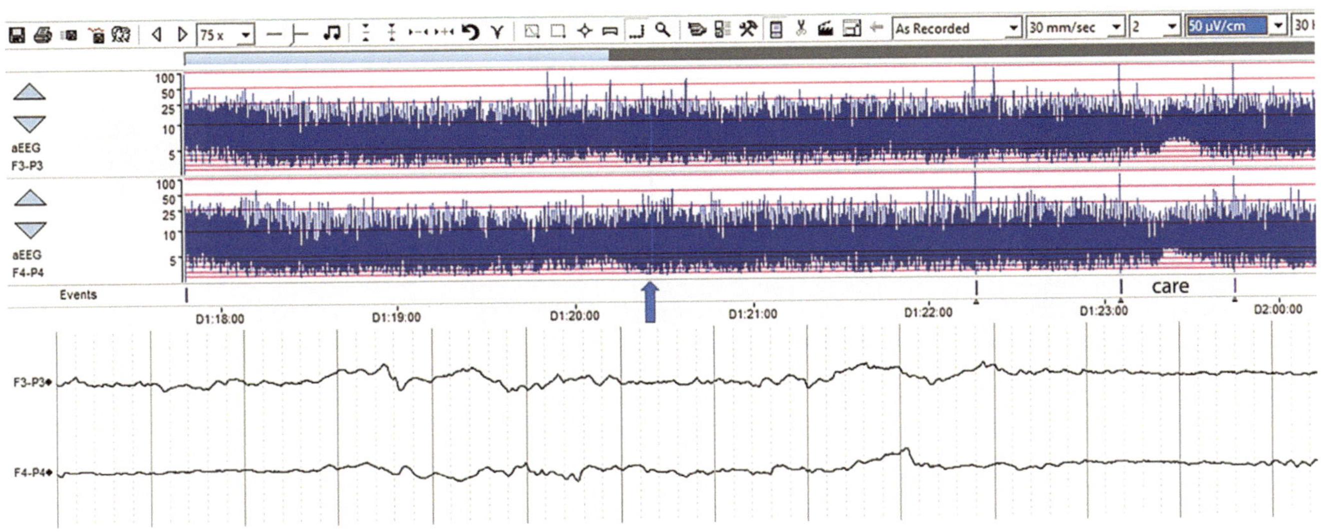

FIGURE 5.1A

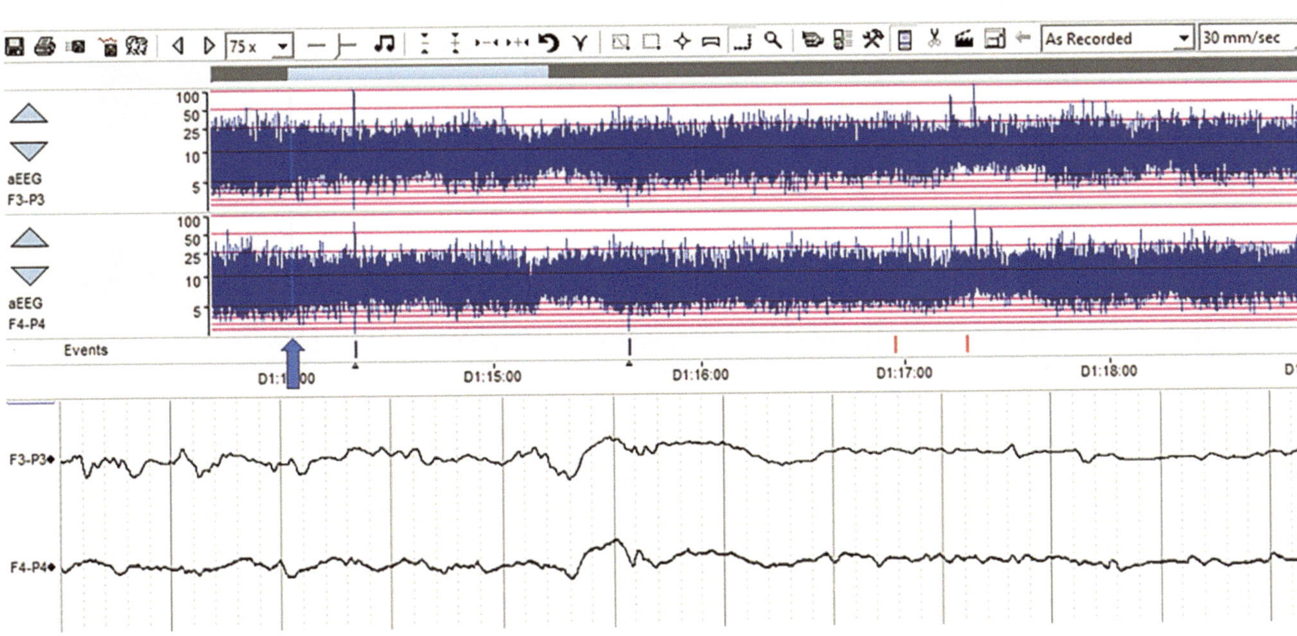

FIGURE 5.1B

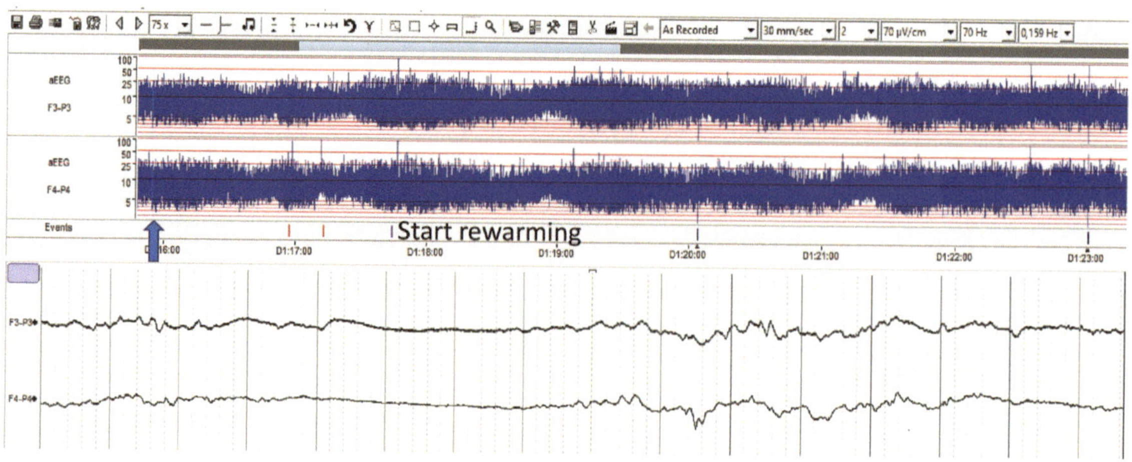

FIGURE 5.1C

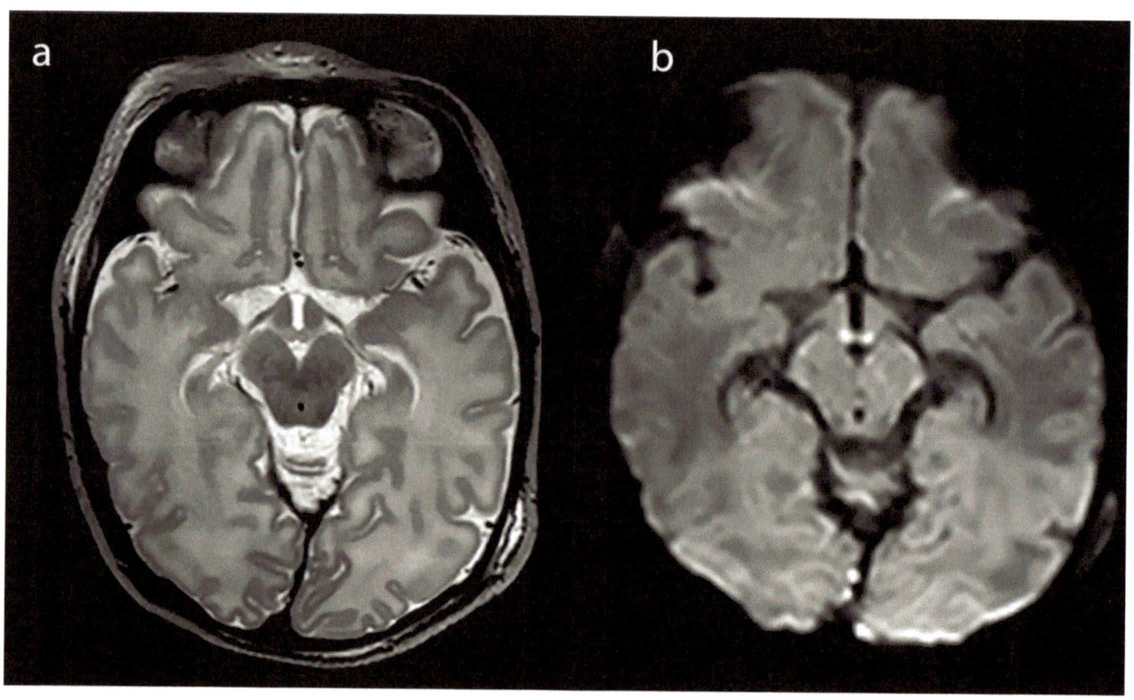

FIGURE 5.1D

Case 5.2 Mild Encephalopathy with Evolution to Moderate Encephalopathy

This infant was born at 41 weeks' gestation by ventouse extraction following spontaneous labour and meconium-stained liquor. Apgar scores were 6, 8 and 8 at 1, 5 and 10 minutes, respectively. The arterial umbilical pH was 6.96 and base excess was −19.7 mmol/L. As the Thompson score was 1, the infant was considered to have a rapid recovery and was not referred for hypothermia. At 24 hours of age, apneas with desaturation developed, and as these were considered suspected seizures, a loading dose of phenobarbital (20 mg/kg iv) was given. Transfer for neuromonitoring followed.

Following the start of the *aEEG* monitoring, a CNV background pattern was present but interrupted by repetitive seizures (*,*) and phenobarbital was administered twice (10 mg/kg iv each) (Figure 5.2A). In Figure 5.2B, 36 h later, there is CNV with clear SWC.

The *MRI* (Figure 5.2C) showed diffusion restriction in the right posterior watershed region (a), and a repeat MRI performed 5 weeks later still showed increased signal intensity in this region (b).

The child had a normal outcome on the BSID-III at 24 months with a composite cognitive score of 96 and motor score of 92.

See also:

Montaldo P, Puzone S, Caredda E, et al. Magnetic resonance biomarkers and neurological outcome of infants with mild hypoxic-ischaemic encephalopathy who progress to moderate hypoxic-ischaemic encephalopathy. *Neonatol.* 2023;120(1):153–160.

Parmentier CEJ, Steggerda SJ, Weeke LC, et al. Outcome of non-cooled asphyxiated infants with under-recognised or delayed-onset encephalopathy. *Arch Dis Child Fetal Neonatal Ed.* 2022;107(4):364–370.

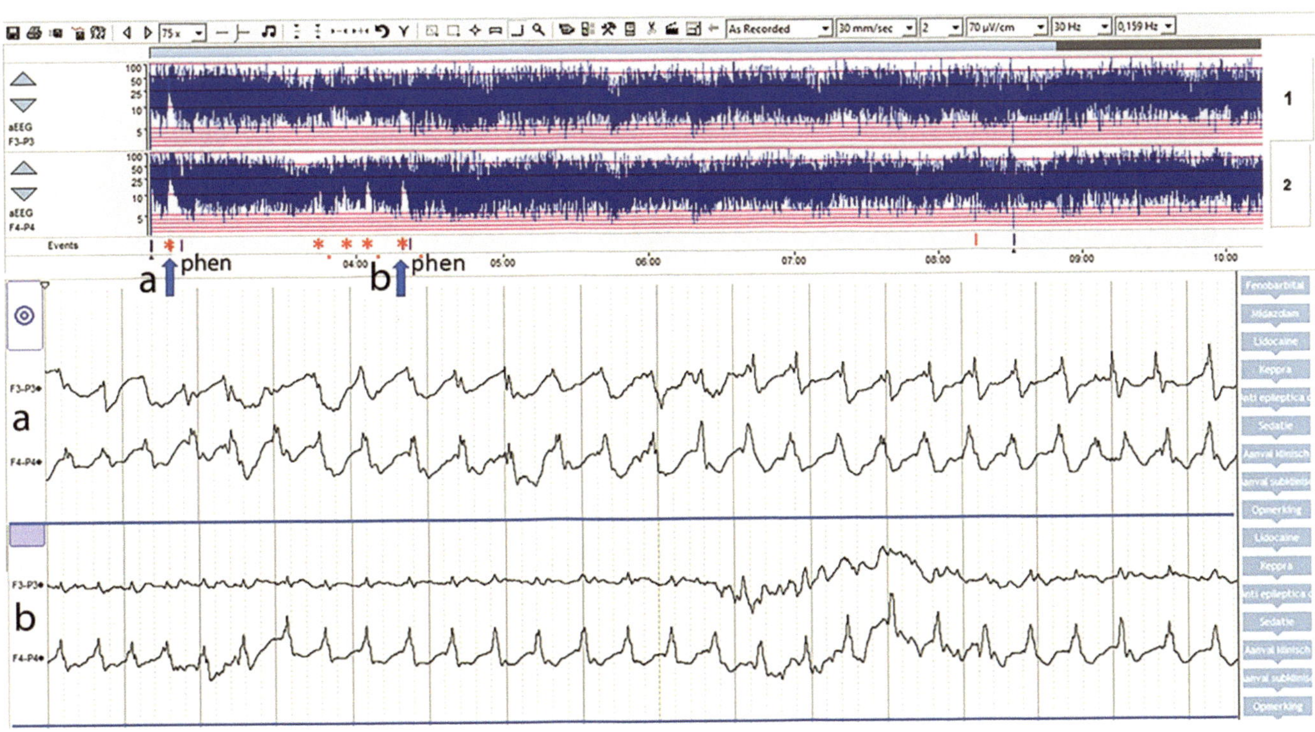

FIGURE 5.2A

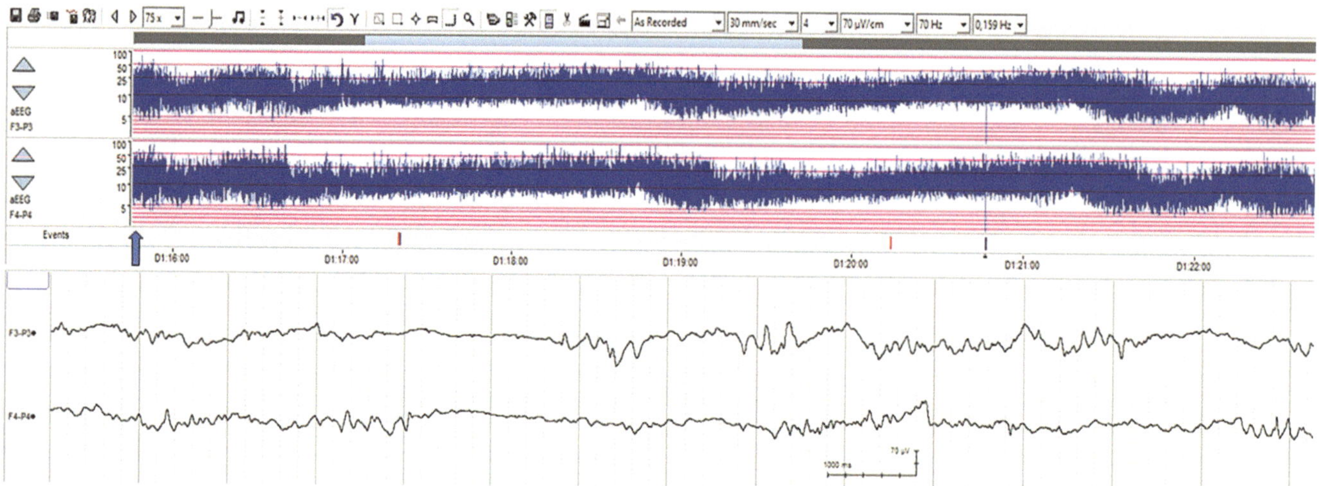

FIGURE 5.2B

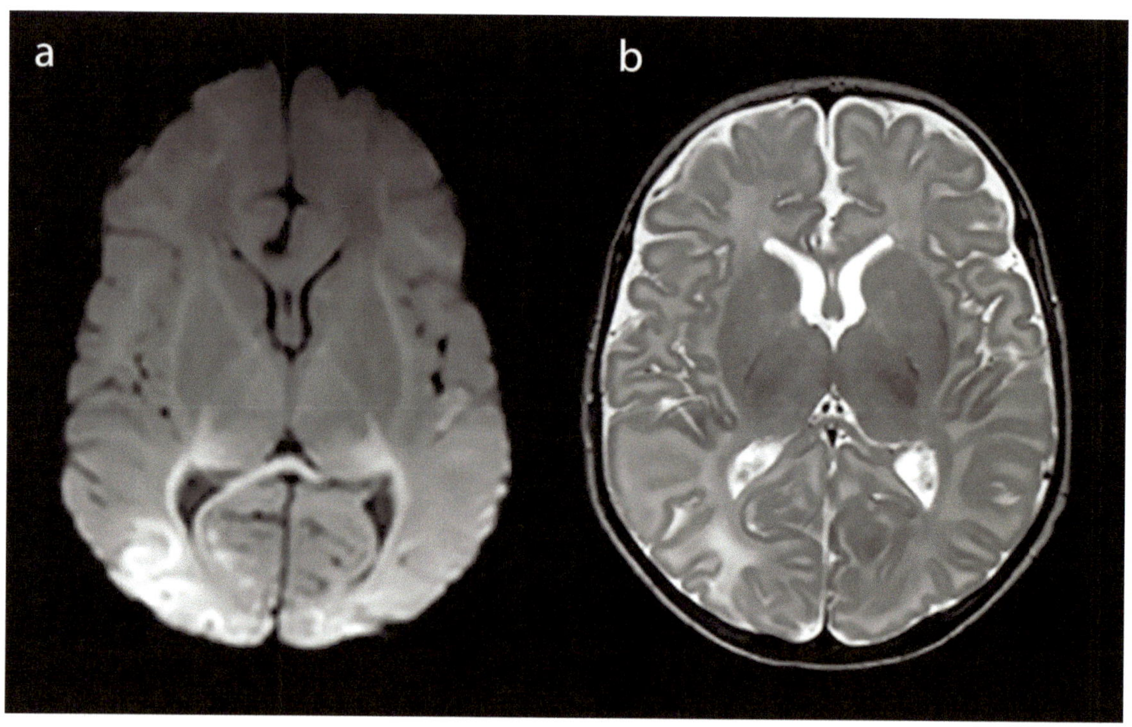

FIGURE 5.2C

Case 5.3 Full-Term Infant, Mild HIE with Evolution to Moderate HIE

This infant was born at 41 weeks' gestation by emergency caesarean section following decelerations on the CTG and a fetal blood gas indicating severe acidosis (pH 6.90 and base excess −14 mmol/L). Apgar scores were 1, 7 and 8 at 1, 5 and 10 minutes, respectively. The first blood glucose was 1.1 mmol/L. As the Thompson score was reported to be 0, and the infant showed a rapid recovery, it was decided not to start hypothermia. However, in view of the cranial ultrasound findings seen at 10 hours of age, the infant was admitted to the NICU for aEEG monitoring.

Clinical seizures were noted at 10 hours of age, confirmed on the *aEEG*. The seizures were also detected with the seizure detection algorithm (Figure 5.3A). The initial background pattern was CNV on the left side but could not be assessed on the right side due to the repetitive seizures. A loading dose of phenobarbital (20 mg/kg iv) was given at marker 1, and after that, a transient depression (DNV) was seen on both sides. The recording was continued with bilateral aEEG and an eight-channel EEG and bilateral aEEG (note that the right side is now the upper aEEG trace) (Figure 5.3B). Seizures dominated on the right side, as seen in the aEEG and in C4-Cz in the EEG. Another loading dose of phenobarbital (20 mg/kg iv) was given at *. Repeated seizures (status epilepticus) occurred in the 1.5-hour period highlighted in red. The background pattern was mainly DNV without clear SWC. At 72 hours, a predominantly CNV pattern with immature SWC was seen (Figure 5.3C). The seizure-suspected discharges at the end of the aEEG screen were not confirmed as seizures on the raw EEG.

Cranial *ultrasound* (Figure 5.3D), coronal (a), performed at 10 hours of age, showed diffuse increased echogenicity in the white matter and to a lesser degree in the thalami.

The *MRI* on day 4, showed findings compatible with predominantly right-sided watershed pattern of injury. The axial T2-weighted sequence (b) showed loss of the cortical ribbon, especially in the right frontal lobe as well as increased signal intensity in both frontal lobes. Using DWI (c), restricted diffusion is seen in both frontal lobes, but most marked on the right, as well as the corpus callosum (not shown). There are also a few punctate white matter lesions.

Outcome was well within the normal range at 3½ years of age.

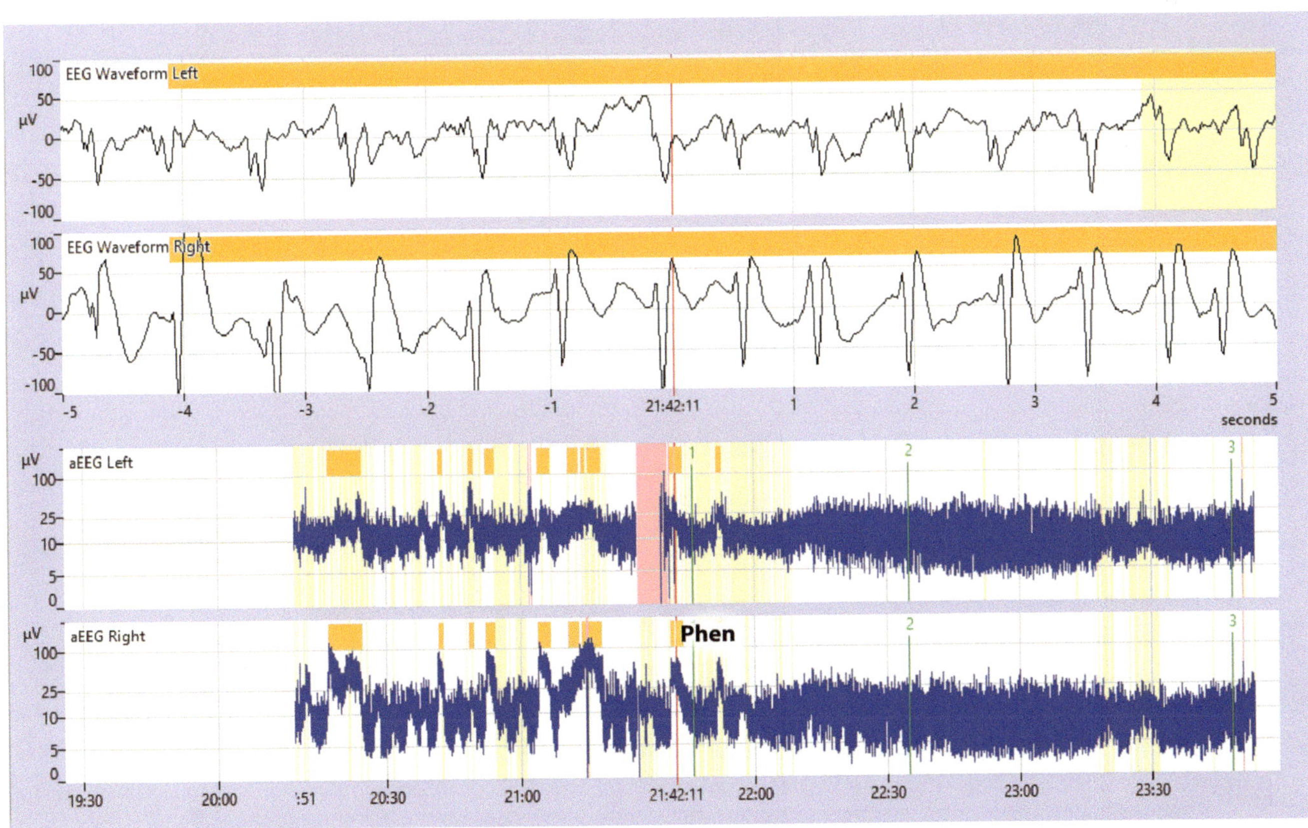

FIGURE 5.3A

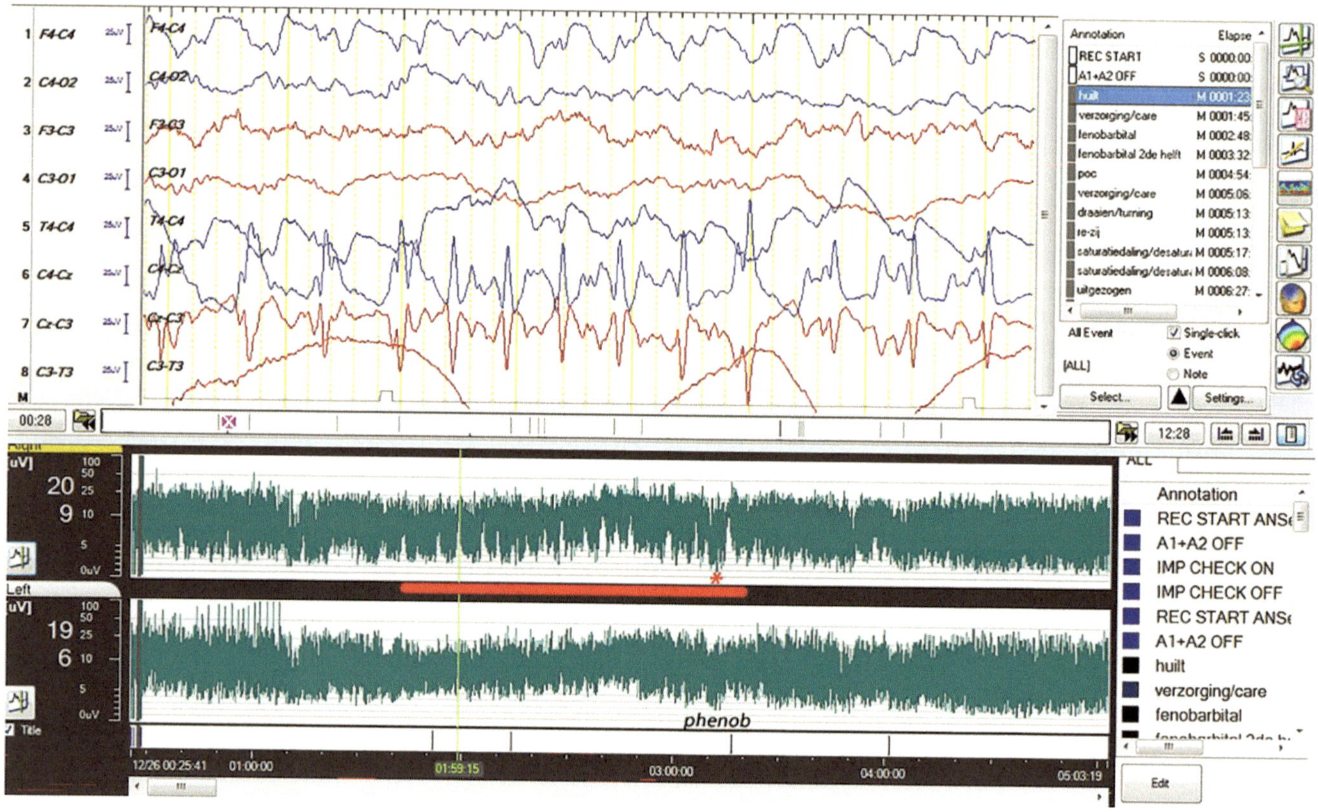

FIGURE 5.3B

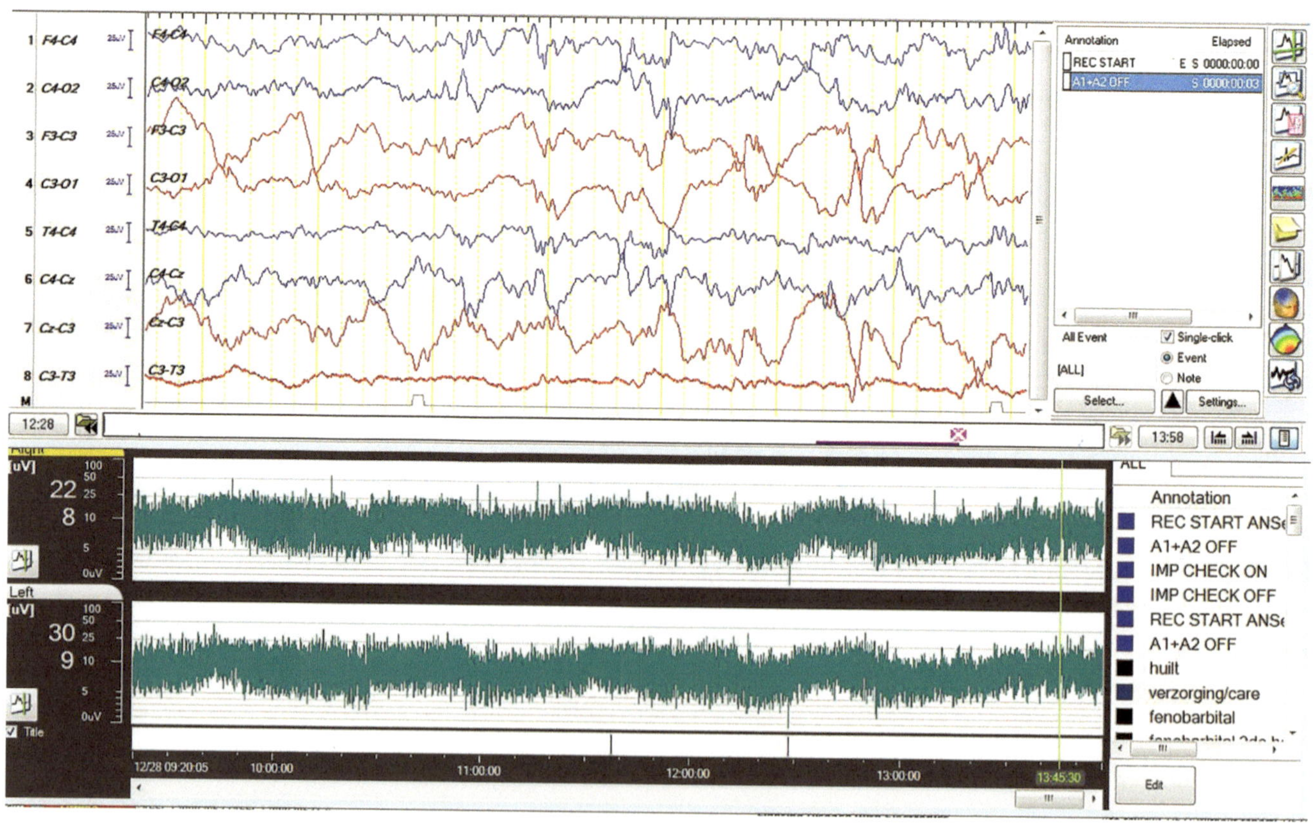

FIGURE 5.3C

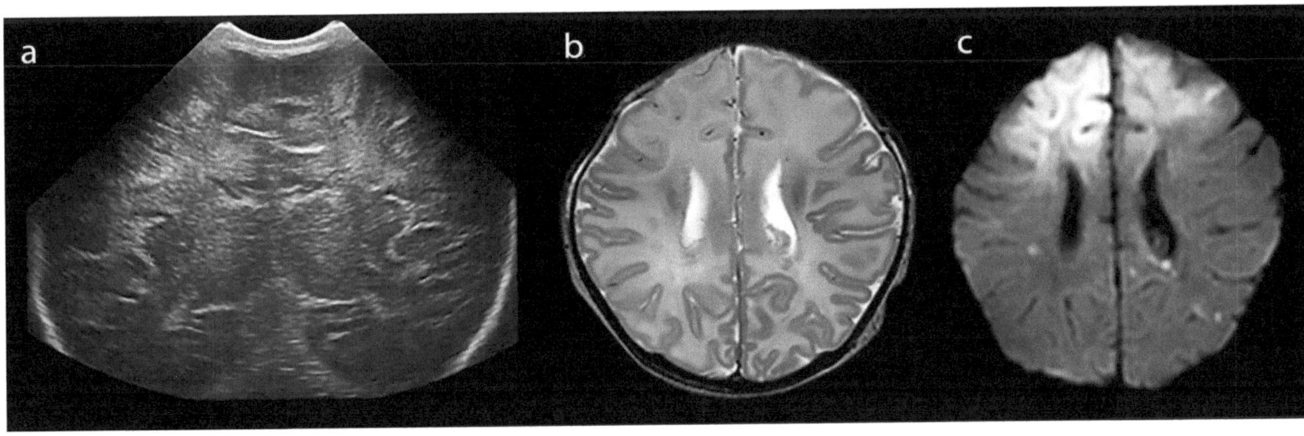

FIGURE 5.3D

Case 5.4 Full-Term Infant with Moderate HIE and Predominant Injury to the Thalami

This infant was born at 36 gestational weeks by caesarean section because of concerns for placental abruption and non-reassuring fetal heart tracing. The Apgar score was 2 and 4 at 1 and 5 minutes, respectively. Respiratory support provided included CPAP and positive pressure ventilation. Neurologic examination showed hypotonia and absence of Moro reflex and encephalopathy. Arterial umbilical cord pH revealed a pH of 7.20 and a base excess of −7.1. Lactate was 9.8 mmol/L. The infant received therapeutic hypothermia starting from 4 hours after birth.

The *aEEG* was started at 8 hours of life, showing rather sparse BS pattern (Figure 5.4A). At 24 hrs of life, the background pattern improved to a DNV pattern but no SWC (Figure 5.4B). At 48 hrs, the DNV pattern is more established, but there is still no SWC present (Figure 5.4C). The last figure (Figure 5.4D) is taken 5 hrs after rewarming, showing further improvement with imminent SWC. Based on the longitudinal analysis published by Meder et al. 2022, the probability of a good outcome would be 55.6% (36.2%, 73.4%).

An *MRI* (Figure 5.4E) was performed on day 4 and again on day 12. On the first MRI, there is restricted diffusion in the basal ganglia (a). On the second MRI (T1-weighted sequence), areas of signal abnormality are seen in the posterior lentiform nuclei and ventrolateral thalami bilaterally without myelination of the posterior limb of the internal capsule (PLIC).

Even though this infant did not develop any seizures, there was insufficient recovery of the background activity during the hypothermia period. Using the longitudinal aEEG analysis by Meder et al. can be helpful for the prediction for outcome. The infant should be followed closely, as there is a risk of subsequent development of dyskinetic cerebral palsy in view of the MRI abnormalities.

Reference

Meder U, Cseko AJ, Szakacs L, et al. Longitudinal analysis of amplitude-integrated electroencephalography for outcome prediction in hypoxic-ischemic encephalopathy. *J Pediatr*. 2022;246:19–25.e5.

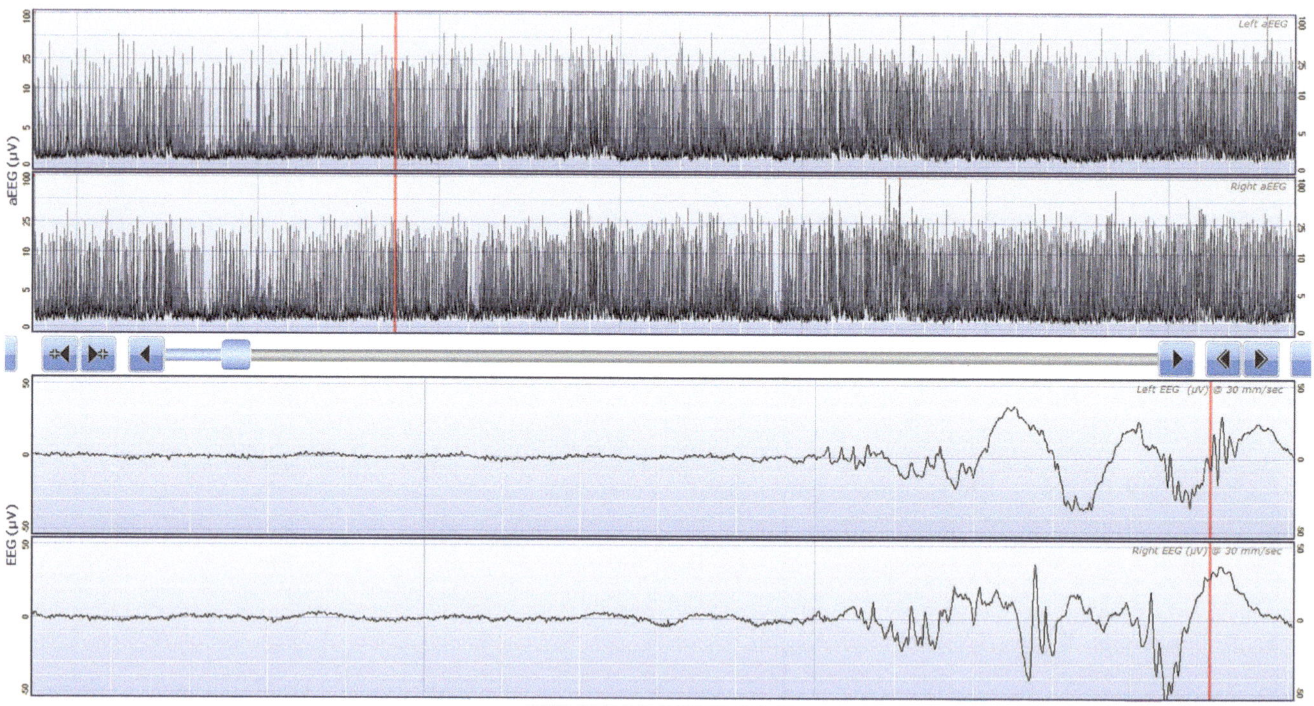

FIGURE 5.4A

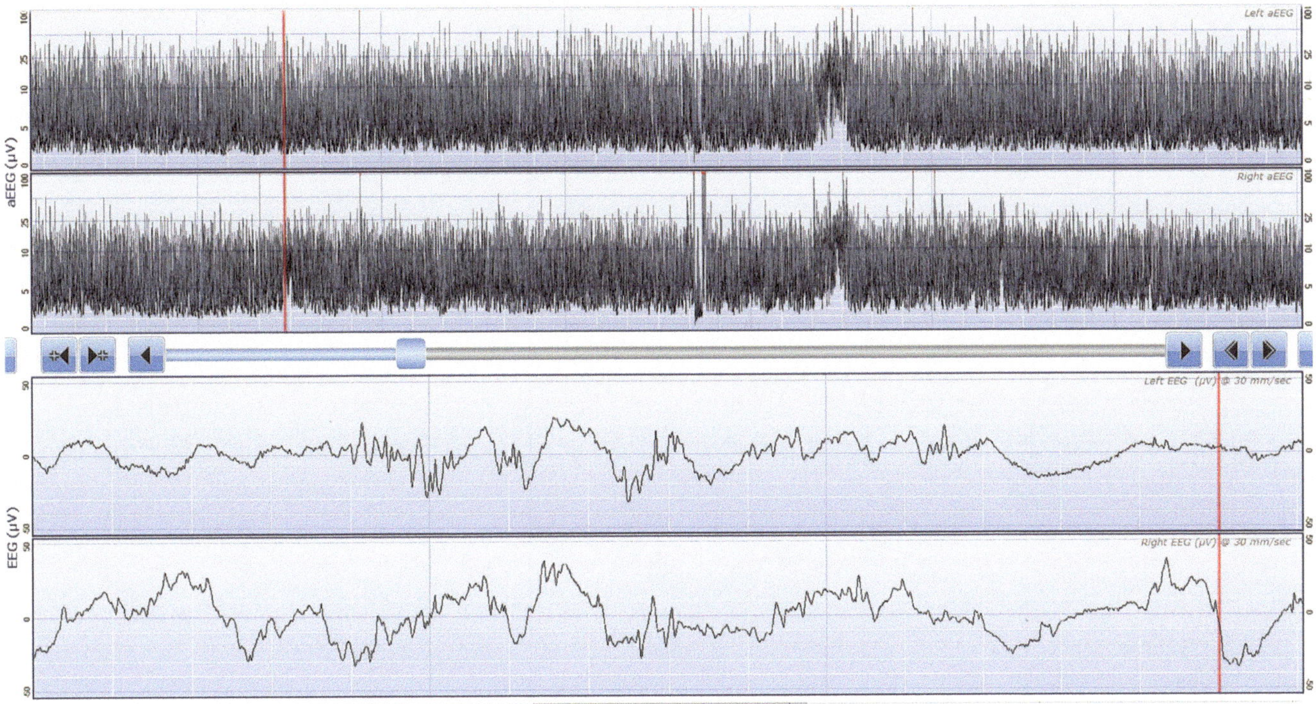

FIGURE 5.4B

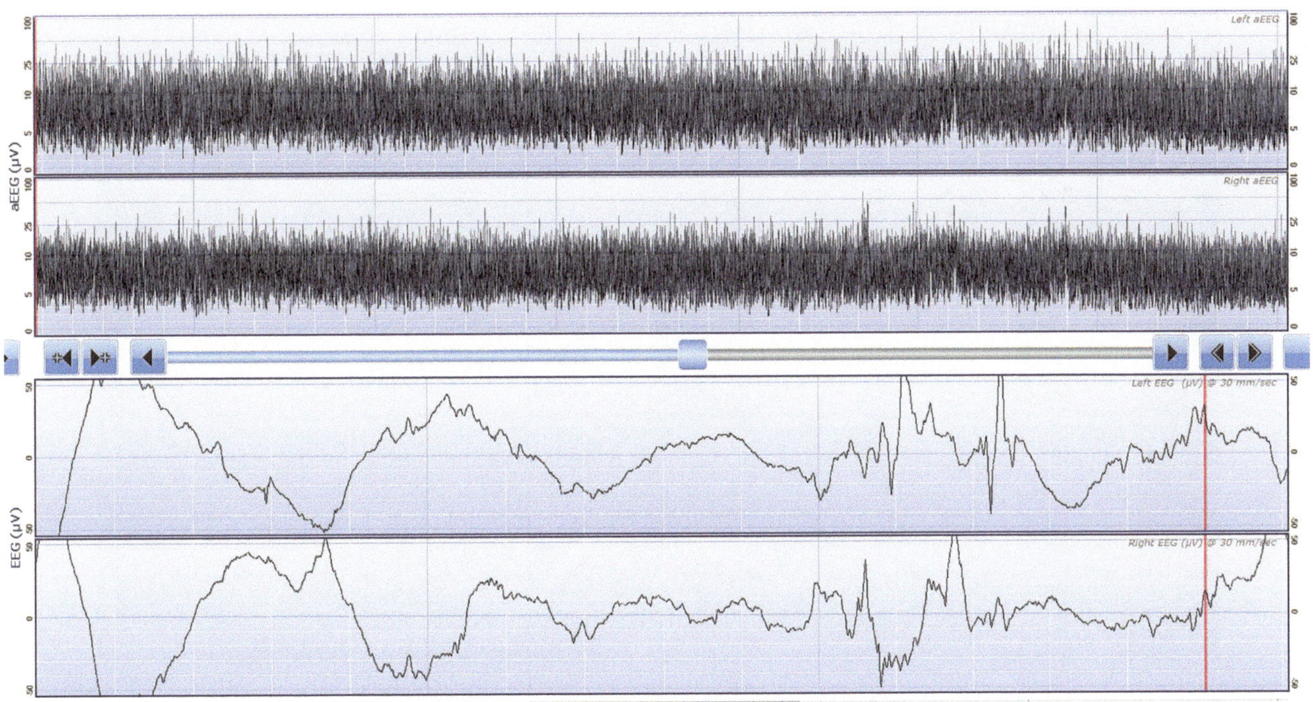

FIGURE 5.4C

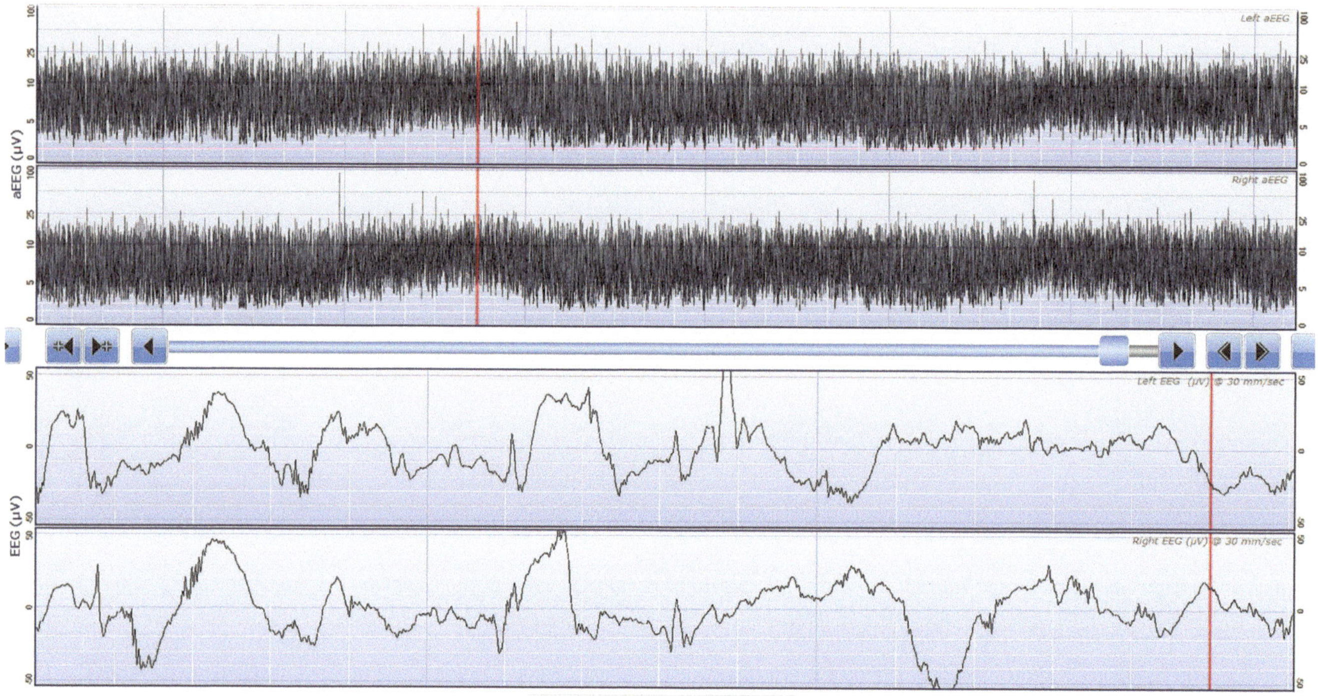

FIGURE 5.4D

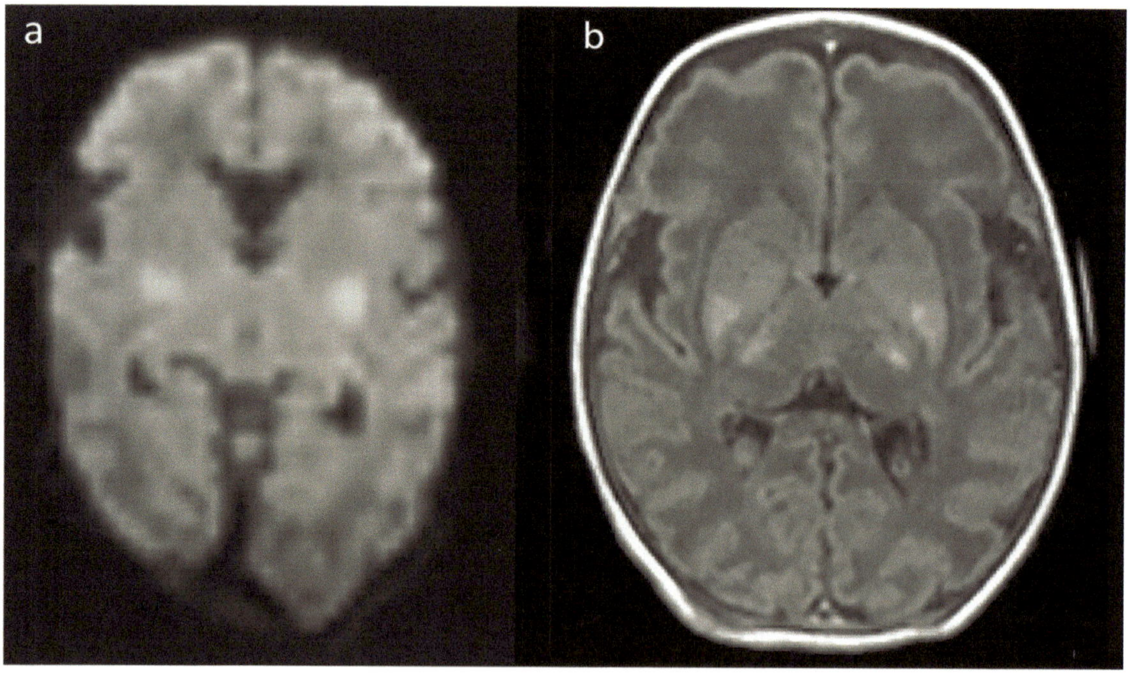

FIGURE 5.4E

Case 5.5 Full-Term Infant with Moderate HIE and Predominant Injury to the Thalami

This full-term infant was born at 41 + 4 weeks' gestation. The delivery was induced, and there was fetal distress. The infant was born by ventouse extraction complicated by severe shoulder dystocia. Apgar scores were 0, 0 and 2 at 1, 5 and 10 minutes, respectively.

The initial *aEEG*, prior to transport from the level 2 hospital to the neonatal intensive care unit, was mainly flat (not shown). Hypothermia treatment was started at 5 hours of age, and Figure 5.5A shows an initially flat background activity, but after around 1 hour, a sparse burst-suppression pattern is seen and thereafter successively increasing burst density. The green markers show procedures, (4) dopamine, both (5) and (6) are during care. The yellow markers above the aEEG trace indicates that the system recognized EEG waveforms that could be associated with seizures. No seizures were confirmed on the raw EEG.

Figure 5.5B shows how the background activity continuously recovered with increasing burst density and also showing a seizure marker (11); phenobarbital was given at marker 12. Figure 5.5C was recorded 5 hours after the start of rewarming, showing recovery of the electrocortical background activity to a discontinuous background with repetitive seizures. A standard EEG was performed (green marker 32), confirming the aEEG/EEG findings on the monitor, but did also reveal several brief seizures that were not seen with the two-channel EEG. Here, the raw EEG displays two seizures (at red asterisks in the aEEG) dominating on the left side, picked up by the waveform alert. Phenobarbital was given at marker 33. The last figure (Figure 5.5D) was recorded at the end of rewarming, showing recovery to a CNV pattern with imminent SWC.

An *MRI* [axial plane; T2-weighted sequence (a), DWI sequence (b)] was performed during hypothermia when the infant was 48 hours old and showed diffusion restriction in the thalami (Figure 5.5E). This infant survived but developed cerebral palsy, GMFCS level II–III.

It is important to confirm suspected seizures in the aEEG by evaluation of the corresponding raw EEG. In this case, many suspected seizures were not confirmed by the two-channel EEG (Panel C). However, the standard EEG recognized more seizures than were recognized by the aEEG and the two-channel EEG.

It is not uncommon to see a recurrence of seizures during or after rewarming, especially in infants with an initially depressed electrocortical background activity and seizures during hypothermia. It is, therefore, important to continue the monitoring until after completion of the rewarming period.

Bibliography

Chalak LF, Pappas A, Tan S, et al.; Eunice Kennedy Shriver National Institute of Child Health and Human Development Neonatal Research Network. Association between increased seizures during rewarming after hypothermia for neonatal hypoxic ischemic encephalopathy and abnormal neurodevelopmental outcomes at 2-year follow-up: A nested multisite cohort study. *JAMA Neurol.* 2021;78(12):1484–1493.

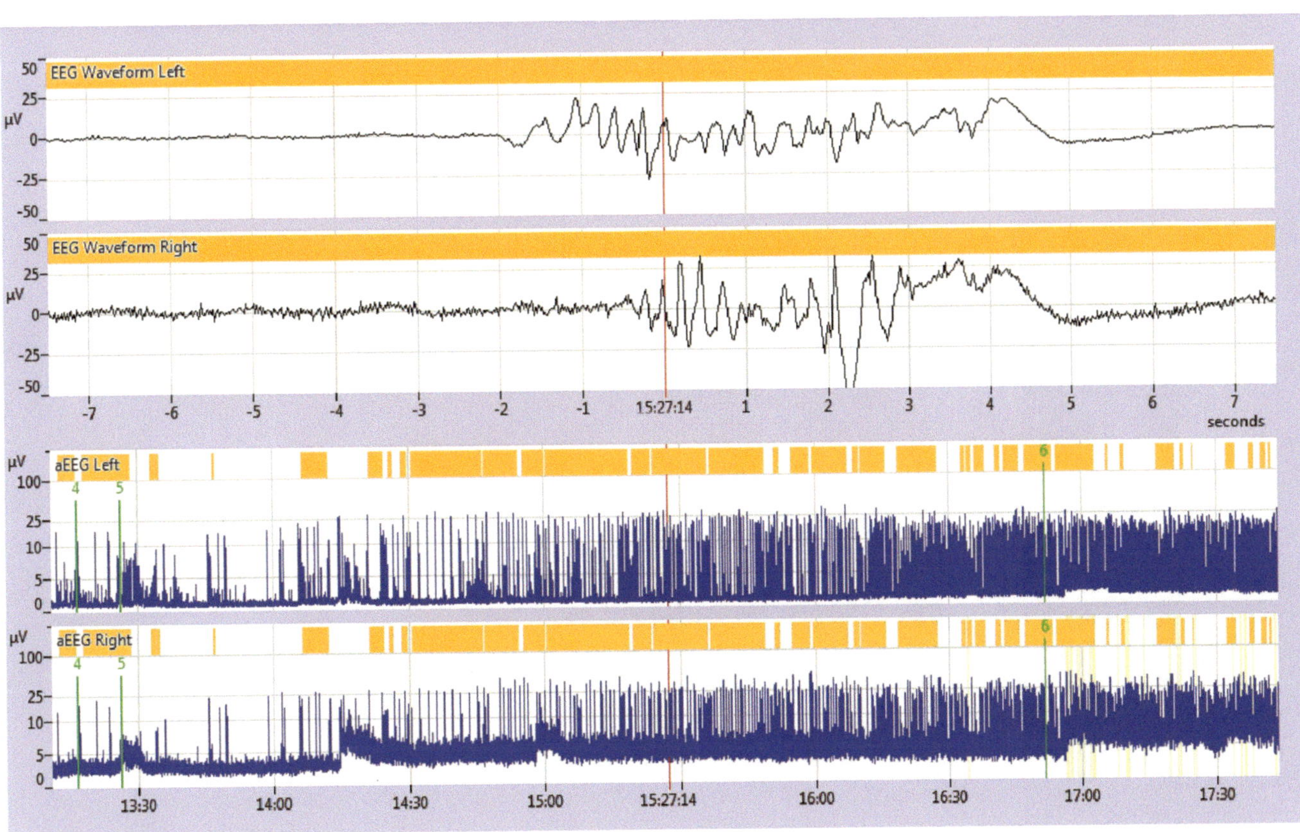

FIGURE 5.5A

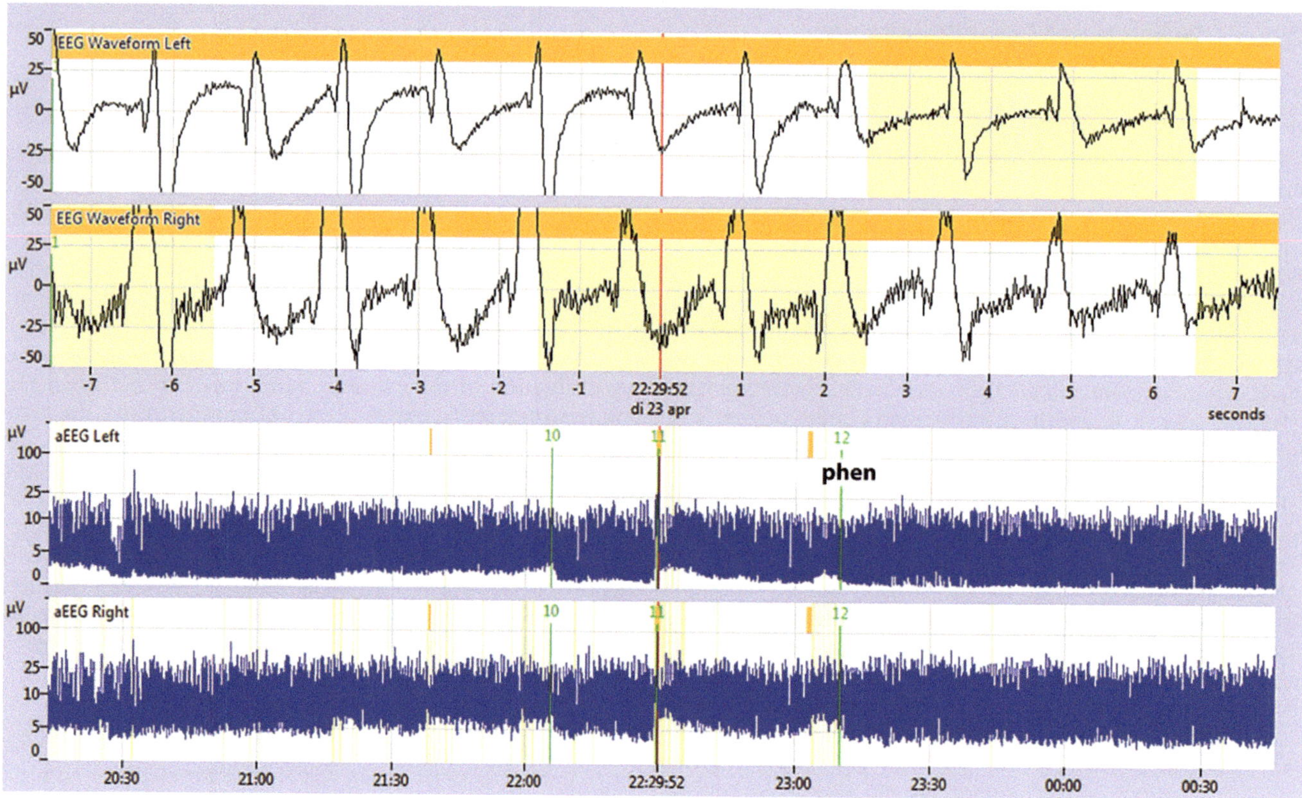

FIGURE 5.5B

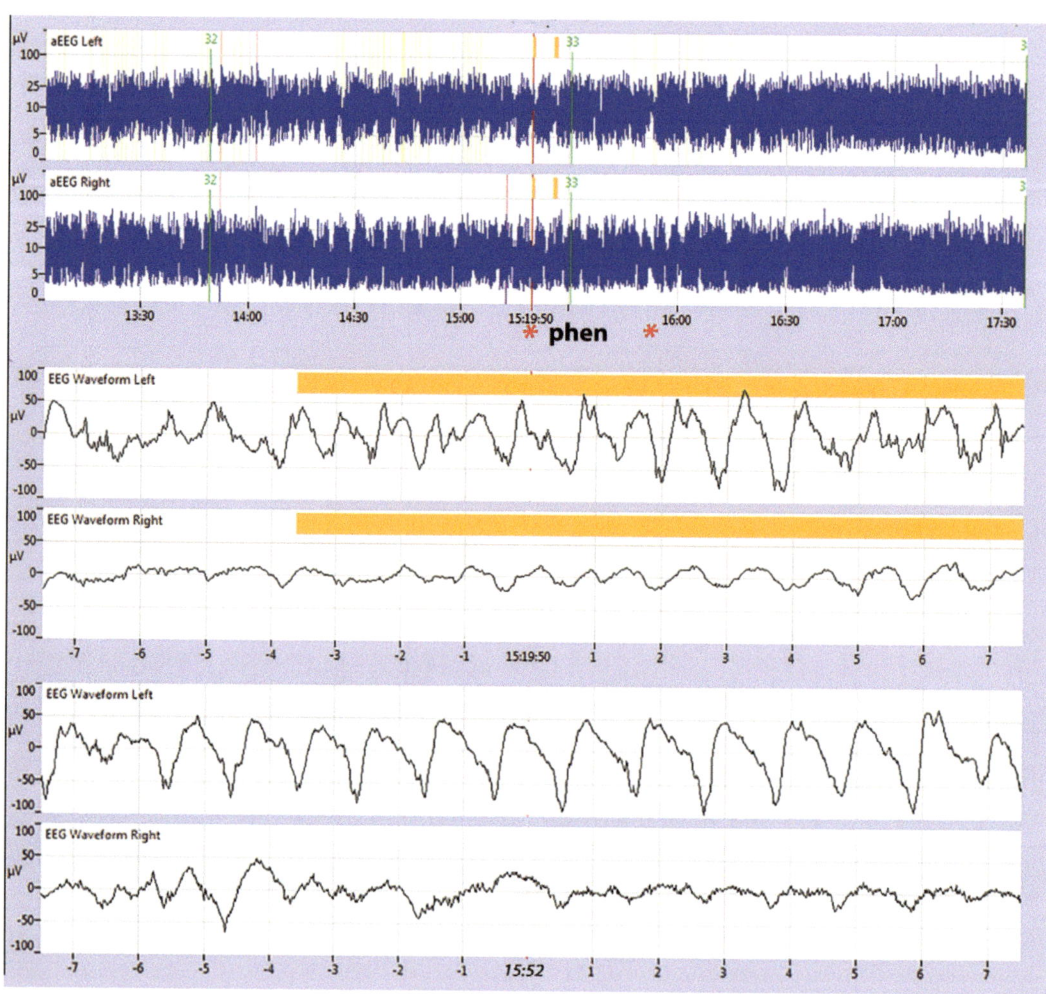

FIGURE 5.5C

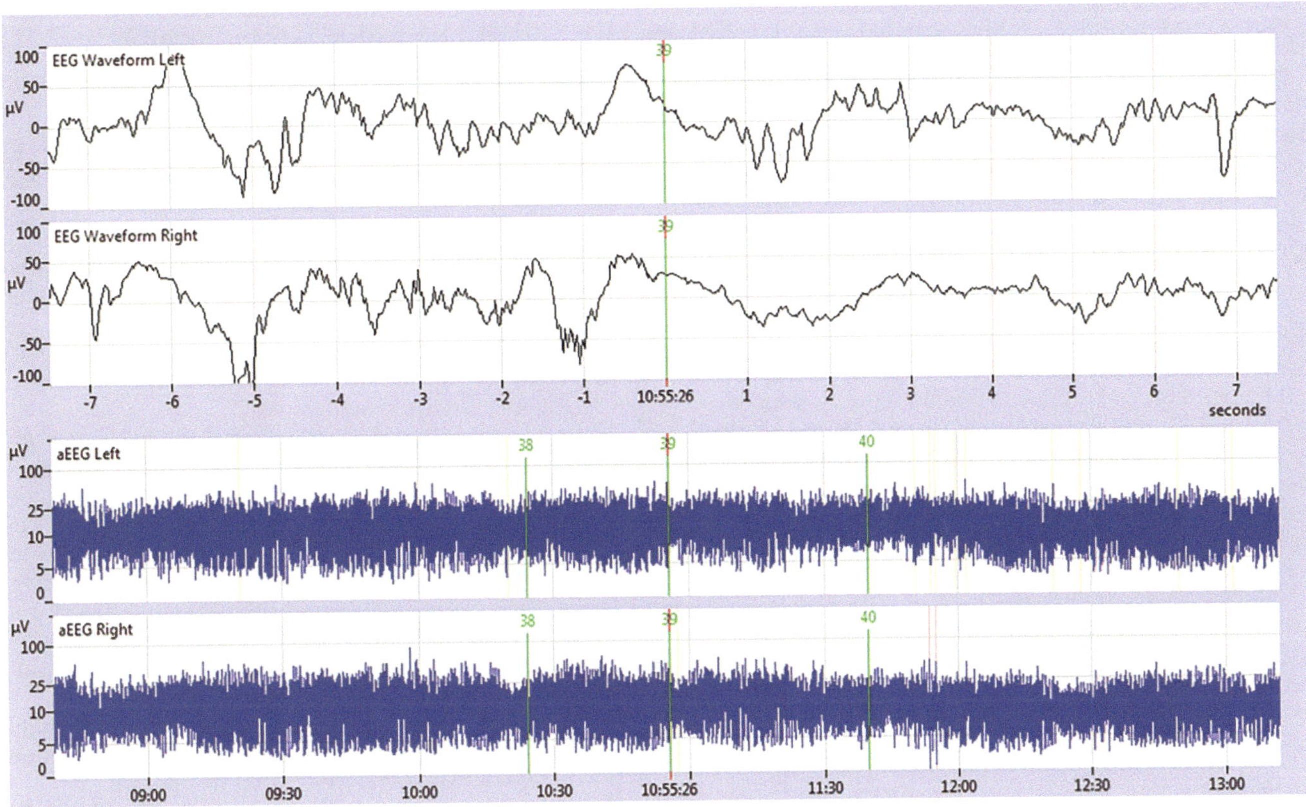

FIGURE 5.5D

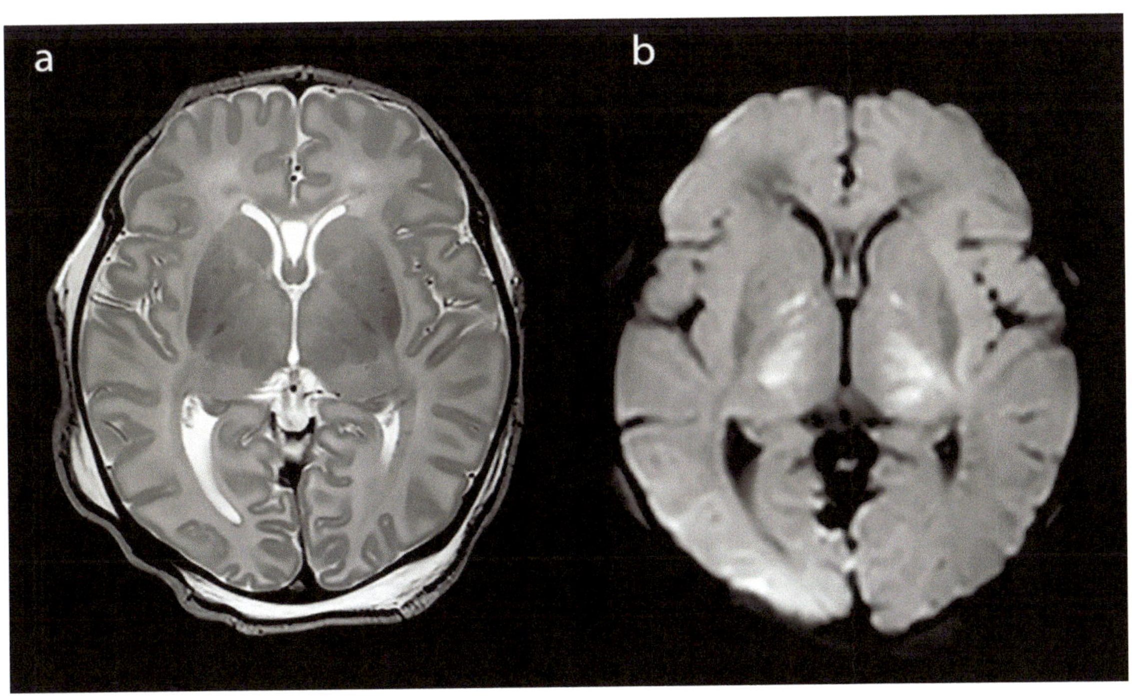

FIGURE 5.5E

Case 5.6 Full-Term Infant with Severe HIE after Acute Intrapartum Event

This infant was born at term with a birthweight of 3330 g. There was vaginal blood loss and fetal bradycardia due to placental abruption, and delivery was by an emergency caesarean section. The arterial umbilical pH was 6.91, and Apgar scores were 2, 5 and 8 at 1, 5 and 10 minutes, respectively. The first arterial lactate was 7.6 mmol/L. Hypothermia was started at 3 hours of age.

Figures 5.6A and B show the same 4 hours of *aEEG* recordings, from around 5 hours after birth, when a loading dose of phenobarbital was given for an EEG-verified seizure (not shown here). Two hours later, at time 23:00, a new seizure appeared, and Figures 5.6A and B show 15 and 60 seconds, respectively, of the raw EEG from that seizure. In Figure 5.6B, the full development of a typical seizure (dominating on the right side) can be seen, which is reassuring for the seizure diagnosis. Please note also the difference in amplitude scales of the displayed EEGs, in Figure 5.6A +/–50 µV and in Figure 5.5 6 +/–100 µV. The viewing scales of both aEEG and EEG can be adjusted to show the best displays in most monitors.

The seizures were better controlled following lidocaine, midazolam and another loading dose of phenobarbital and also resulting in a more depressed background activity. Figure 5.6C shows a mainly flat trace on the second day, but the automated seizure detection (orange markers) still recognizes some seizures. The right-sided aEEG is displayed, with seizure detection on a tiny "spike" in the trace, and the corresponding and continuous display of the EEG later shows around 30 seconds of a seizure pattern with a change in frequency and amplitude over time. Please also note the very low voltage of this seizure, with the EEG panel showing +/–20 µV.

During the following days, brain activity recovered slowly to a sparse burst-suppression pattern (not shown) first and then, at 36 hrs of age, a dense burst-suppression pattern without seizures (Figure 5.6D).

There was, however, no clear improvement of the background pattern, and seizures recurred on day 6, 2 days after rewarming (Figure 5.6E). Seizures were difficult to control in spite of additional antiseizure medication (including levetiracetam and diazepam). The background activity recovered slowly and was still depressed on day 7.

As the infant was unstable and on HFO, the *MRI* was postponed and was performed on day 8 (Figure 5.6F). The T2 (a) shows a widespread increased signal intensity with loss of the cortical ribbon posteriorly. The signal is also increased in the thalami and parts of the internal capsule in agreement with the areas of diffusion restriction (b). A repeat MRI at 6 weeks of age showed cystic evolution in the parietal and occipital lobes (c). The outcome was poor with cerebral palsy (GMFCS level IV), cerebral visual impairment and development of postneonatal epilepsy.

This example shows that aEEG monitoring preferably should be continued until after rewarming is completed due to the increased risk of seizures during that period.

This case also shows typical recovery of a severely depressed electrocortical background, which is often associated with development of seizures.

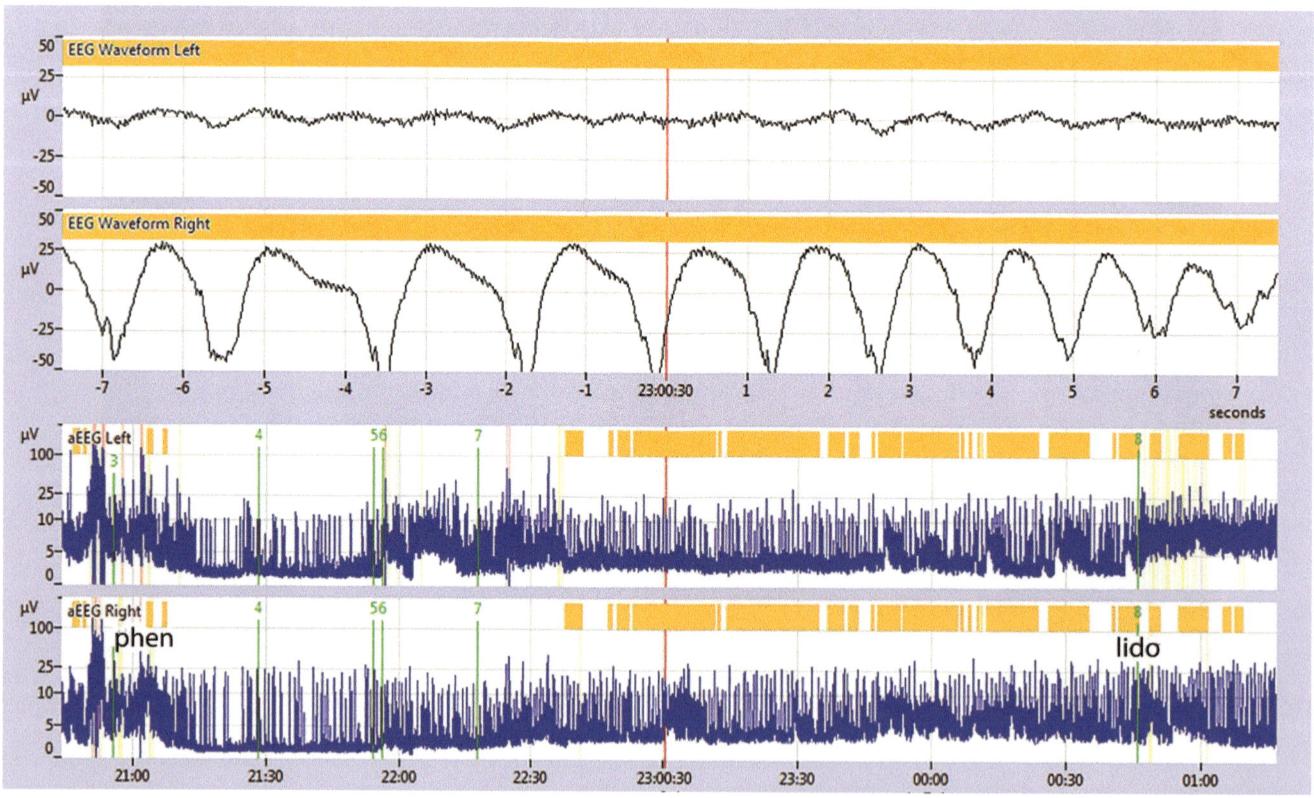

FIGURE 5.6A

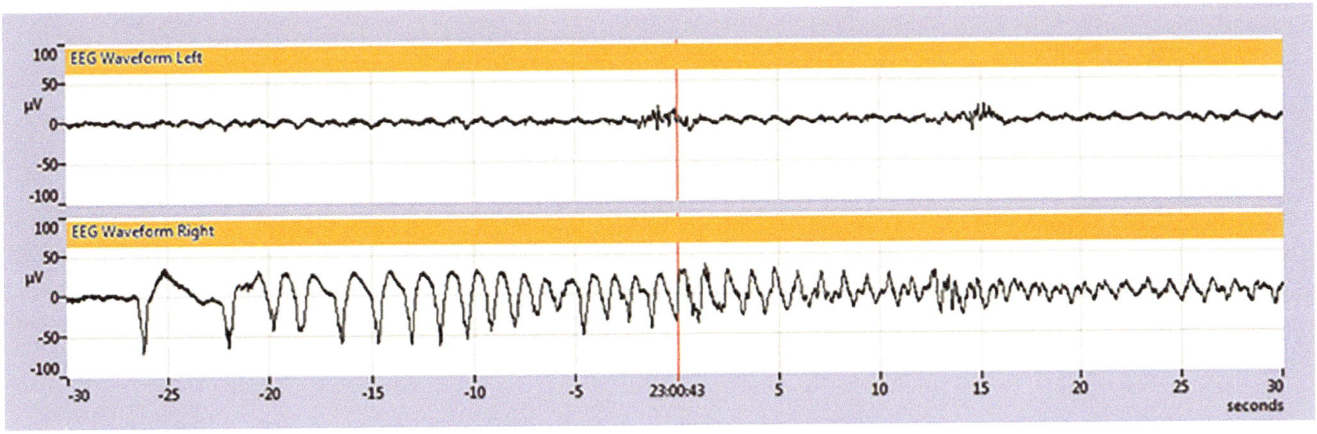

FIGURE 5.6B

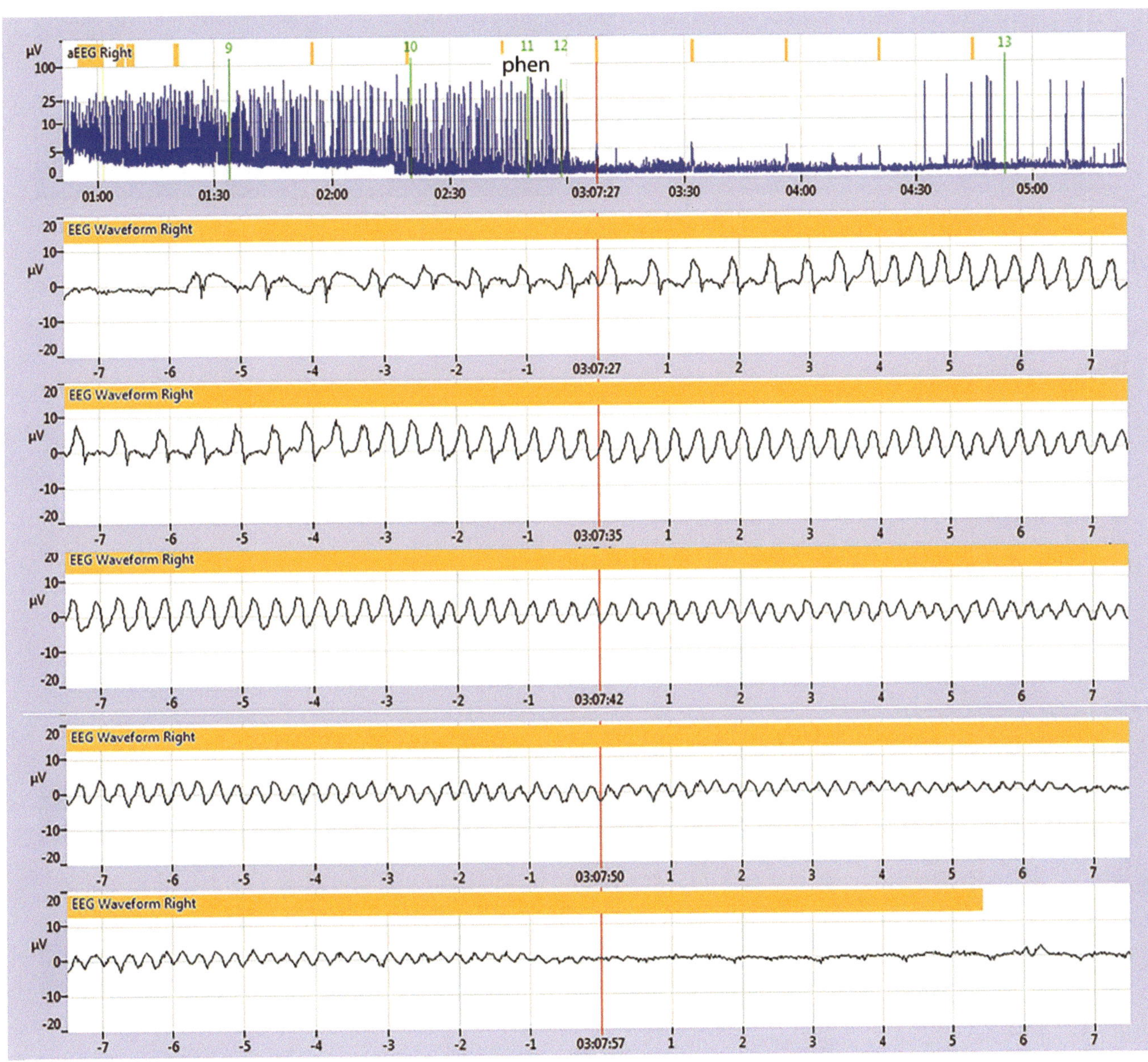

FIGURE 5.6C

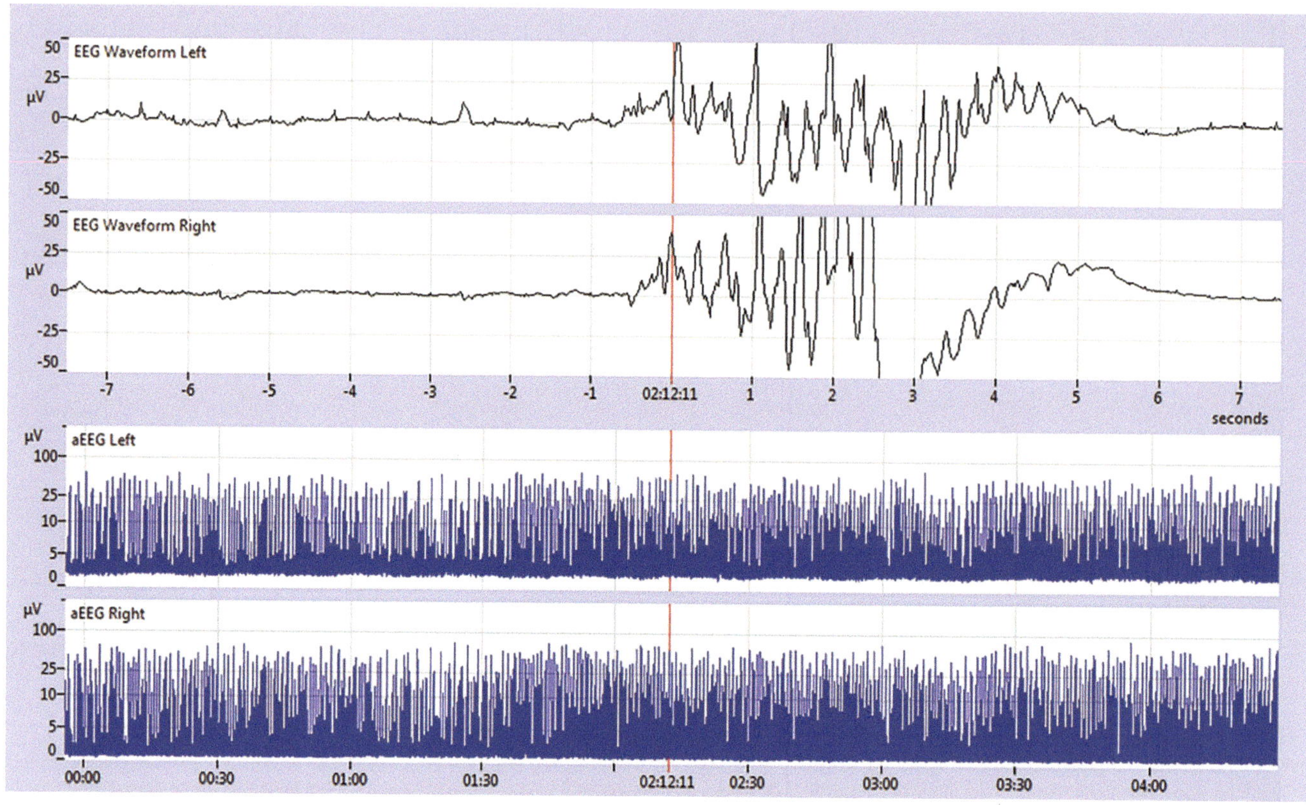

FIGURE 5.6D

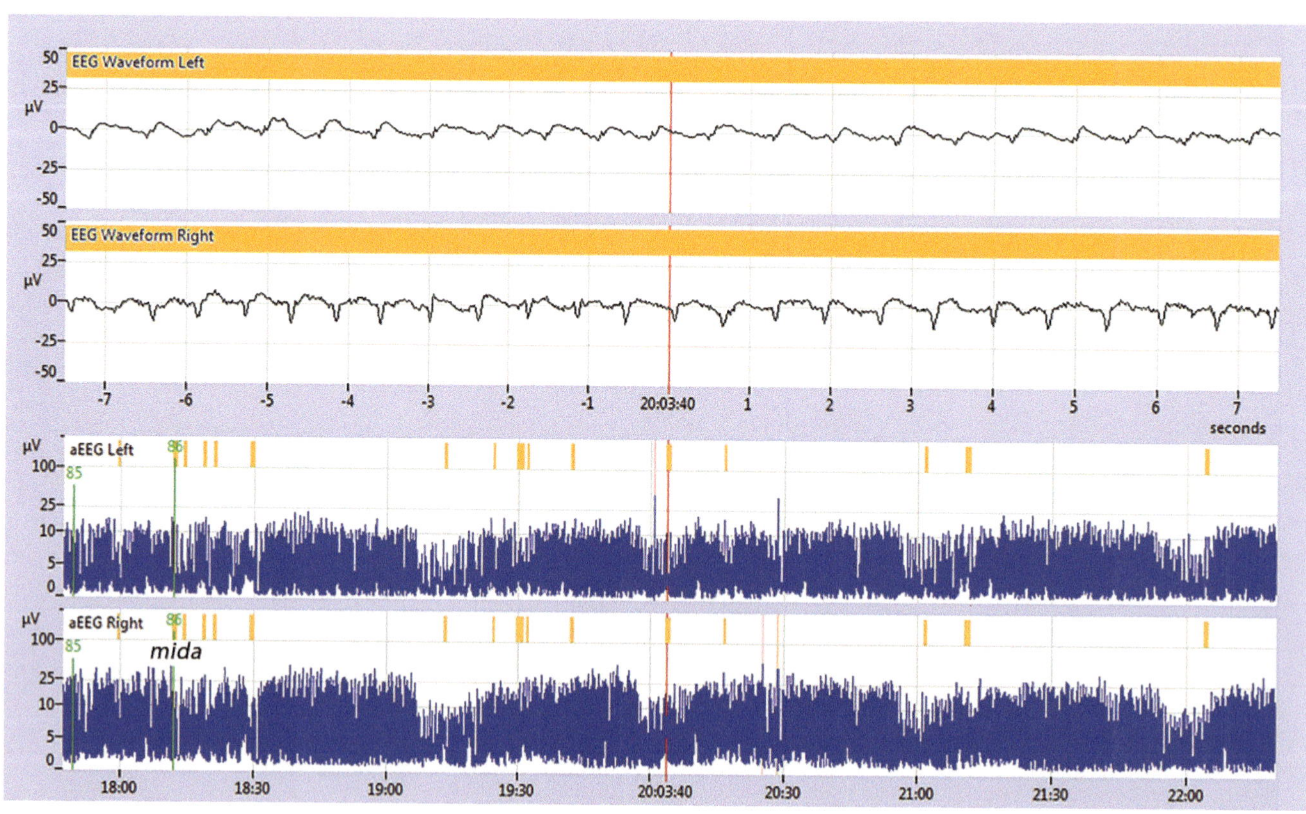

FIGURE 5.6E

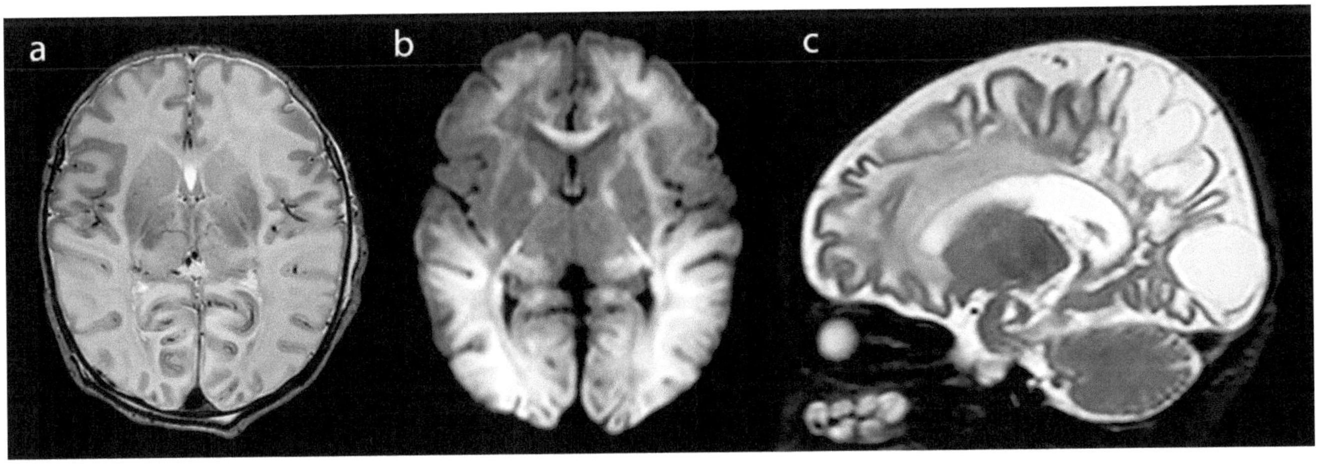

FIGURE 5.6F

Case 5.7 Full-Term Infant with Postnatal Collapse Who Was Treated with Hypothermia

Term infant, born by caesarean section because of fetal distress. Apgar scores were 8 and 10 after 1 and 5 minutes, respectively. The infant did well and was discharged home on day 2. On day 5, the infant suffered a postnatal collapse and was resuscitated at home. The first capillary blood gas showed a capillary pH of 6.86. Lactate was 17 mmol/L. Hypothermia was started 5 hours later.

The *aEEG* [Nihon Kohden device, showing roughly 5.5 hours of bilateral aEEG and 7 seconds of raw EEG at (a), i.e. the grey vertical marker]. The recording (Figure 5.7A) started 7 hours after the postnatal collapse, and the aEEG/EEG showed a burst-suppression pattern with an ECG artefact. Between markers (a) and (b), the background pattern changed, but it didn't look like a typically recovering burst-suppression pattern. The infant was gasping on the ventilator, and at (b), muscle paralysis was given. This resulted in an immediate response, the infant stopped gasping, and the aEEG/EEG background pattern became flat, indicating that the recorded activity had been respiratory movements and that the cerebral activity was severely depressed.

Thirty hours after the postnatal collapse, the aEEG still showed a mainly flat trace (Figure 5.7B). Suspected seizures began to appear around 48 hours. Regional oxygen saturation, monitored with NIRS, was initially 65% but increased at this time to 90–95%, further indicating severely depressed brain function. During rewarming after 72 hours, the aEEG pattern improved from flat to burst-suppression, and repetitive seizures developed (Figure 5.7C). Phenobarbital (10 mg/kg iv) was administered at (a). On day 5 (106 hrs) after the postnatal collapse, seizures recurred and midazolam was started (not shown).

Monitoring was continued with another device (Figure 5.7D, BrainZ) and showed, on day 6 (130 hrs), repeated seizures and a burst-suppression pattern with increasing burst activity. Levetiracetam was given at marker 11 (Figure 5.7D), and more phenobarbital was given later (not shown).

On day 7 after the postnatal collapse, background activity was more discontinuous, i.e. the lower border of the aEEG trace has variability and is lifted to 2–4 μV in the aEEG. A few seizures were recognized with the seizure-detection algorithm, along with a few additional EEG-confirmed seizures (marked *) with clear seizure-suspected appearance in the aEEG trend, but were not marked by the waveform algorithm (Figure 5.7E). On days 7 and 8, the aEEG background showed a DNV pattern, with no confirmed seizures and no SWC (Figure 5.7F). The background pattern remained abnormal and was affected by care (Figure 5.7G). The infant was extubated 10 days after the postnatal collapse but was unable to breathe without support.

Cranial ultrasound (Figure 5.7H), 3 days after the collapse (a) showed increased echogenicity in the thalami. The *MRI* (DWI), performed 3 days after the collapse, showed extensive diffusion restriction, most pronounced in the thalami as well, but when looking at the signal intensity of the cerebellum, this is the only part of the brain showing a normal signal (b, c). This is a near-total pattern of injury and also referred to as "the white brain" (Vermeulen et al. 2003). The infant died following redirection of care.

This very long recording shows the initially severely depressed brain activity after the collapse and poor recovery of the electrocortical background activity during cooling. Seizures occurred during rewarming and recurred several days later.

Reference

Vermeulen RJ, Fetter WPF, Hendrikx L, et al. Diffusion-weighted MRI in severe neonatal hypoxic ischaemia: The white cerebrum. *Neuropediatrics*. 2003;34(2):72–76.

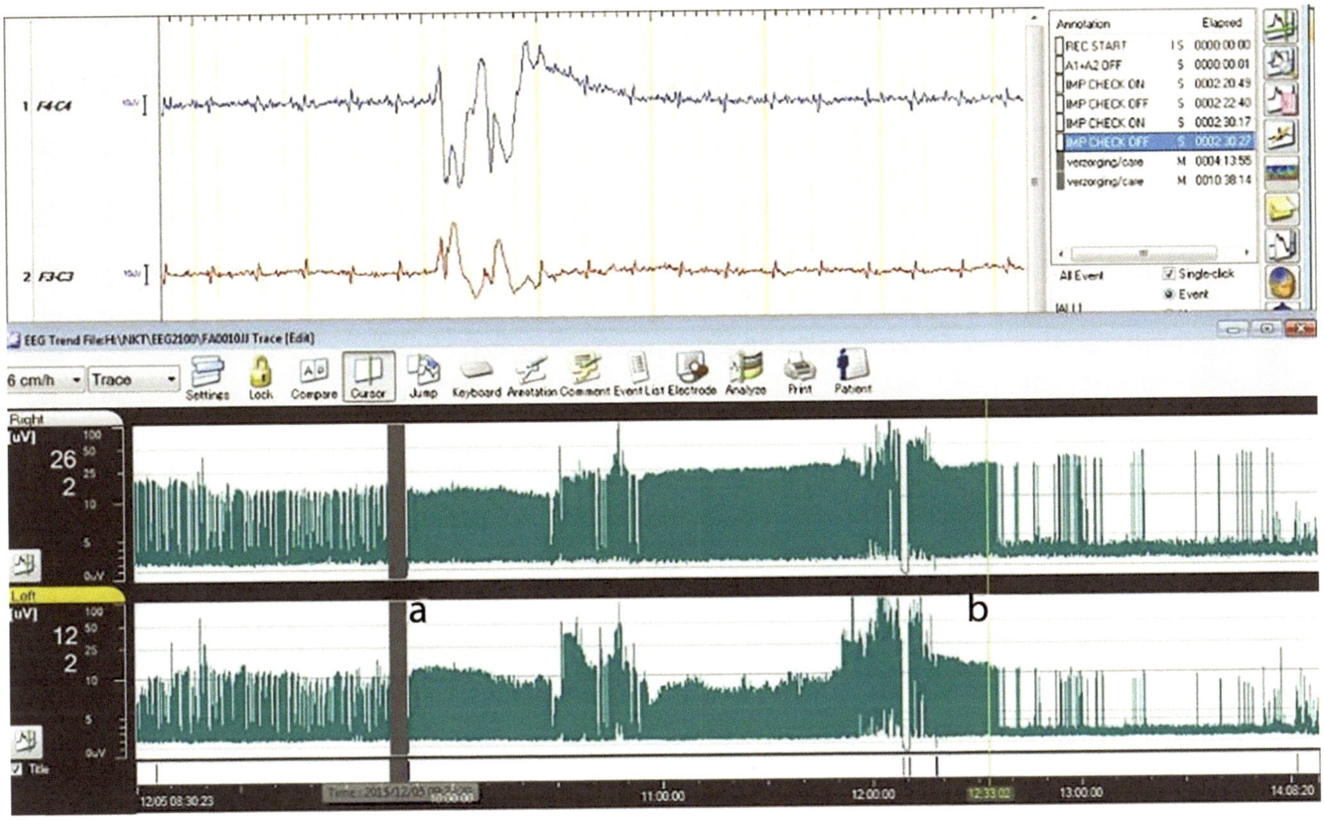

FIGURE 5.7A

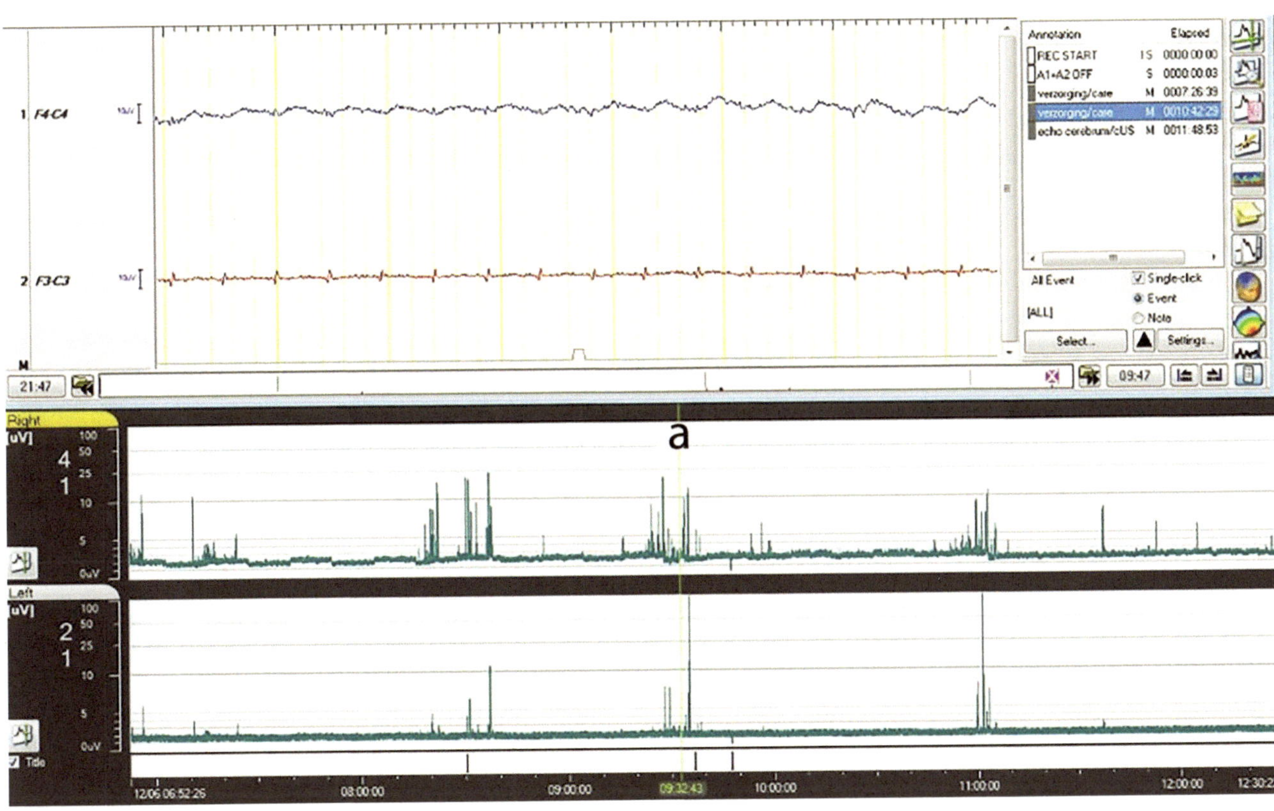

FIGURE 5.7B

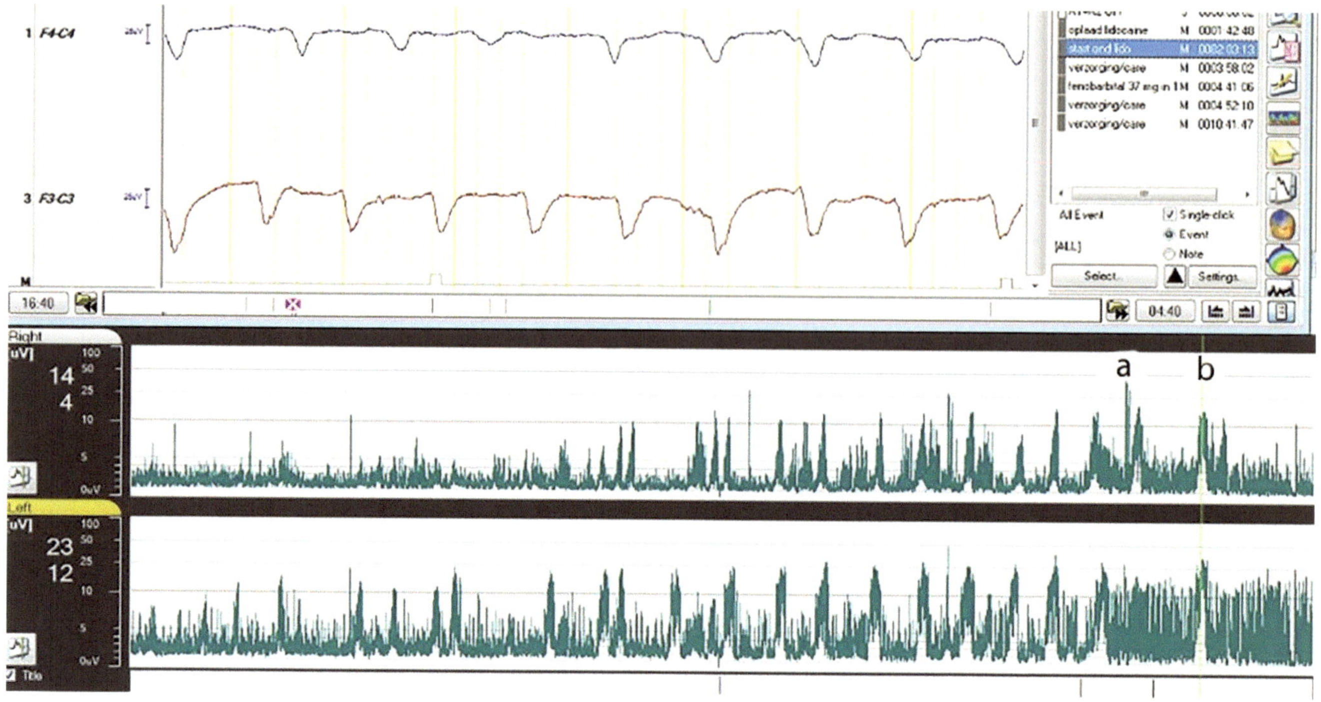

FIGURE 5.7C

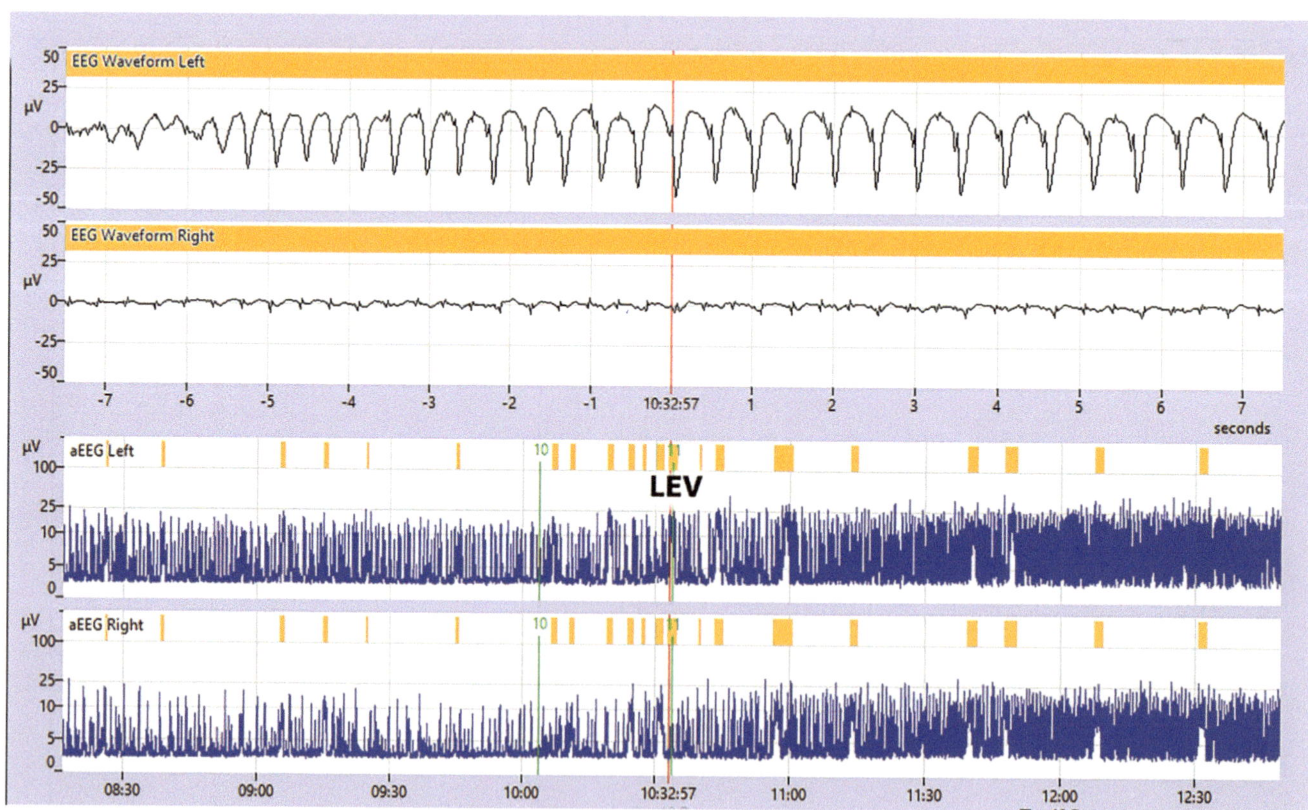

FIGURE 5.7D

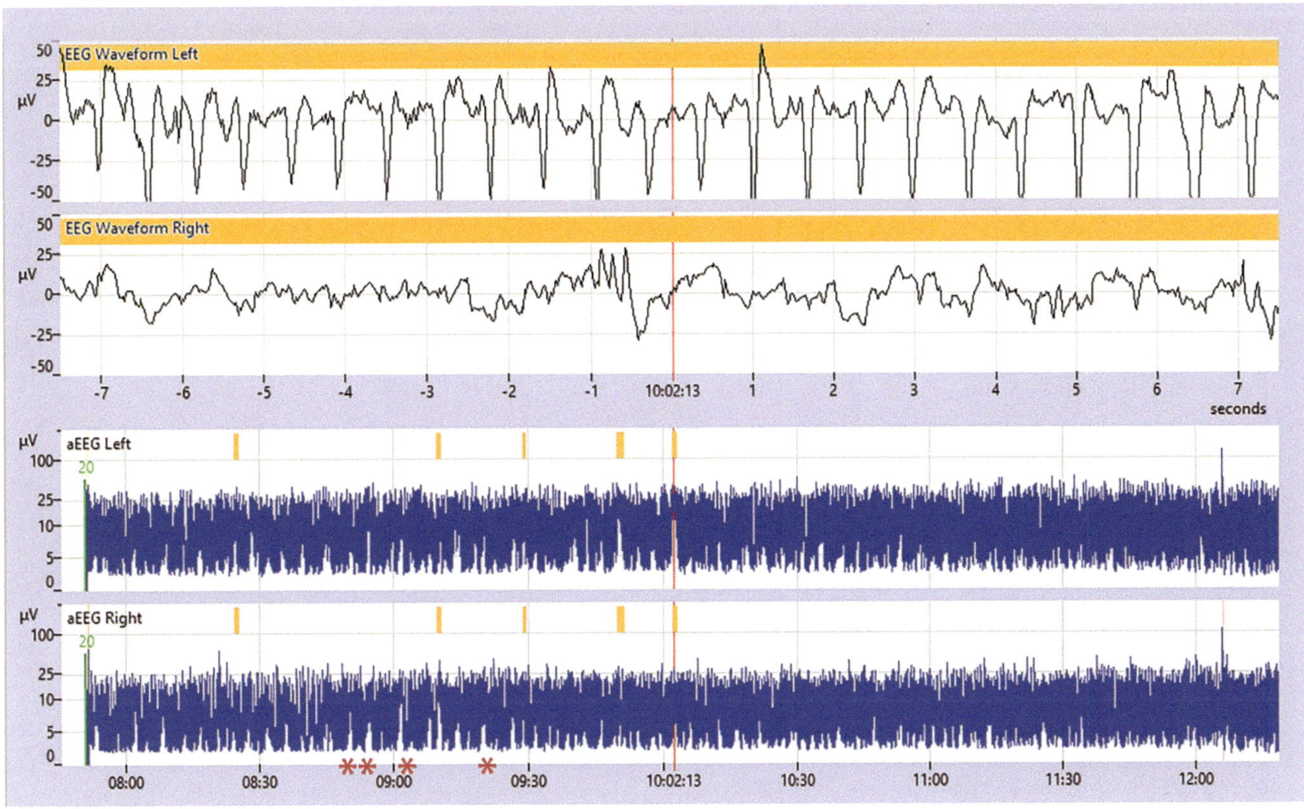

FIGURE 5.7E

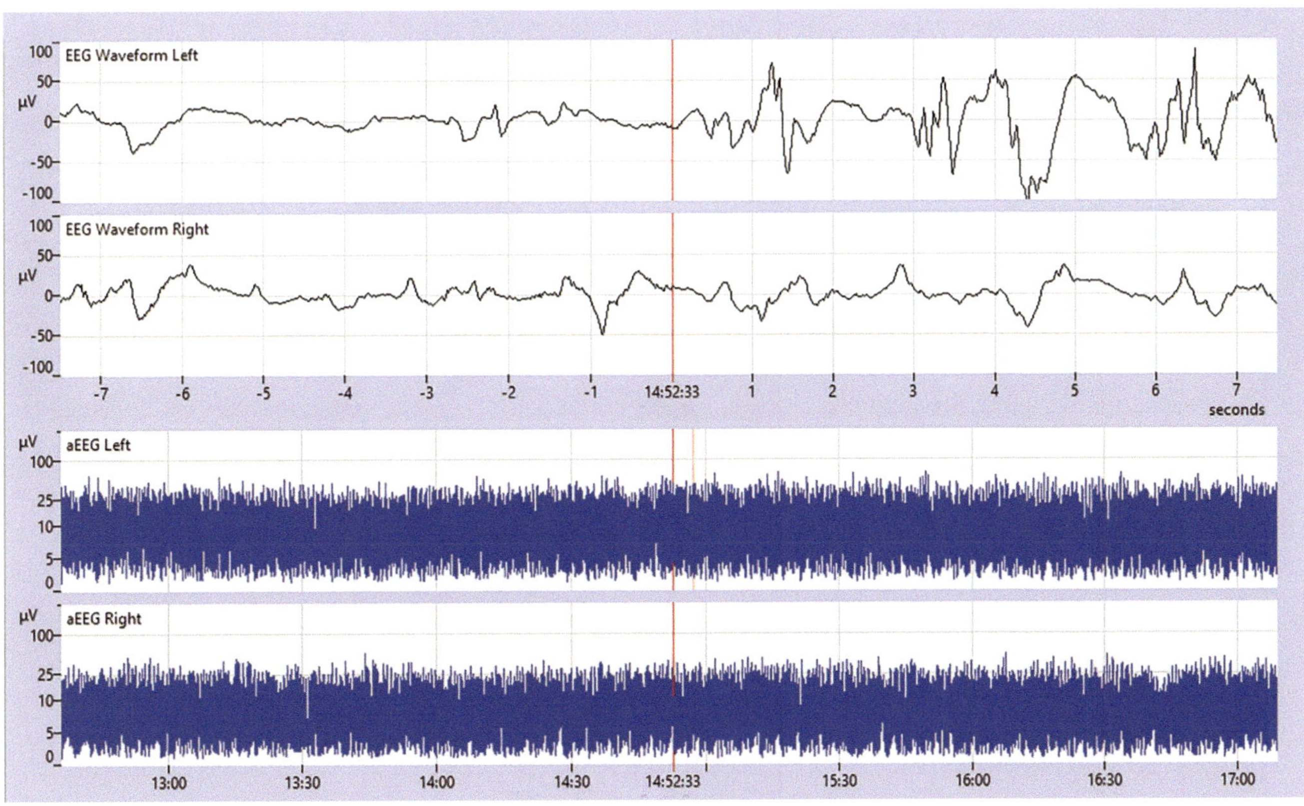

FIGURE 5.7F

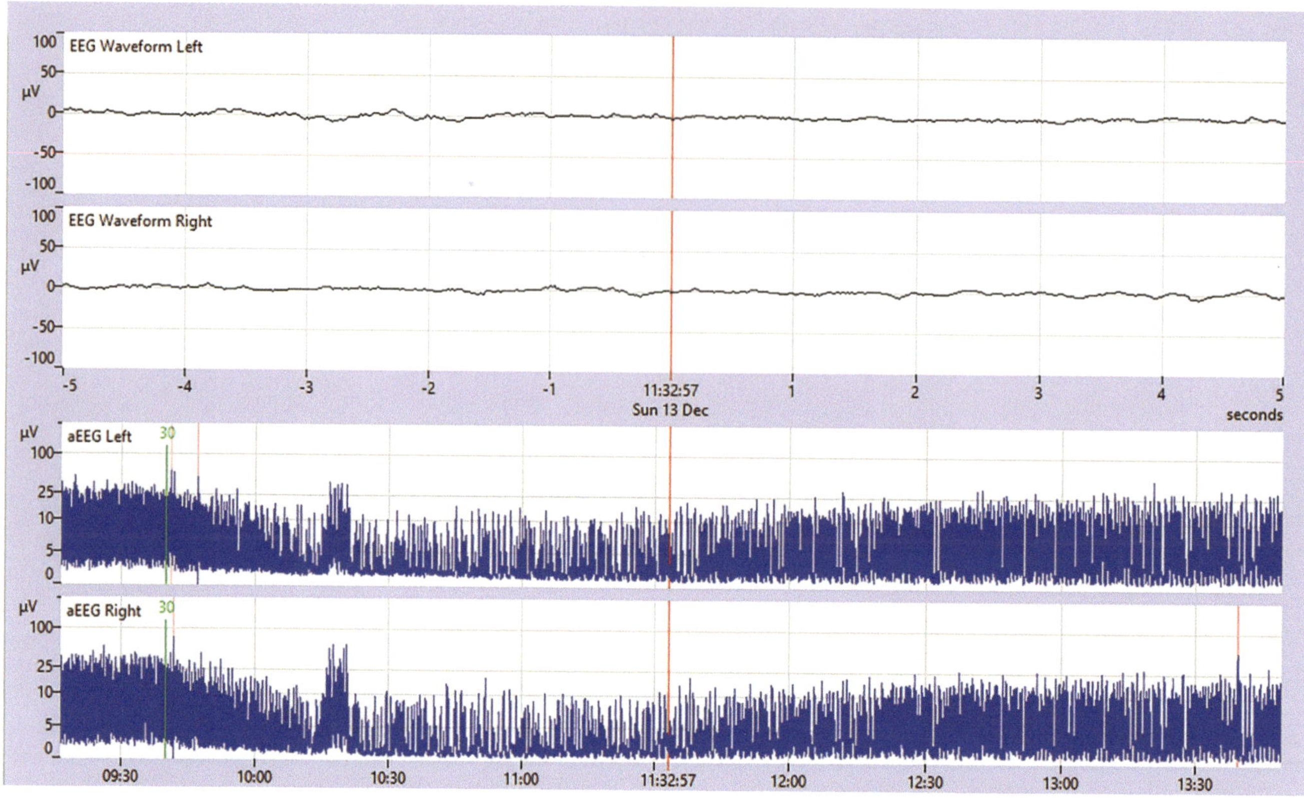

FIGURE 5.7G

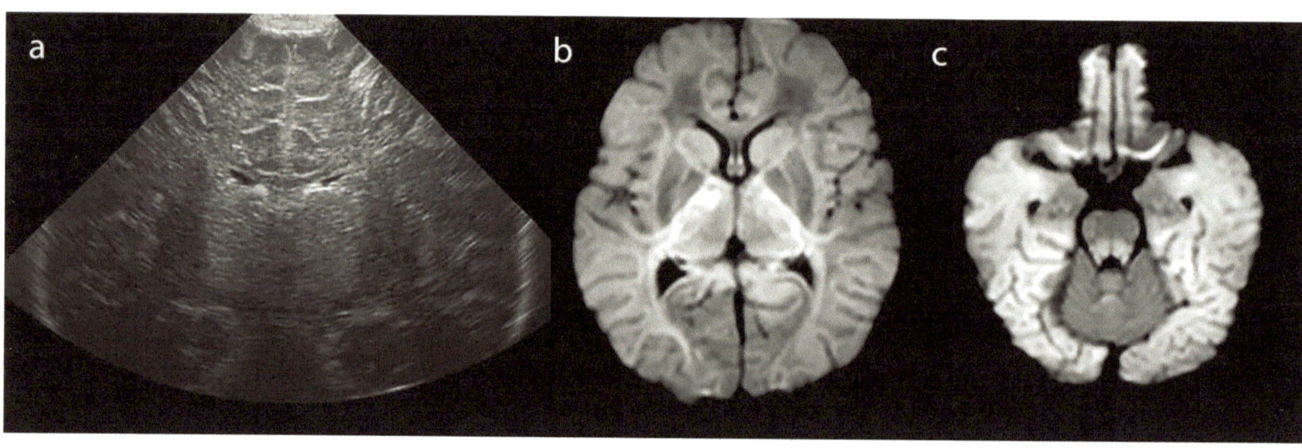

FIGURE 5.7H

Case 5.8 Full-Term Infant with Severe HIE

This infant was born by emergency caesarean section for placental abruption at 39 weeks' gestation with a birthweight of 3900 g. Apgar scores were 0, 0 and 2 at 1, 5 and 10 minutes, respectively. The umbilical artery pH was 6.56 with a BE of –32 mmol/L. The infant was intubated and ventilated and was given cardiac massage. Heart rate was > 100/min at 9 minutes. The Thompson score was 10 at one hour after birth, and hypothermia was started.

The *aEEG* was started at 6 hrs of age. Figure 5.8A shows a drift of the baseline, which appears to be due to artefacts, as seen on the raw EEG during the first 4 hours of recording. Monitoring was probably stopped, and the electrodes reattached between 1 and 2 AM (Day 2:01.00; part B). There were no clinical notes, and the aEEG and EEG were very depressed, flat or low voltage with seizures. A loading dose of phenobarbital (20 mg/kg iv) was given at around 3:30 AM (phen) (Figure 5.8A and see Video 5.8). In Figure 5.8B, the overall background is mainly flat (< 5 μV) with repeated very low-voltage seizures. Another dose of phenobarbital (10 mg/kg, phen) was given followed by midazolam (mida), but seizures continued. After lidocaine administration, seizures stopped (Figure 5.8C). There was no recovery of the background activity, which is flat and only showing electrocardiogram (ECG) artefacts (Figure 5.8D). Recovery to a sparse BS pattern is seen at 60 hrs of age (Figure 5.8E). The rhythmic change seen is less than 10 seconds and could be referred to as a brief rhythmic discharge (BRD). In the last panel, there is recurrence of short ictal discharges after rewarming, shown at 96 hrs of age (Figure 5.8F). There is still a BS pattern that has now become dense.

MRI (Figure 5.8G; see also H) was performed on day 6, and the DWI showed extensive restriction in the thalami, caudate nuclei, white matter and cortex, a near-total pattern of injury. 1H-magnetic resonance spectroscopy (MRS) shows reduced N-acetyl asparate (NAA) and a very high lactate peak. Care was withdrawn.

This case shows that, in infants with severe HIE, even after a long period of a flat trace, some recovery is often seen but, in this case, not beyond a BS pattern and without any SWC indicating the severe prognosis.

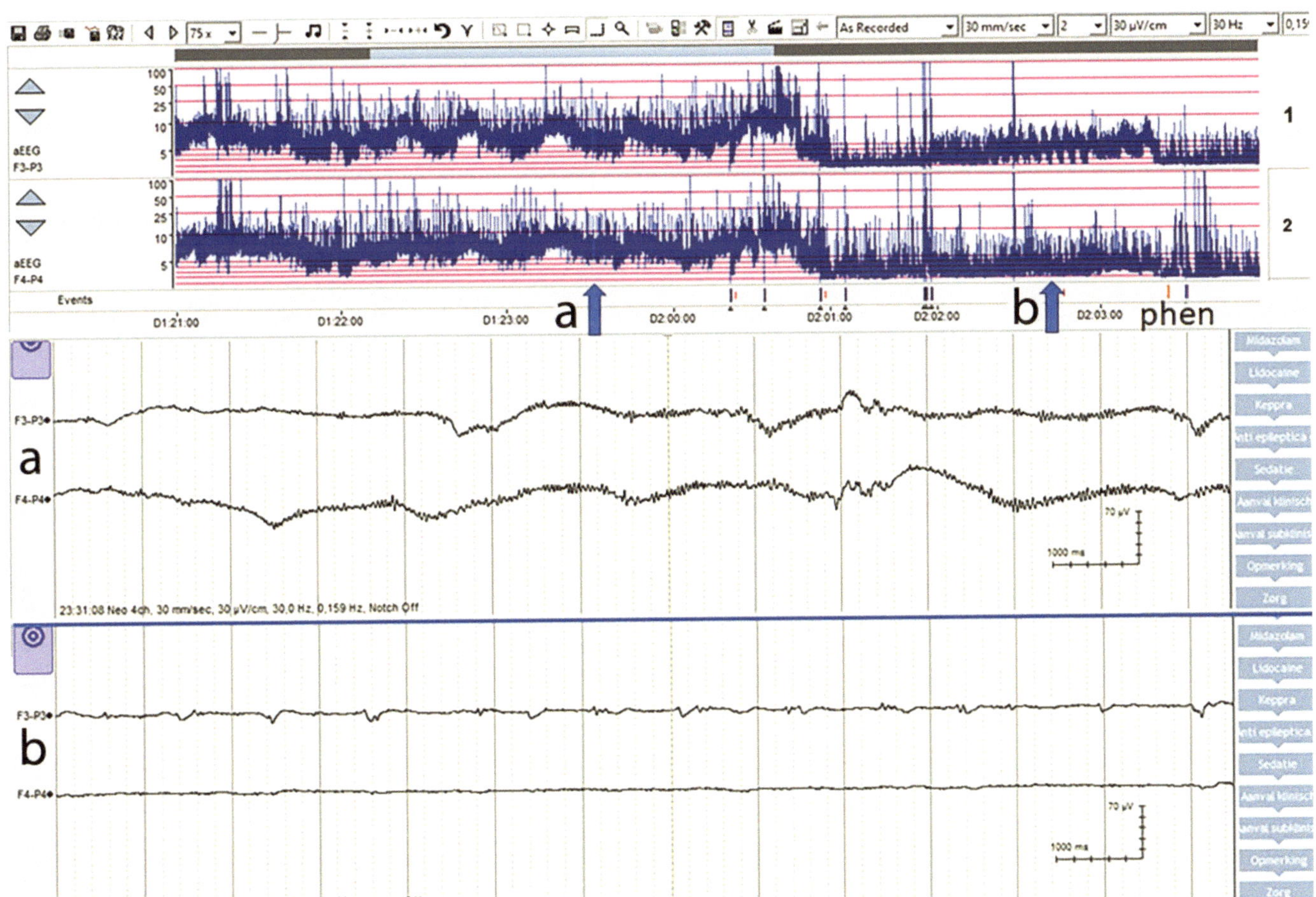

FIGURE 5.8A

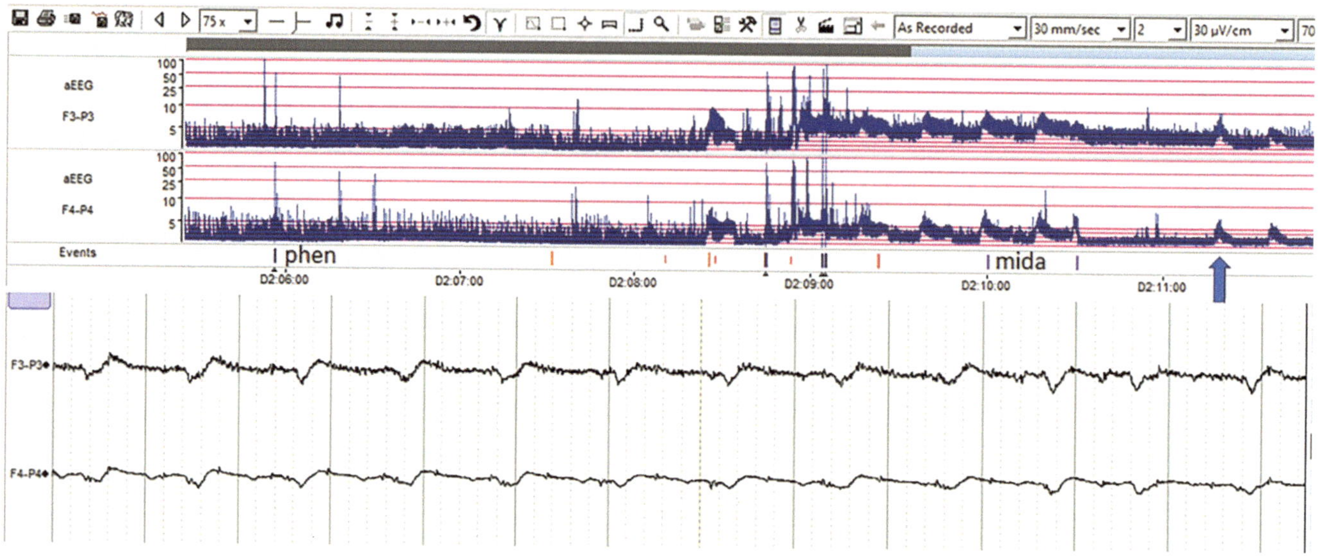

FIGURE 5.8B

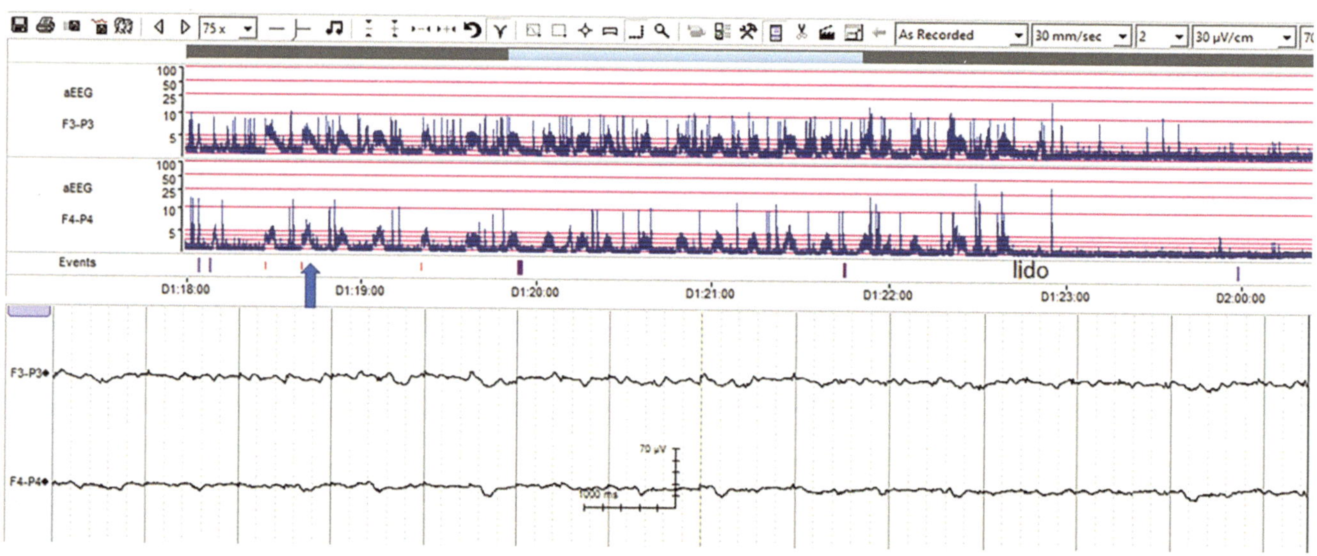

FIGURE 5.8C

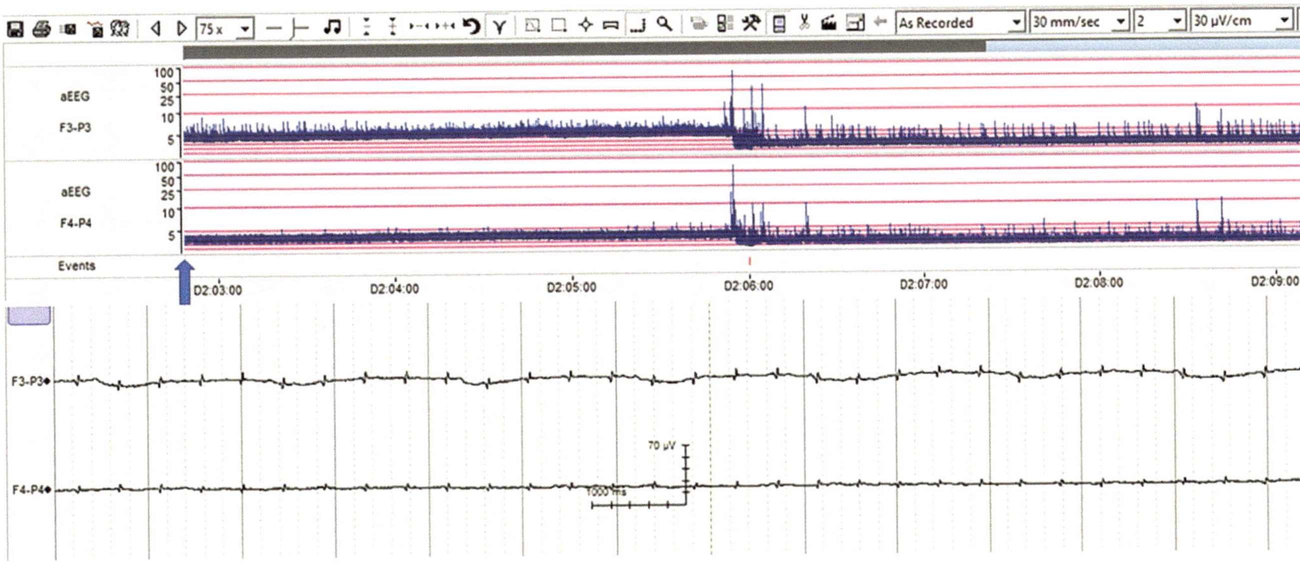

FIGURE 5.8D

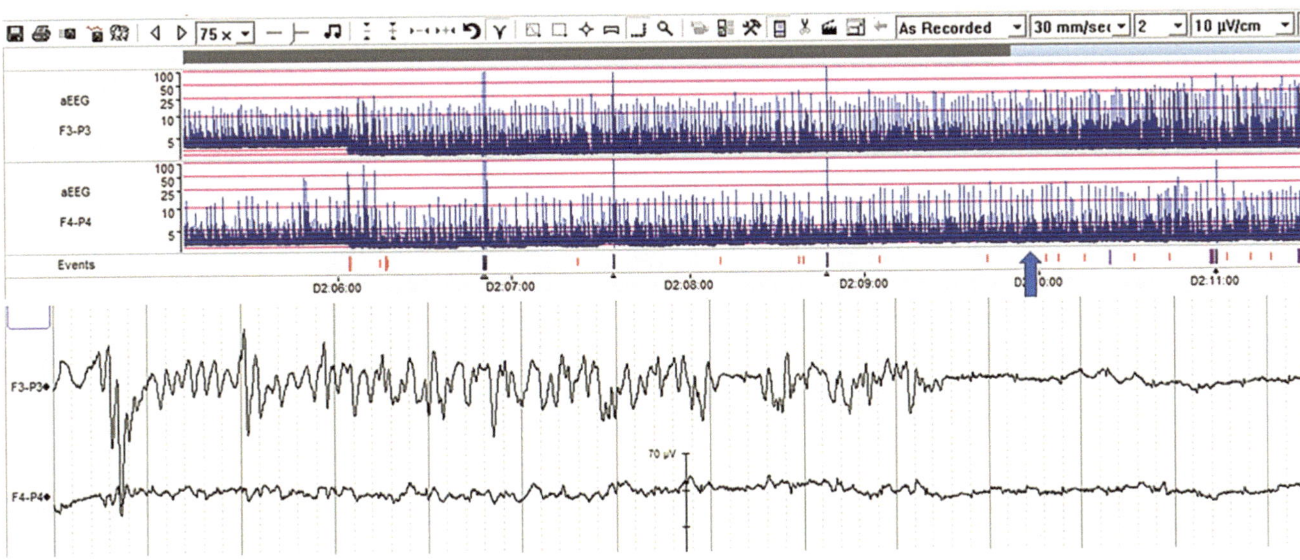

FIGURE 5.8E

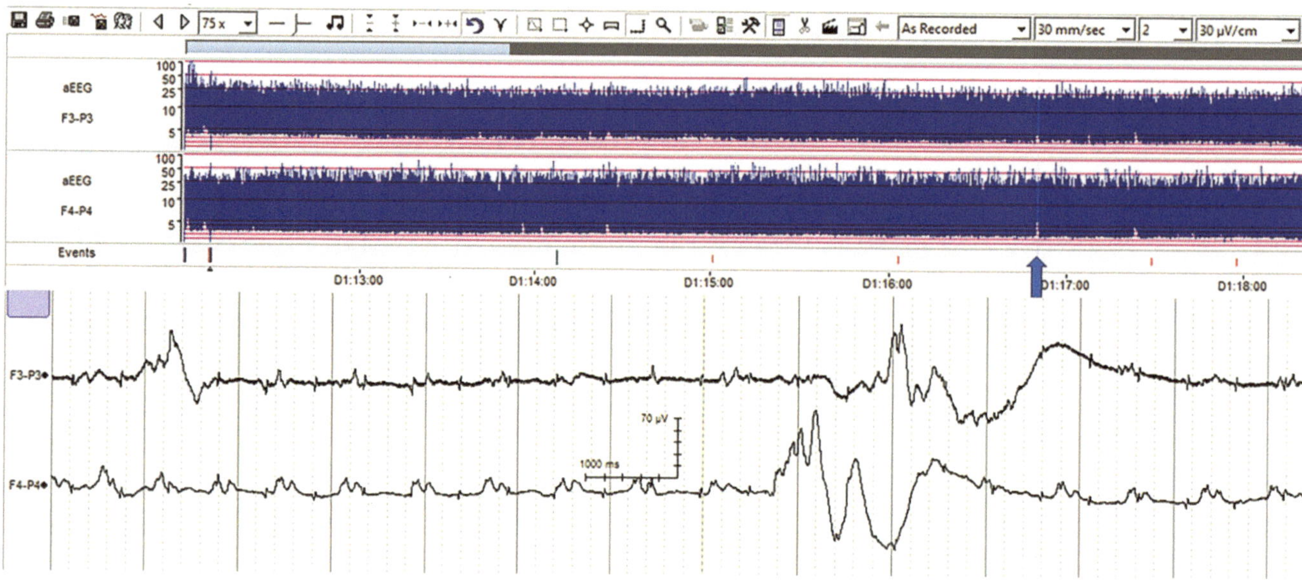

FIGURE 5.8F

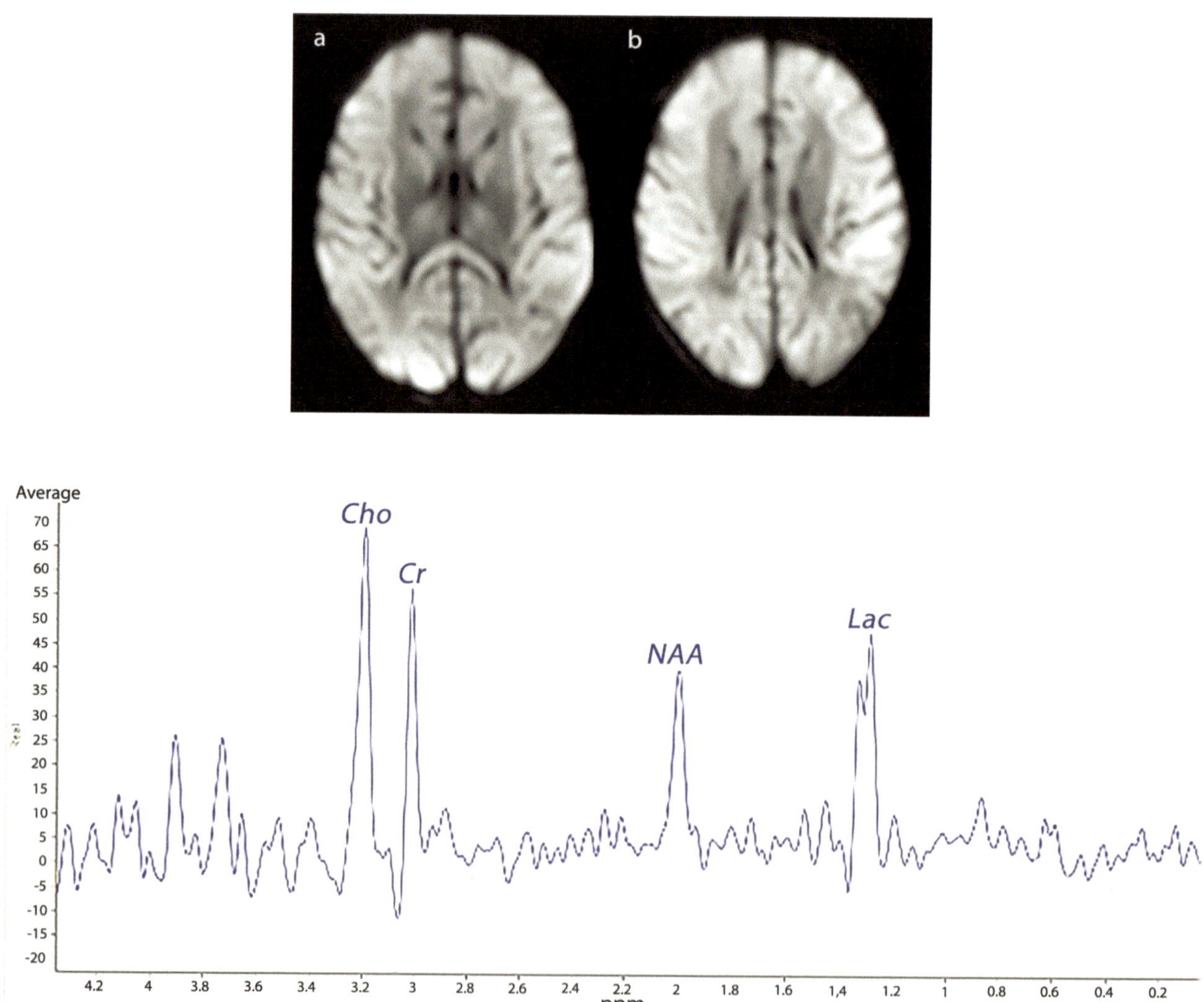

FIGURE 5.8G AND H

Case 5.9 Term Infant with Severe HIE Following a Sentinel Event

This infant was born at 38 weeks' gestation with a normal birthweight, following a normal pregnancy. The delivery was initially uneventful, but just before birth, there was a placental abruption. The infant was very pale, and Apgar scores were 1, 1 and 1 at 1, 5 and 10 minutes, respectively. Umbilical arterial pH was 6.9, BE was −11 mmol/L and first Hb was 50 g/L after blood transfusion. The infant stabilized after repeated blood transfusions but was lethargic with hypotonia. Therapeutic hypothermia was initated at 2 hours. Breathing was assisted with mechanical ventilation. The clinical course was complicated by coagulation problems, hypotension, hypoglycemia, and seizures that were difficult to control. On day 3, the encephalopathy progressed with a bulging fontanel and stupor.

Cranial ultrasound and MRI showed evidence of severe ischaemic brain injury and cerebral edema, and it was decided to redirect care.

The *aEEG* traces show 12 hours of aEEG from left (F3-P3) and right (F4-P4) electrodes in contrast to 6 hours in other cases in this chapter. There are four channels of raw EEG (duration 25 or 64 seconds) from F3-P3, F4-P4, F3-P3 and F4-P4.

Figure 5.9A shows the aEEG development from 8 to 20 postnatal hours. The initial aEEG shows a BS pattern with drift of the baseline, for unclear reasons, up to the 5 μV level. The first seizure was confirmed on the raw EEG when the infant was 19 hours old (red arrow). From the EEG, it is clear that the seizure occurred mainly on the right side (F4-P4) and was visible in the cross-cerebral biparietal P3-P4. The seizure frequency increased, and a status epilepticus developed and was present for almost 3 hours before it was stopped by antiseizure medications (Figure 5.9B). The background activity in the aEEG shows a discontinuous pattern that looks somewhat more depressed on the right side than on the left. There was no aEEG recording from the left side during the last 2 hours.

On day 2 (Figure 5.9C), the aEEG/EEG showed a burst-suppression pattern and no asymmetry. Figure 5.9D shows the burst-suppression pattern in the aEEG/EEG from around 69 to 81 hours, during rewarming. There are small differences in the lower border of the aEEG traces, and as judged from the raw EEG, they are probably artefacts; the signal from F4-P4 looks most "clean". Figure 5.9E shows the seizures that developed after rewarming, between 98 and 104 hours, and stopped by lidocaine, which resulted in a very depressed activity (probably a flat pattern but difficult to assess without examining the raw EEG at this time point).

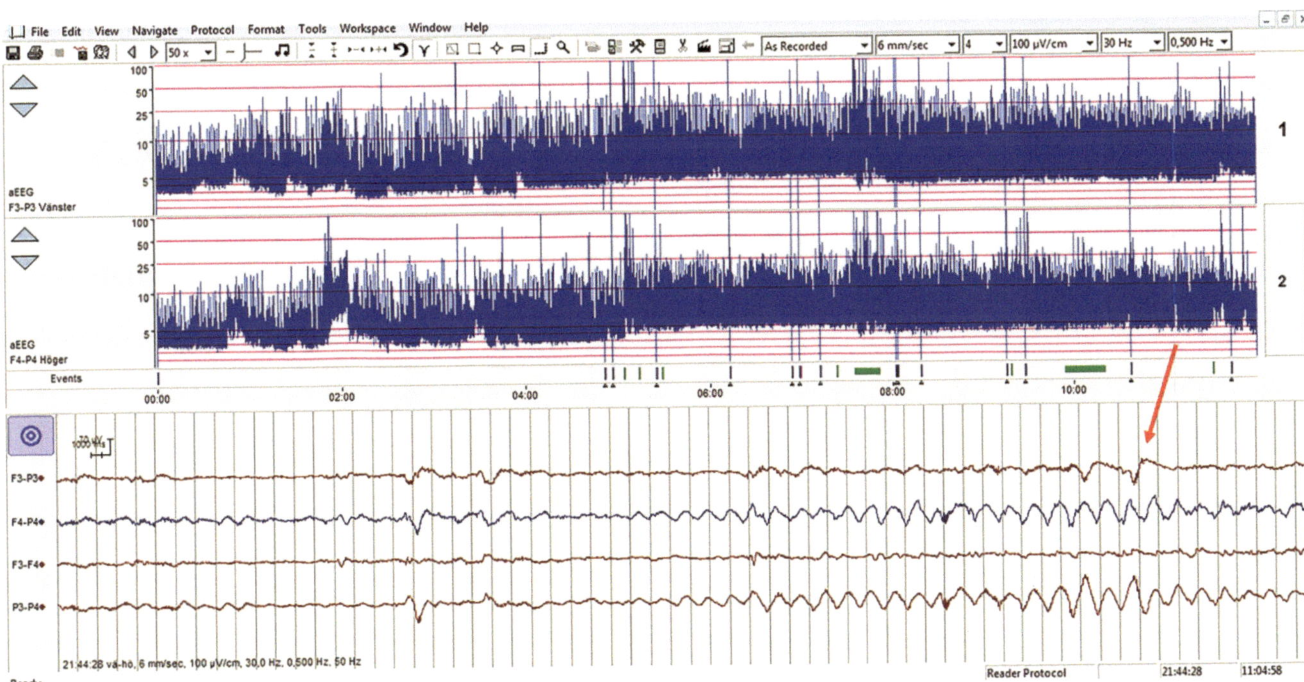

FIGURE 5.9A

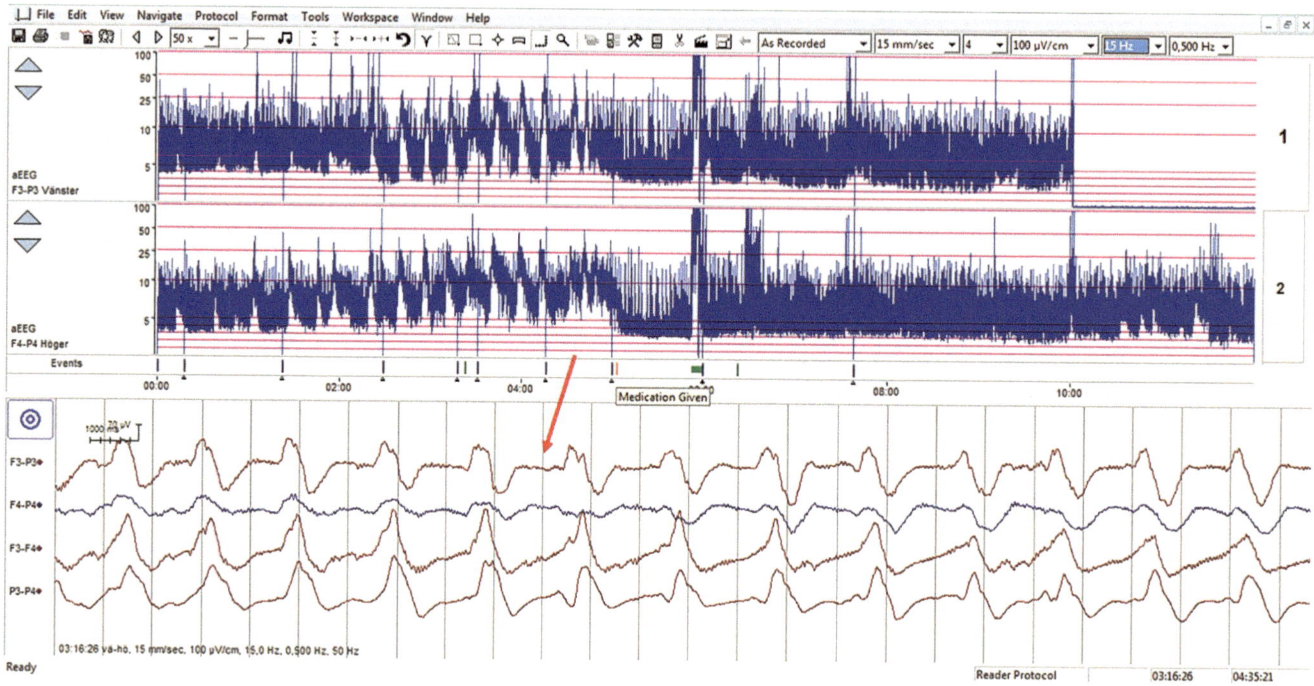

FIGURE 5.9B

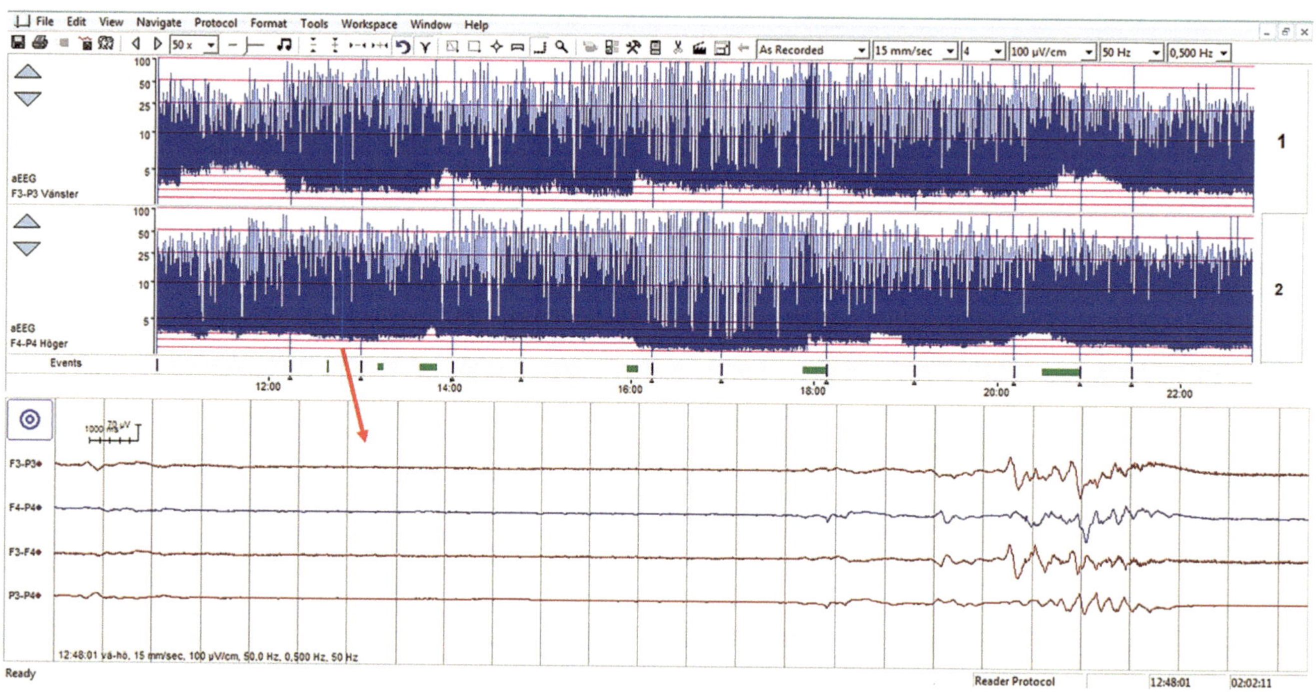

FIGURE 5.9C

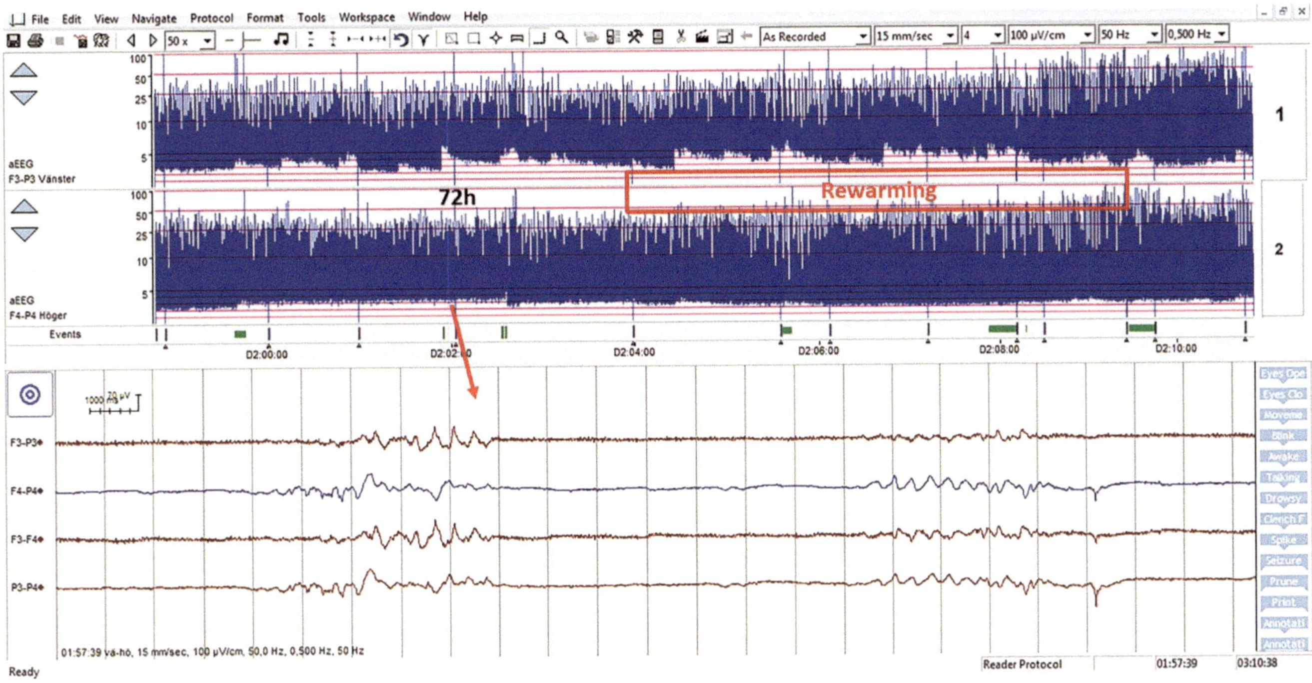

FIGURE 5.9D

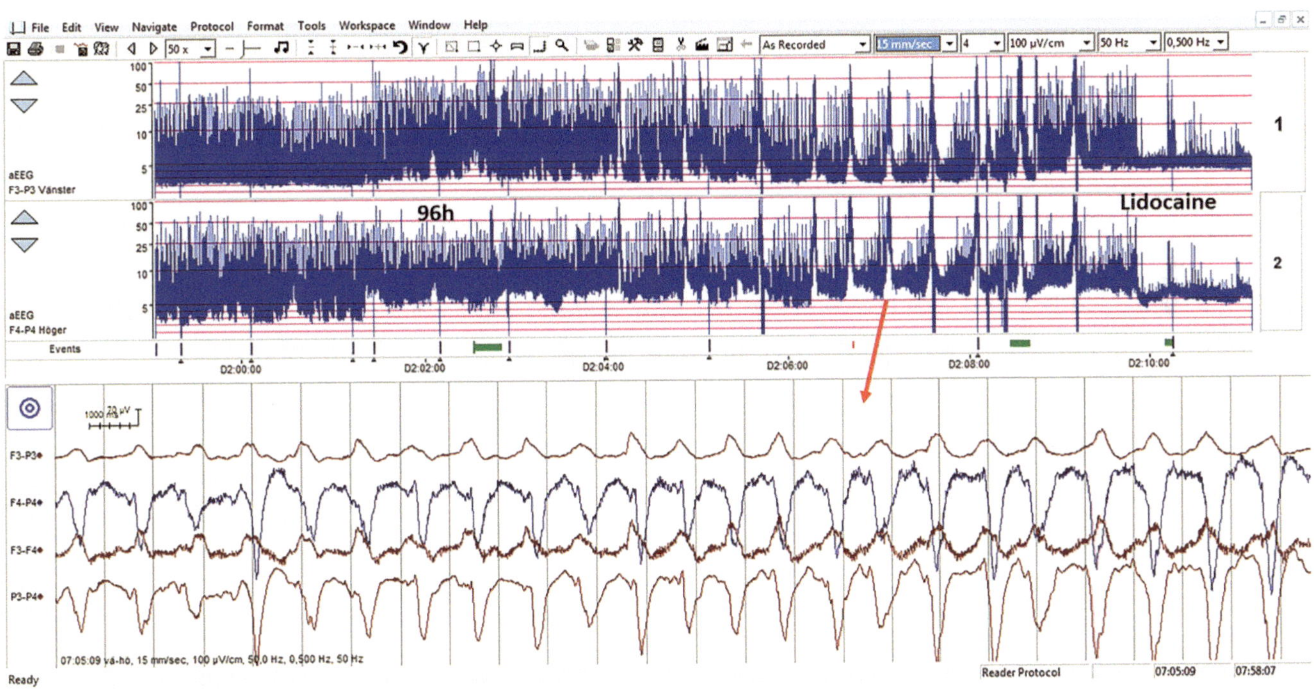

FIGURE 5.9E

Case 5.10 Late Preterm Infant with Moderate Asphyxia and Rapid Recovery

Preterm infant, born at 34 weeks' gestation by emergency caesarean section for placental abruption. Apgar scores were 1, 5 and 7 at 1, 5 and 10 minutes, respectively. Extensive resuscitation was required. Umbilical artery pH was 6.8. The first arterial lactate was 20 mmol/L. The Thompson score was 11, but due to the GA, cooling was not started. Care was taken to control the temperature to 36.5 degrees. The infant developed severe respiratory problems, was on HFO with nitric oxide for pulmonary hypertension and needed inotropes to maintain the blood pressure.

The *aEEG* recording was started within 6 hours after birth and showed a continuous low-voltage pattern, with recovery to the DNV pattern 10 hours after birth (Figure 5.10A). In the second figure (Figure 5.10B), imminent sleep-wake cycling is seen from 12 hours of life onward and is well-established and on a CNV background a day later (Figure 5.10C). No seizures were seen, and the background activity normalized in spite of sedation (midazolam and morphine).

MRI (Figure 5.10D) performed on day 4 (a) showed diffusion restriction of the left optic radiation and corpus callosum. No sequelae were apparent on the second MRI (b) performed 10 weeks later (42 weeks postmenstrual age (PMA)). The infant was doing well at 2 years of corrected age.

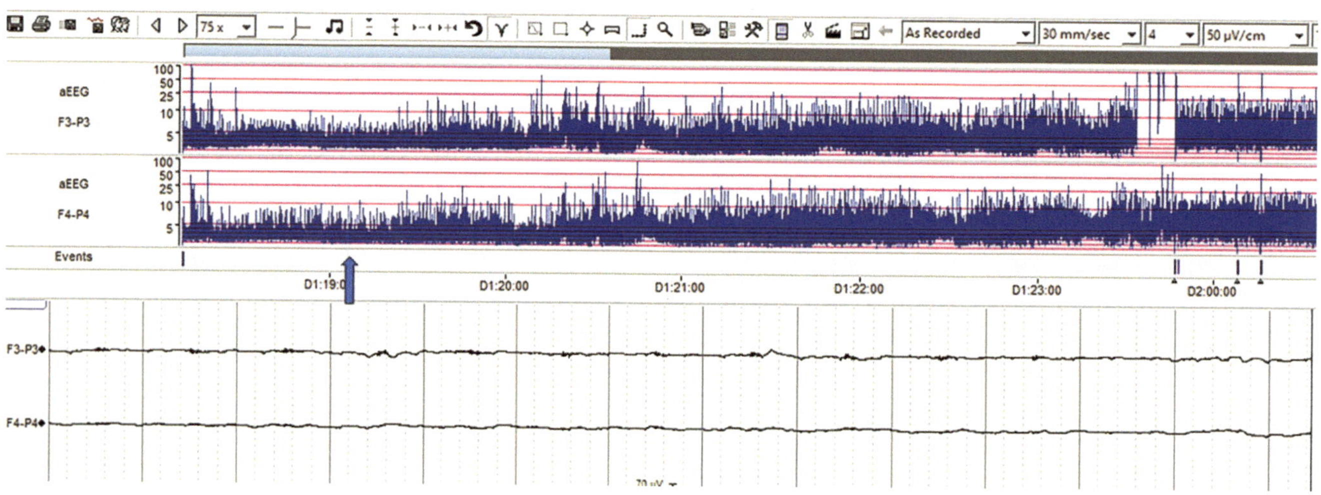

FIGURE 5.10A

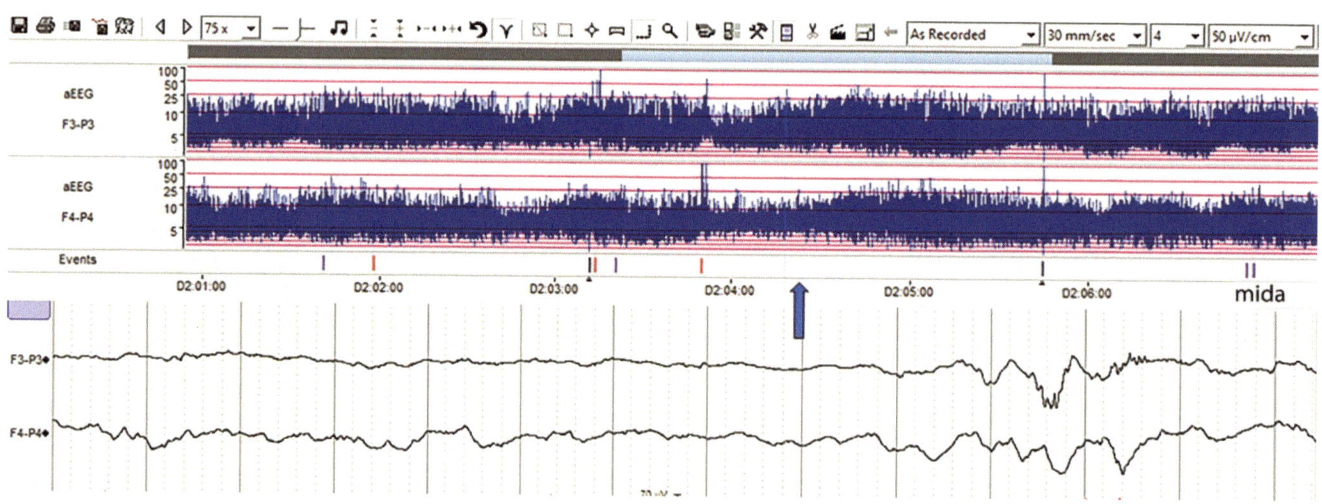

FIGURE 5.10B

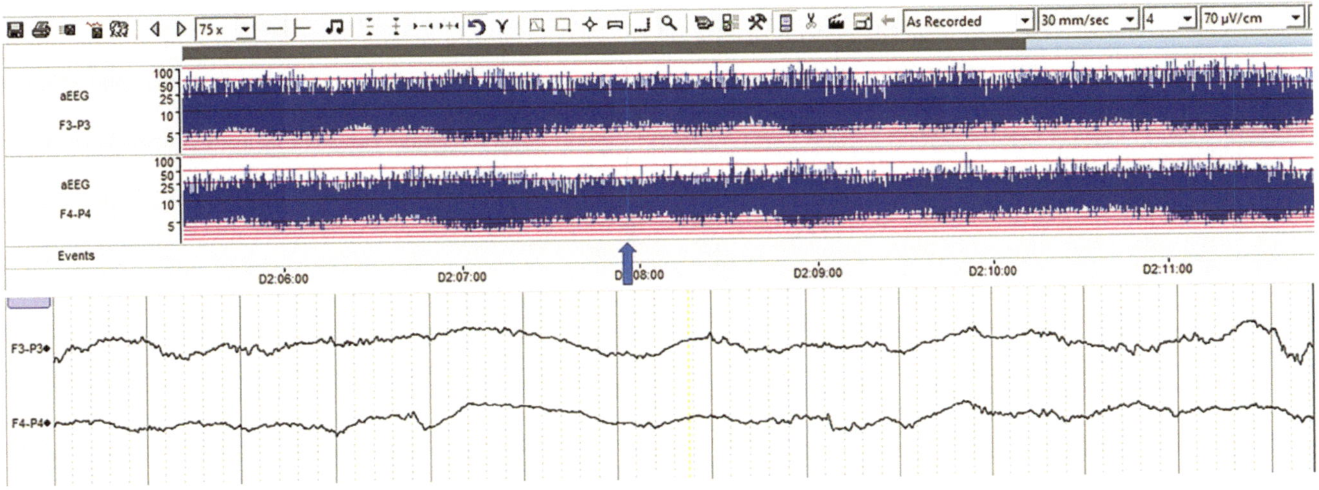

FIGURE 5.10C

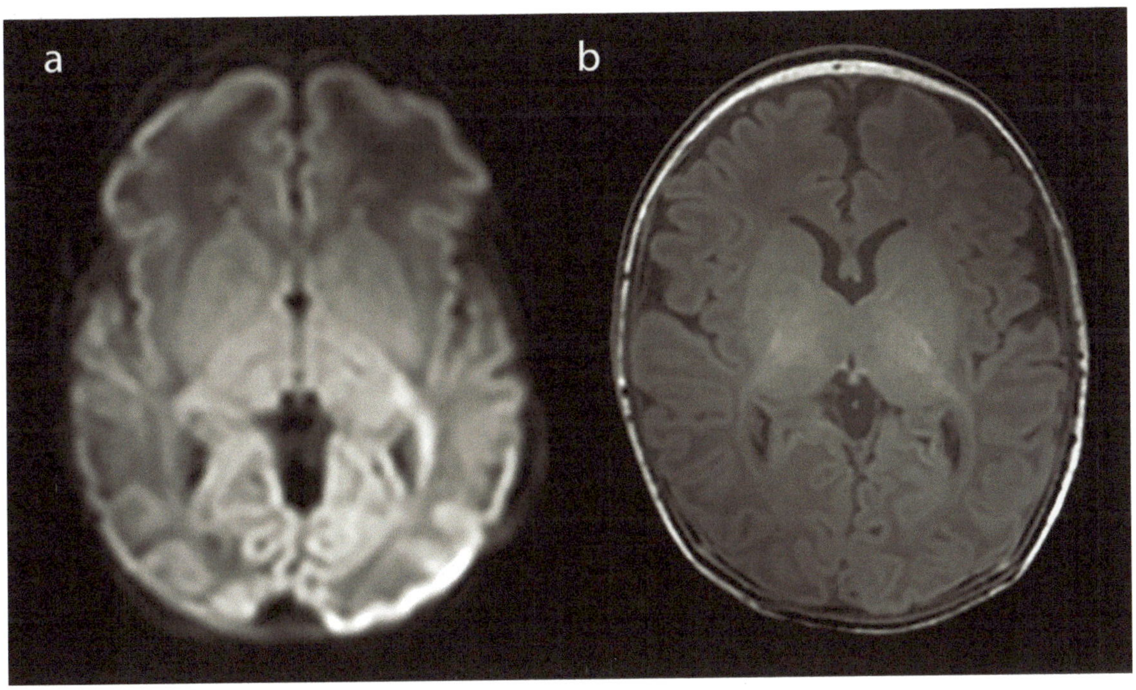

FIGURE 5.10D

Case 5.11 Hemorrhage in the Thalamus in a Late Preterm Infant

This infant was born at 35 weeks' gestation by emergency caesarean section, with a birthweight of 2150 grams. Apgar scores were 2 and 5 at 1 and 5 minutes, respectively. There was rapid recovery, and the infant was admitted to the neonatal unit because of being late preterm. Thompson score was well below 7. A first clinical seizure was seen at 40 hours of age, and a loading dose of phenobarbital was given (20 mg/kg iv). The infant was transferred to the NICU for neuromonitoring.

Shortly after starting the *aEEG* recording, clinical (*) and electrographic seizures were seen on a DNV background, and two further doses of phenobarbital were given (10 mg/kg iv) (Figure 5.11A and see Video 5.11). The evolution of a seizure with a duration of 30 seconds is shown in Figure 5.11B. There are many short interruptions in the background activity in the F3-P3 recording, and most of these showed fast activity but not clear seizures (Figure 5.11C). No further seizures were seen, and SWC is present and fully developed in the next panel when the infant has been recorded for 72 hours (Figure 5.11D).

Cranial ultrasound (Figure 5.11E) on admission (a) showed an IVH and a large hemorrhage in the left thalamus, suggestive of a sinovenous thrombosis, but this was not confirmed on *MRI* (b), including MR venography (not shown). The cause for this large thalamic hemorrhage remains, therefore, unknown.

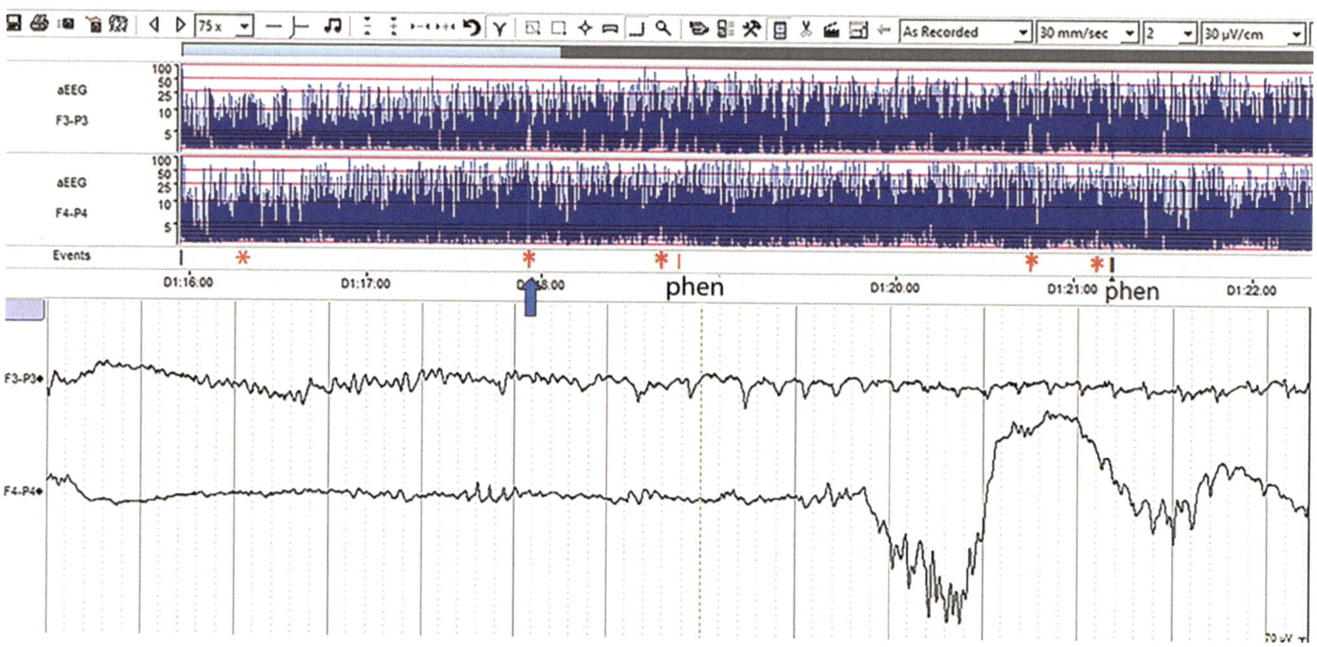

FIGURE 5.11A

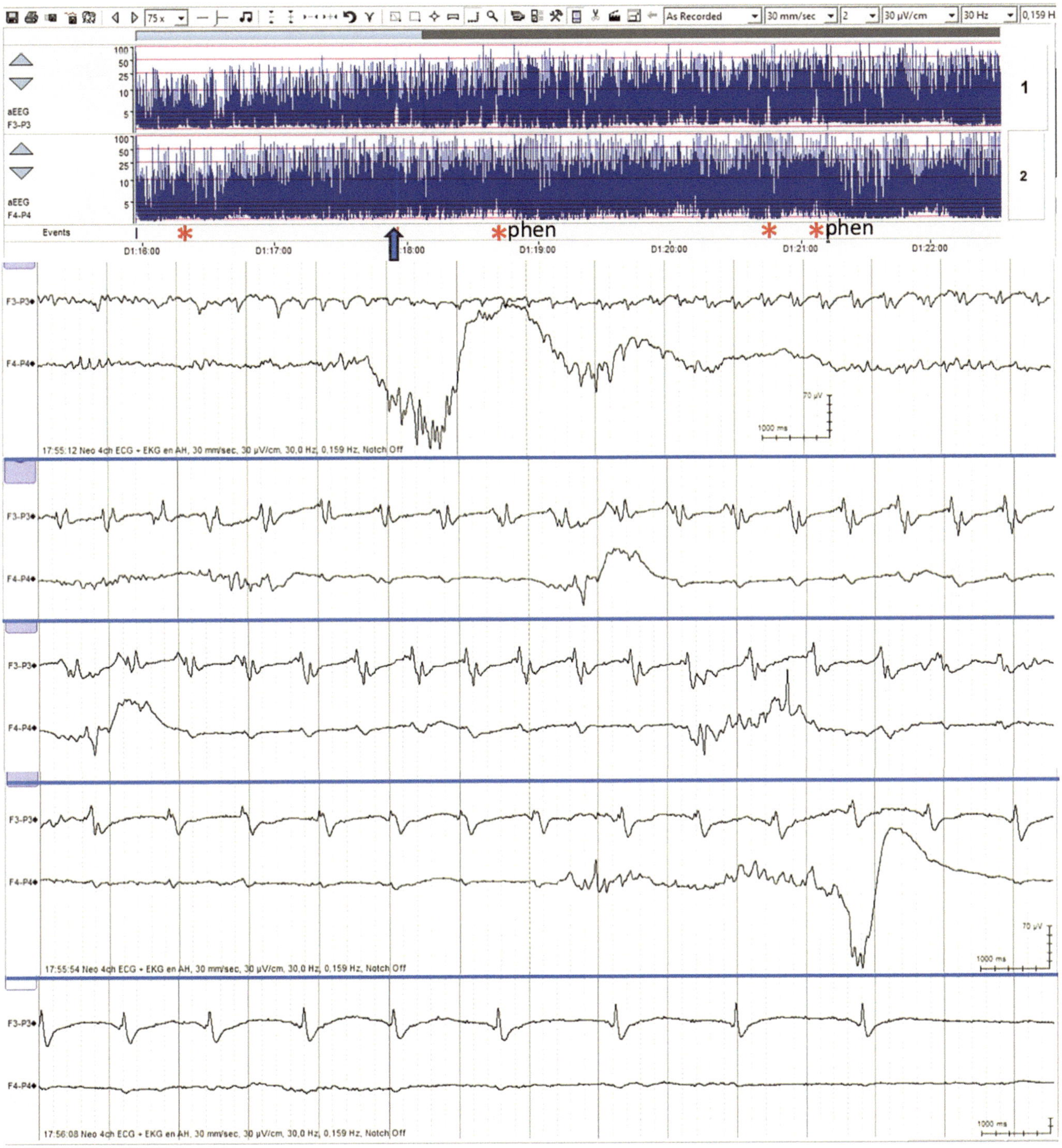
As Recorded
30 mm/sec
30 µV/cm
30 Hz
aEEG F3-P3
aEEG F4-P4
Events
phen
phen
D1:16:00
D1:17:00
D1:19:00
D1:20:00
D1:21:00
D1:22:00
F3-P3
F4-P4

FIGURE 5.11B

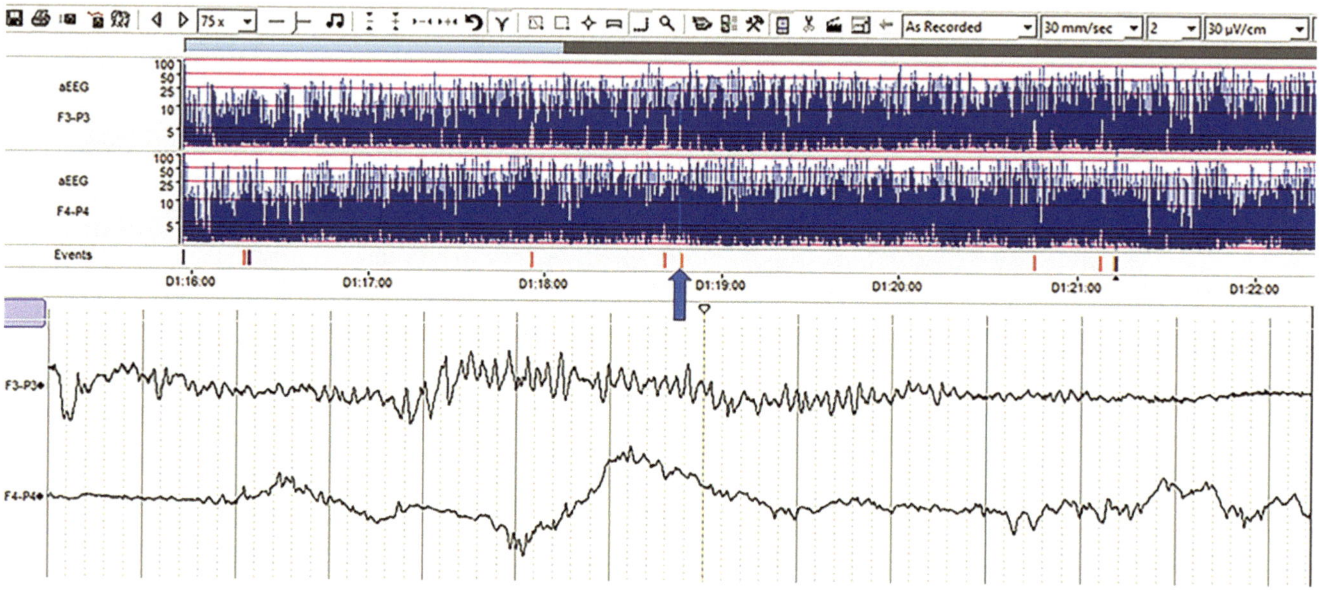

FIGURE 5.11C

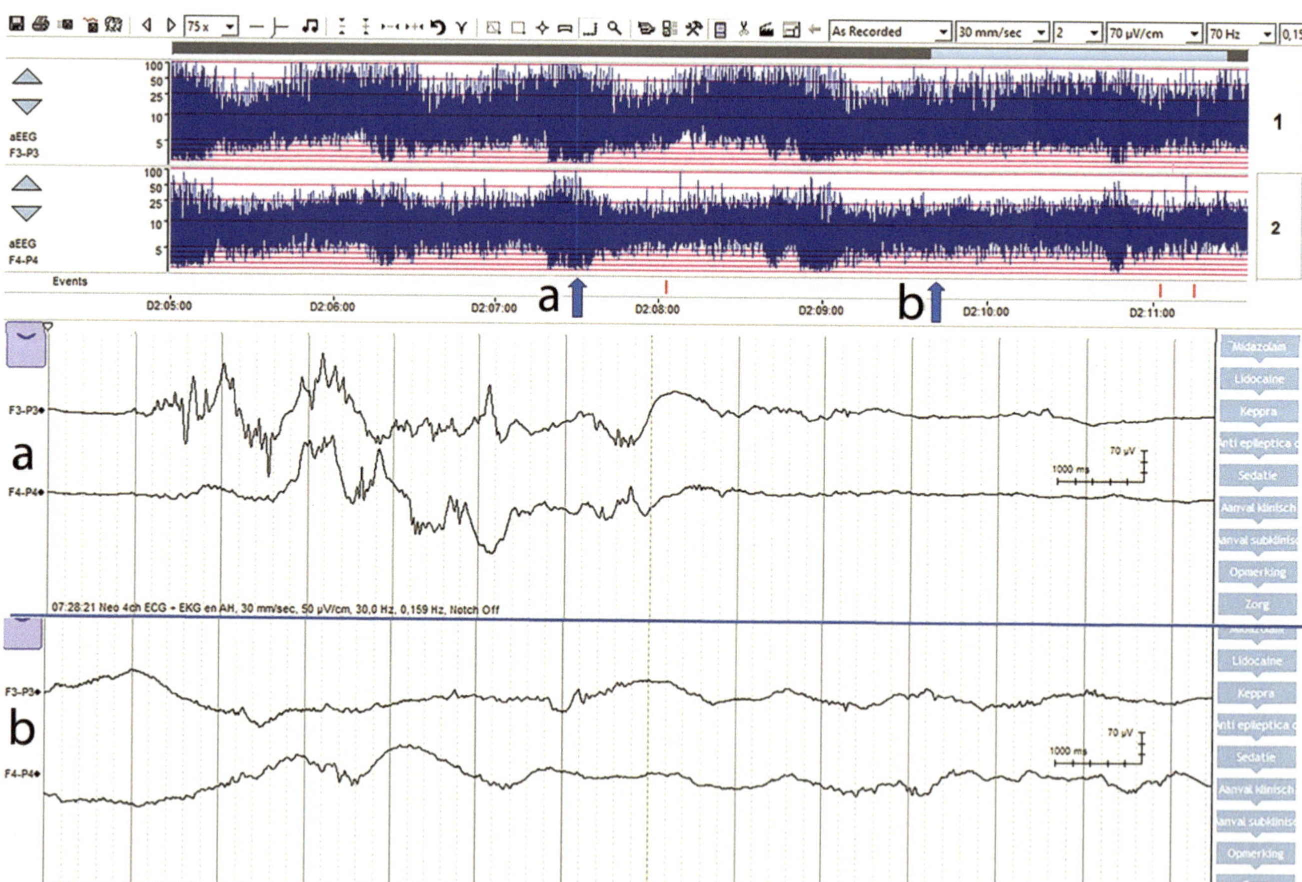

FIGURE 5.11D

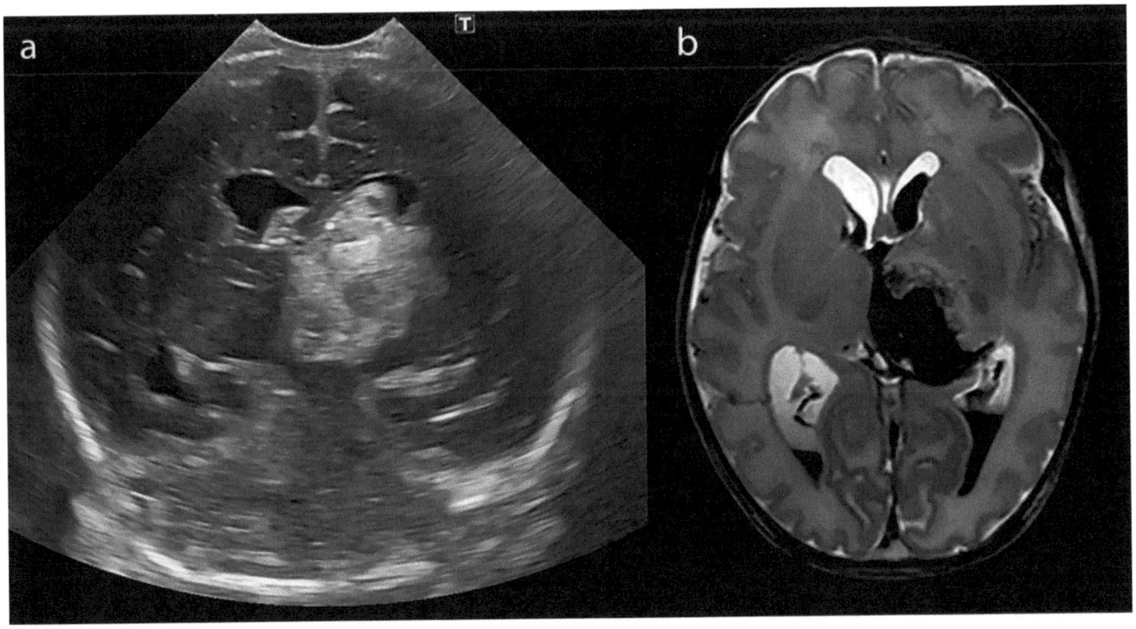

FIGURE 5.11E

Case 5.12 Full-Term Infant with a Temporal Lobe Hemorrhage

This infant was born at 40 weeks' gestation following an uncomplicated vaginal delivery with Apgar scores of 8 and 9 at 1 and 5 minutes, respectively. The birthweight was 3950 grams. At 36 hours of age, the infant was admitted from home because of apneas. The infant was intubated and ventilated.

When the *aEEG* recording was started, apneas were confirmed to be seizures on a predominantly CNV background (Figure 5.12A). All EEG confirmed seizures in Figure 5.12A are marked *. Seizures continued following 40 mg/kg iv of phenobarbital and also after 60 mg/kg iv of levetiracetam (Figure 5.12B). Midazolam was the next antiseizure medication given, and since then, no further seizures were noted (Figure 5.12B). The next day, the background had recovered and SWC was present (Figure 5.12C).

A *cranial ultrasound* (Figure 5.12D) examination was performed (a) and showed a hemorrhage in the right temporal lobe that was also confirmed with *MRI* (b).

At 24 months, development was well within the normal range, with a Bayley-III cognitive composite score of 96 and the combined motor score of 121.

In a previously well full-term infant presenting with apneas, a temporal lobe hemorrhage should always be suspected and cranial ultrasound should be performed on admission.

Bibliography

Hoogstraate SR, Lequin MH, Huysman MA, et al. Apnoea in relation to neonatal temporal lobe haemorrhage. *Eur J Paediatr Neurol.* 2009;13(4):356–361.

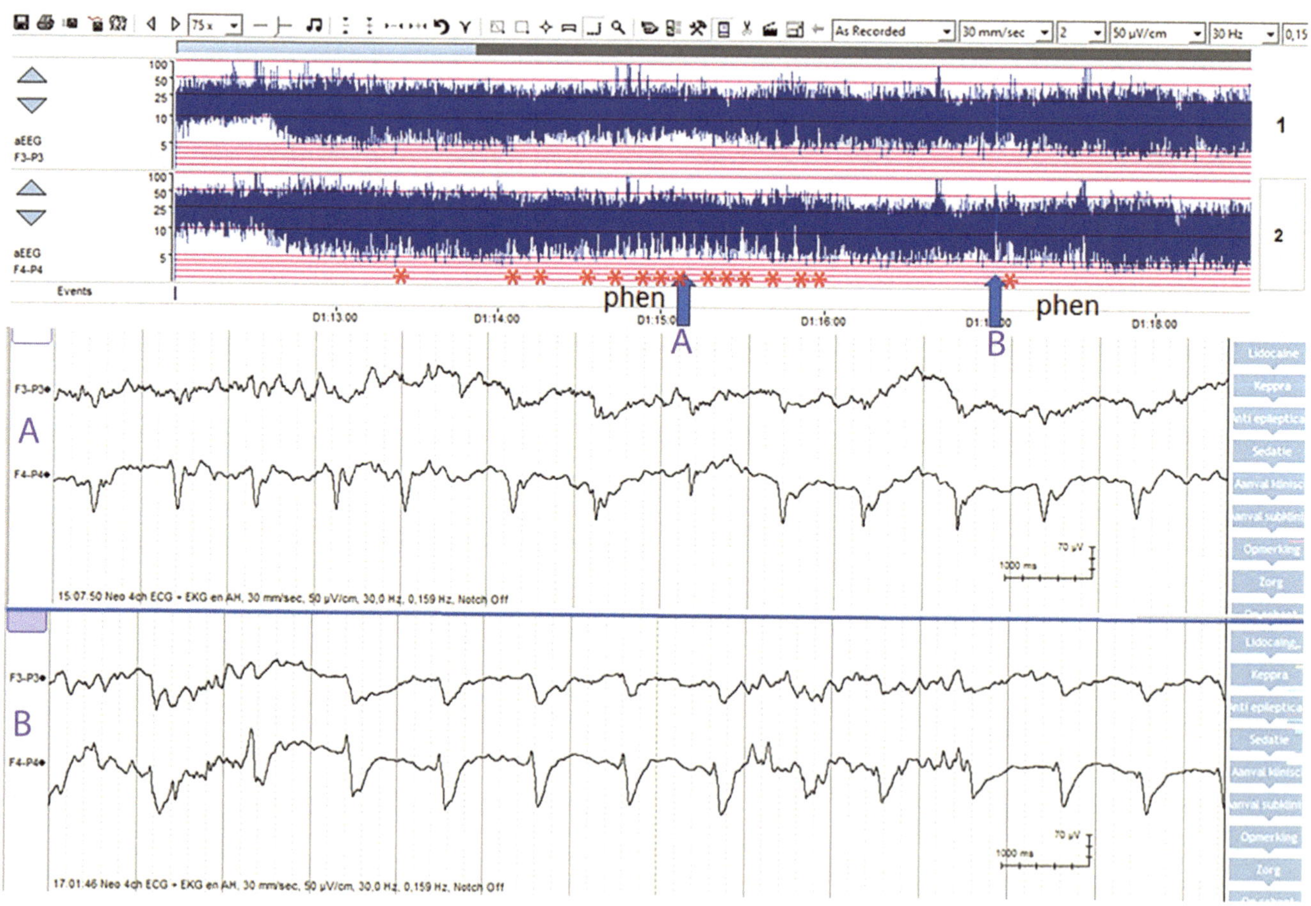

FIGURE 5.12A

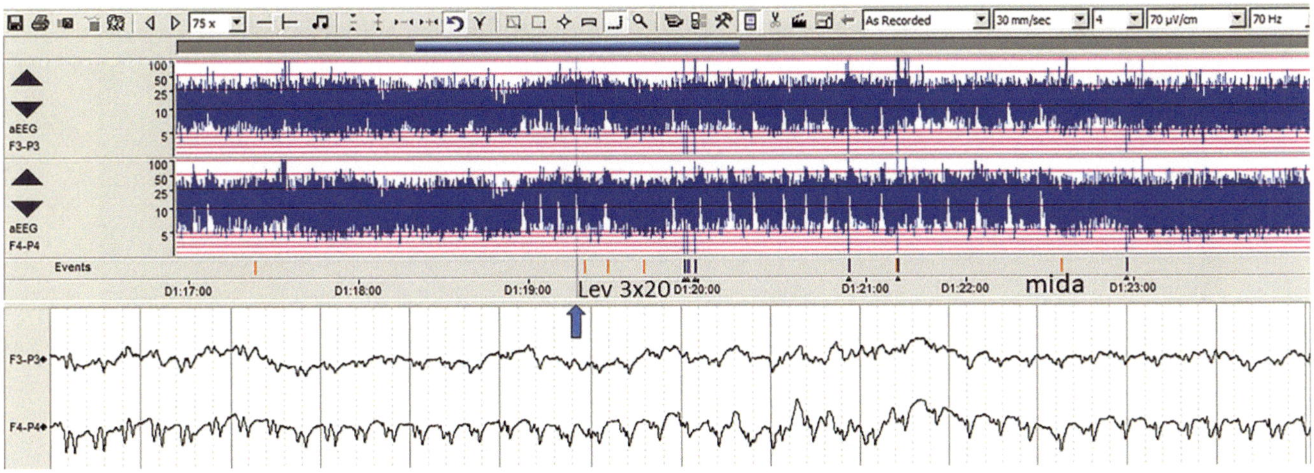

FIGURE 5.12B

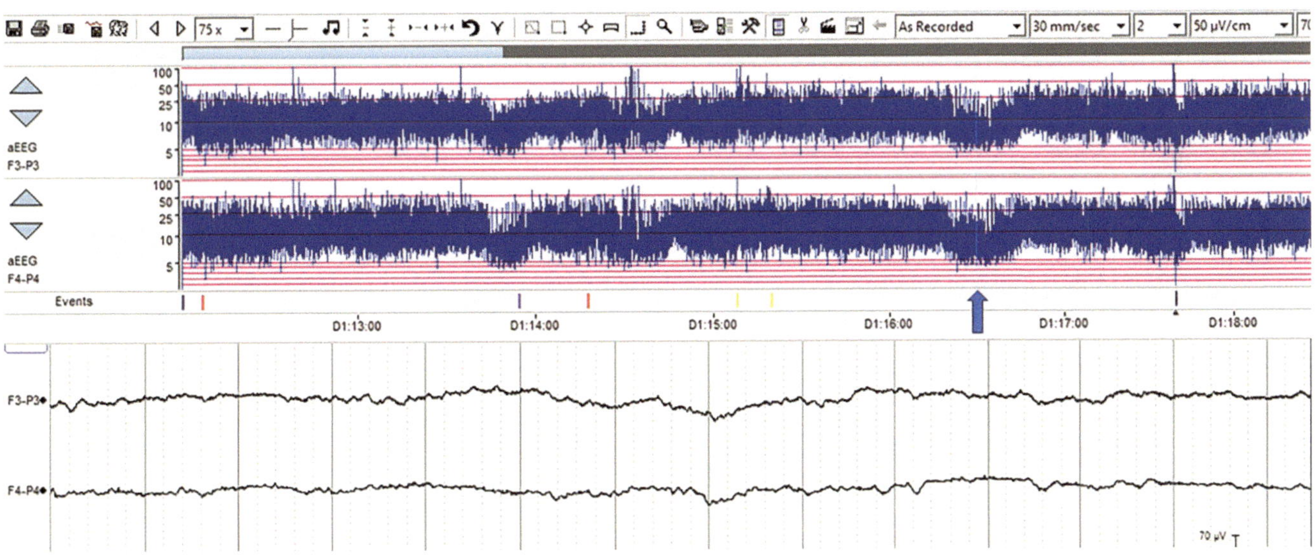

FIGURE 5.12C

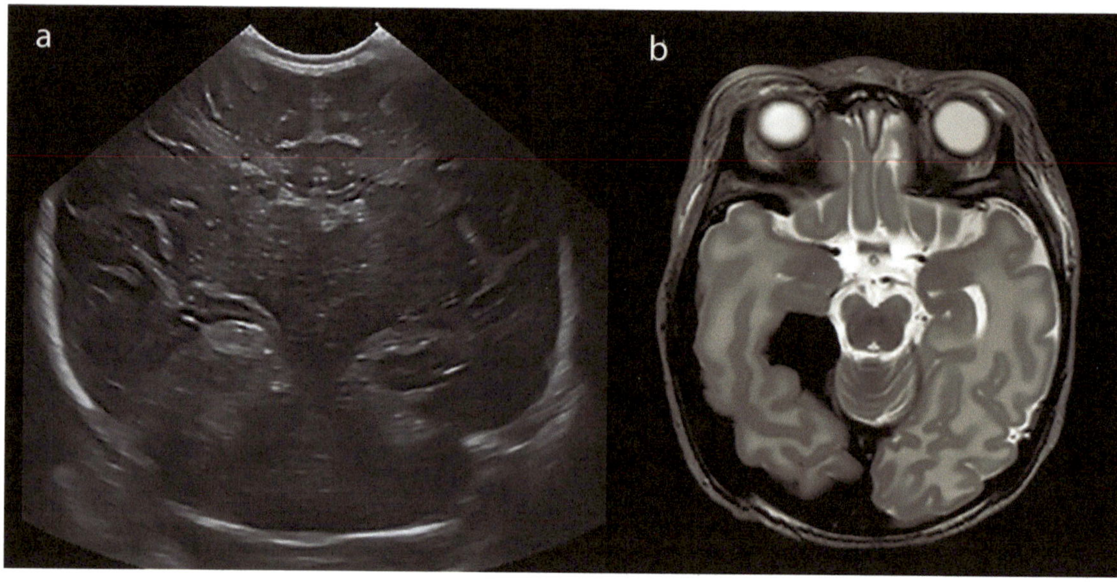

FIGURE 5.12D

Case 5.13 Full-Term Infant with a Frontal Lobe Hemorrhage

This infant was born at 37 weeks' gestation by ventouse extraction. The birthweight was 3500 grams. Apgar scores were 5 and 7 at 1 and 5 minutes, respectively, with an arterial umbilical pH of 7.17. CPAP was needed for a few hours for respiratory distress. Once the CPAP was discontinued, apneas developed and these continued after restarting CPAP. The infant was intubated and ventilated and transferred to a NICU. Apneas were confirmed to be seizures, and four antiseizure medications were needed to control these seizures.

The *aEEG* recording was started at 11 hrs of life and showed a slightly discontinuous background with cyclicity and repetitive seizures (Figure 5.13A). Two doses of phenobarbital (20 mg/kg iv each) were given. Midazolam was given twice and resulted in background depression, but seizures were still not controlled, and a first dose of levetiracetam (20 mg/kg iv) was given (Figure 5.13B). Another two doses of levetiracetam were administered (not shown); in total, there were three doses of levetiracetam (20 mg/kg iv each), but as seizures continued, lidocaine was given, and after that, no further seizures were seen (Figure 5.13C). At this point, the aEEG background activity was severely depressed, showing a burst-suppression pattern. At this time point, it was impossible to tell whether the medication only induced the background depression or if and how brain injury contributed. Recovery of the aEEG background pattern only occurred by 72 hours when a DNV pattern was seen with imminent SWC (Figure 5.13D).

A *cranial ultrasound* on admission (Figure 5.13E) showed a large hematoma in the right frontal lobe. The parasagittal view (a) shows the large hematoma in the right frontal lobe, and this was confirmed on an axial T2 *MRI* the next day (b). There was also blood surrounding the frontal lobe and some blood in the lateral ventricles.

The cause for this large frontal lobe hematoma remained unknown. At 24 months of age, development was within the normal range (Bayley-III cognitive composite score 91, combined motor score 98).

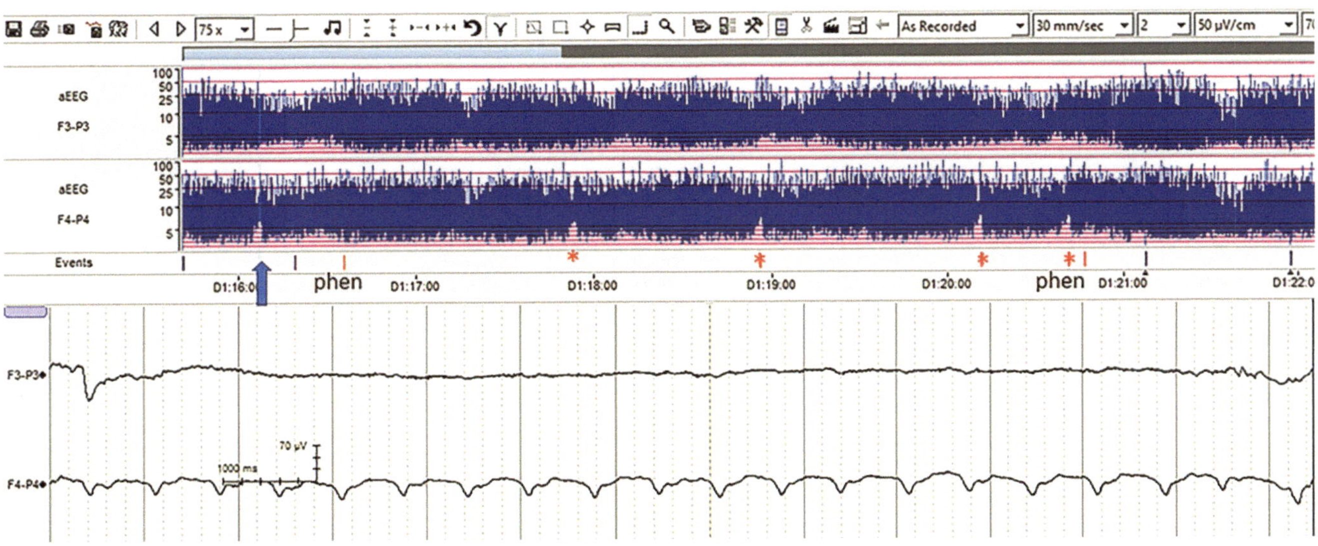

FIGURE 5.13A

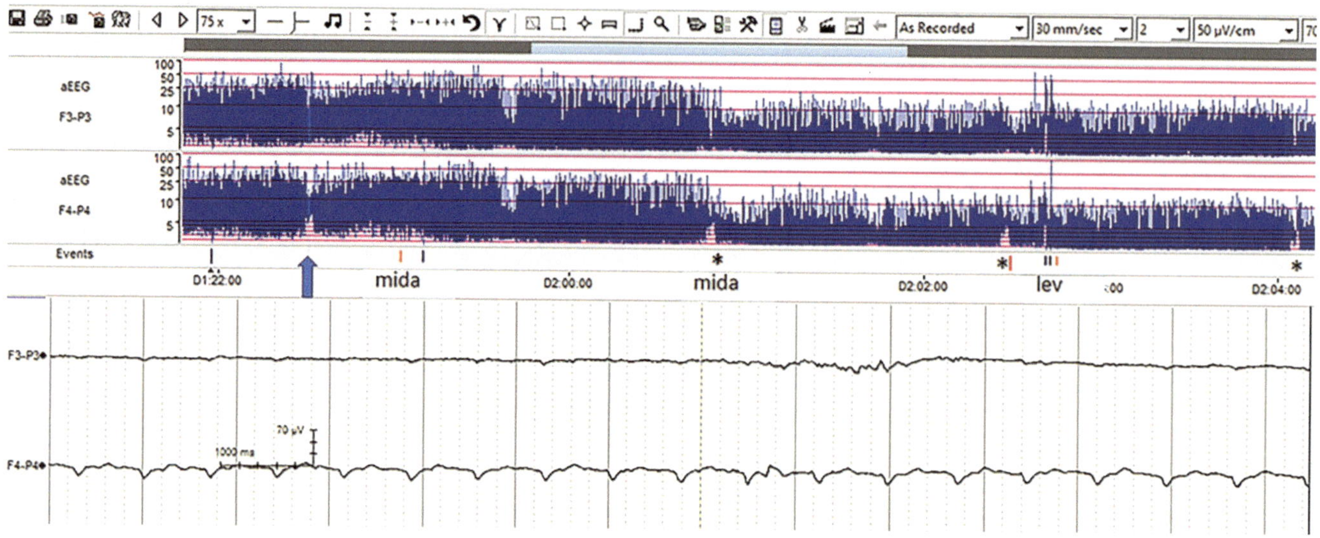

FIGURE 5.13B

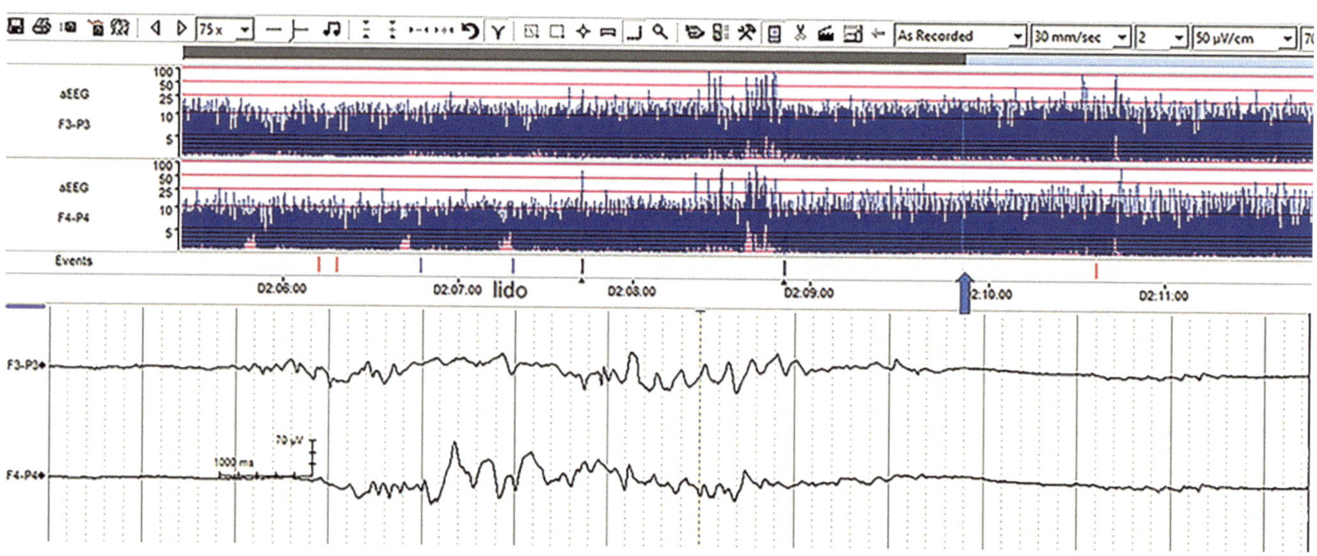

FIGURE 5.13C

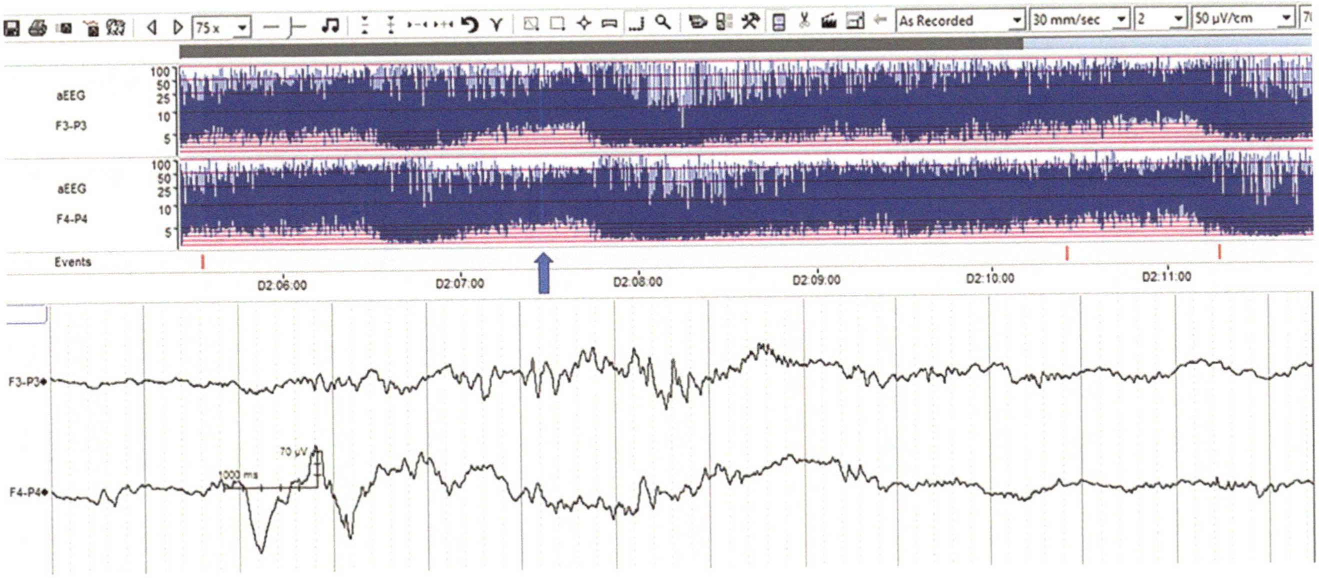

FIGURE 5.13D

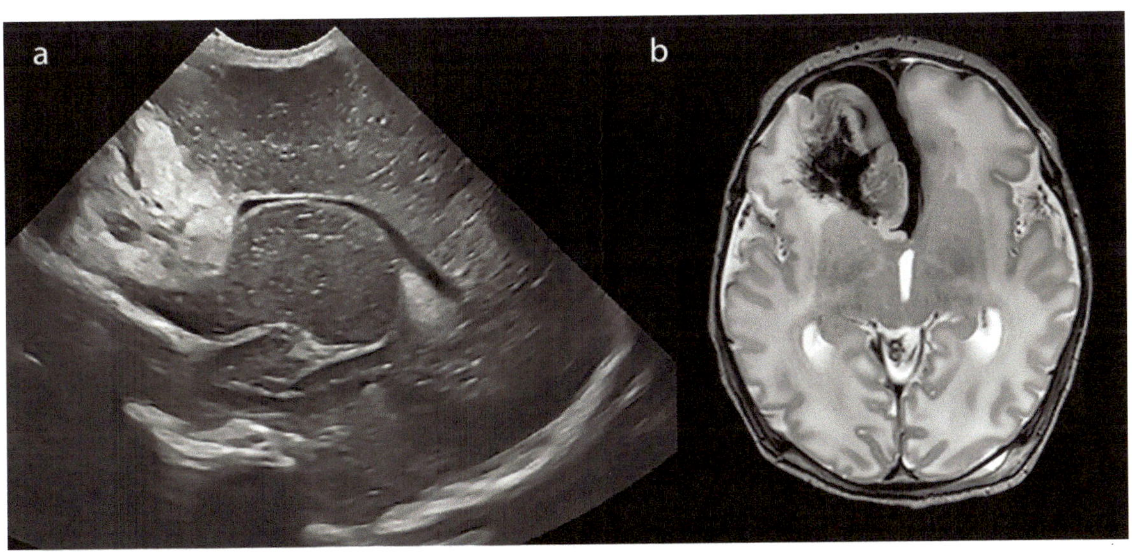

FIGURE 5.13E

Case 5.14 Full-Term Infant with Transposition of the Great Arteries and a Large Subdural Hemorrhage

This infant was born at 41 weeks' gestation with a birthweight of 3900 g. Delivery was uncomplicated, and Apgar scores were 8, 9 and 10 at 1, 5 and 10 minutes, respectively. The infant was cyanotic and needed ventilation for respiratory insufficiency. The infant was diagnosed with transposition of the great arteries (TGA), and a Rashkind procedure was performed to improve oxygenation. cUS was performed after the Rashkind procedure and showed a large subdural hemorrhage and a neurosurgical procedure was performed to reduce the midline shift.

When the *aEEG* recording was started following the neurosurgical procedure, it showed a status epilepticus on the left side with a DNV pattern on the right side. Three doses of phenobarbital were given (20, 10, 10 mg/kg iv), followed by a loading dose of levetiracetam (20 mg/kg iv), but the SE continued (Figure 5.14A; see also Video 5.14). Lidocaine was given next (Figure 5.14B), and the status epilepticus stopped almost immediately. However, 3½ hrs later, repetitive seizures were seen once again (Figure 5.14C), and midazolam was started. A single seizure is still seen in Figure 5.14D. Also note the difference in background pattern between both hemispheres and the effect of ASM on the recording from the right hemisphere especially. Several short discharges were subsequently seen, coming from the other hemisphere, although they were not so easy to confirm on the raw EEG (Figure 5.14E). In the last figure (Figure 5.14F), no discharges are seen anymore, and there is imminent SWC in the right hemisphere but not on the affected side.

cUS was routinely performed after the Rashkind, and a midline shift was noted. A *CT* scan (Figure 5.14G, a) was performed followed by an emergency craniotomy to drain the subdural hemorrhage and reduce the midline shift. An *MRI* performed 3 days later showed marked reduction of the midline shift (b), but there were bilateral areas of diffusion restriction (c) as well as a large parenchymal injury in the left occipital lobe (T2, b). Care was redirected.

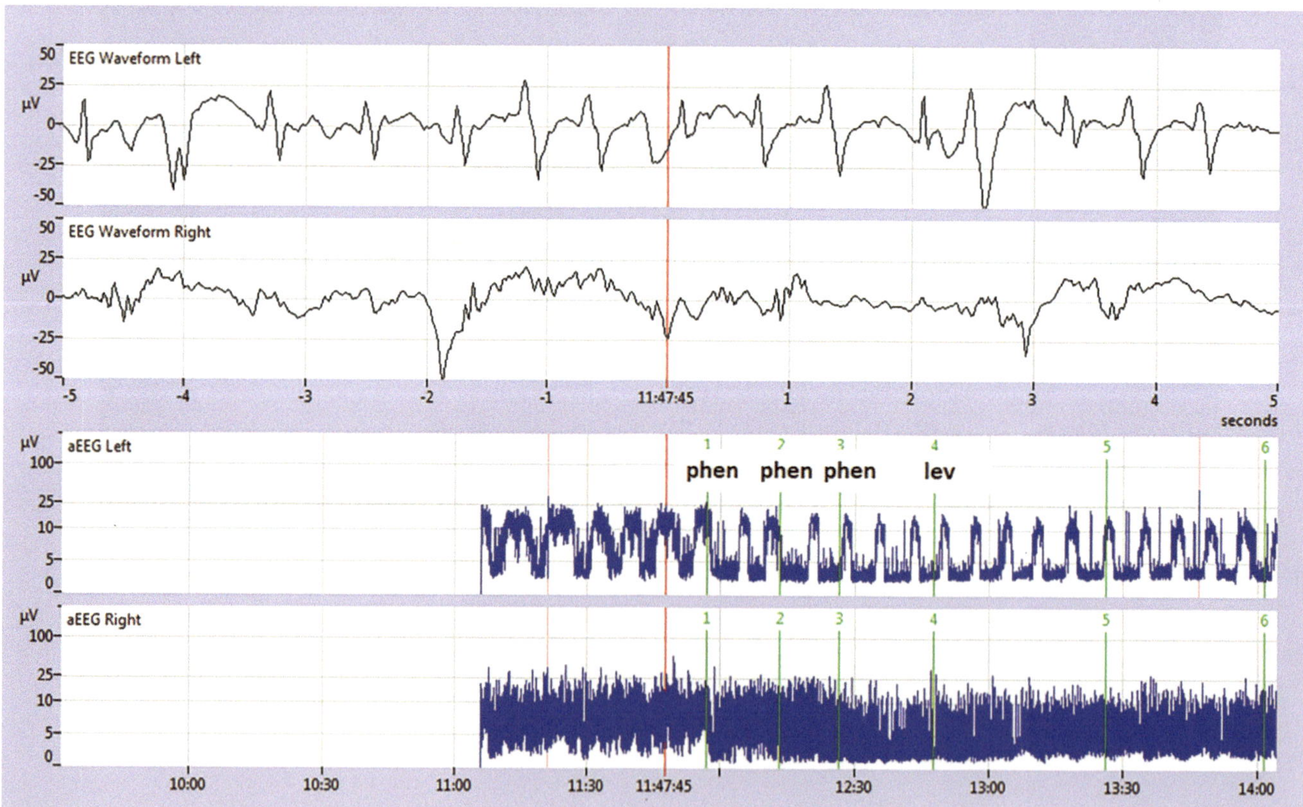

FIGURE 5.14A

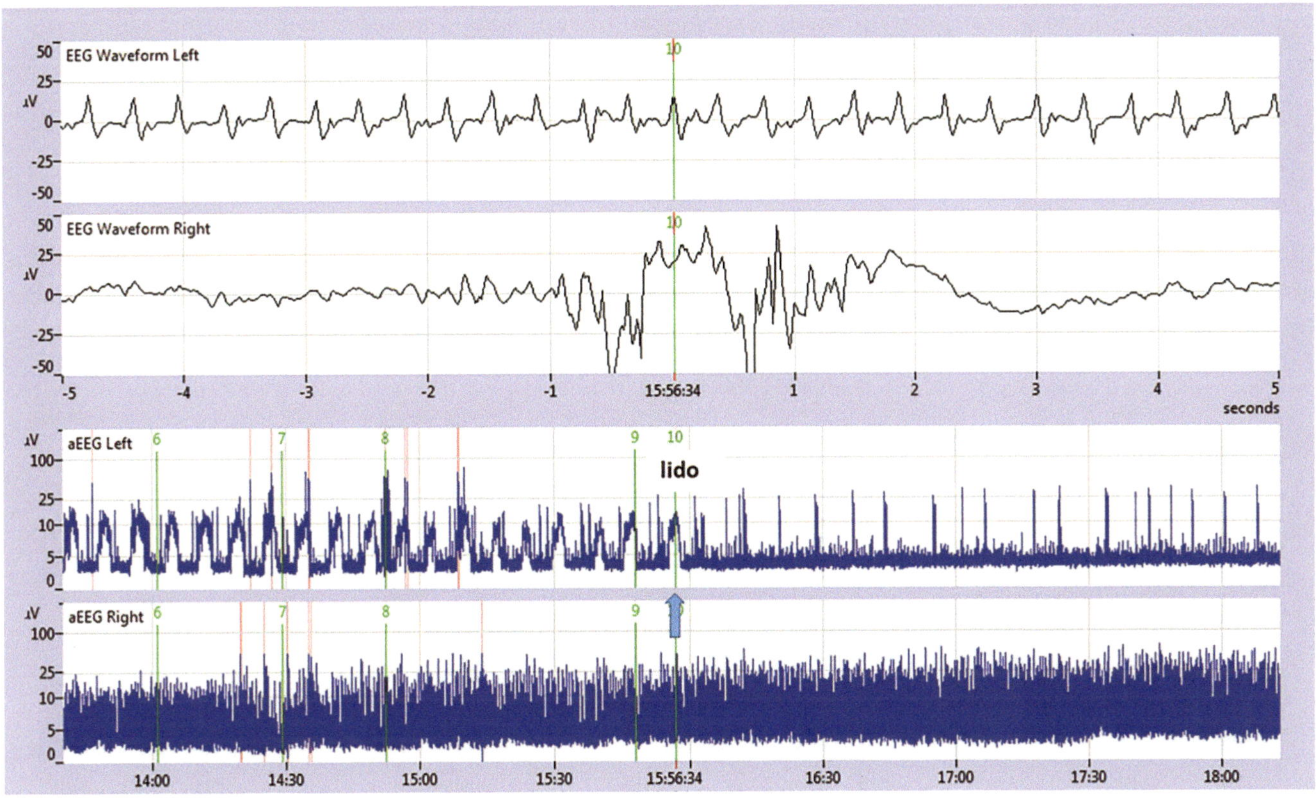

FIGURE 5.14B

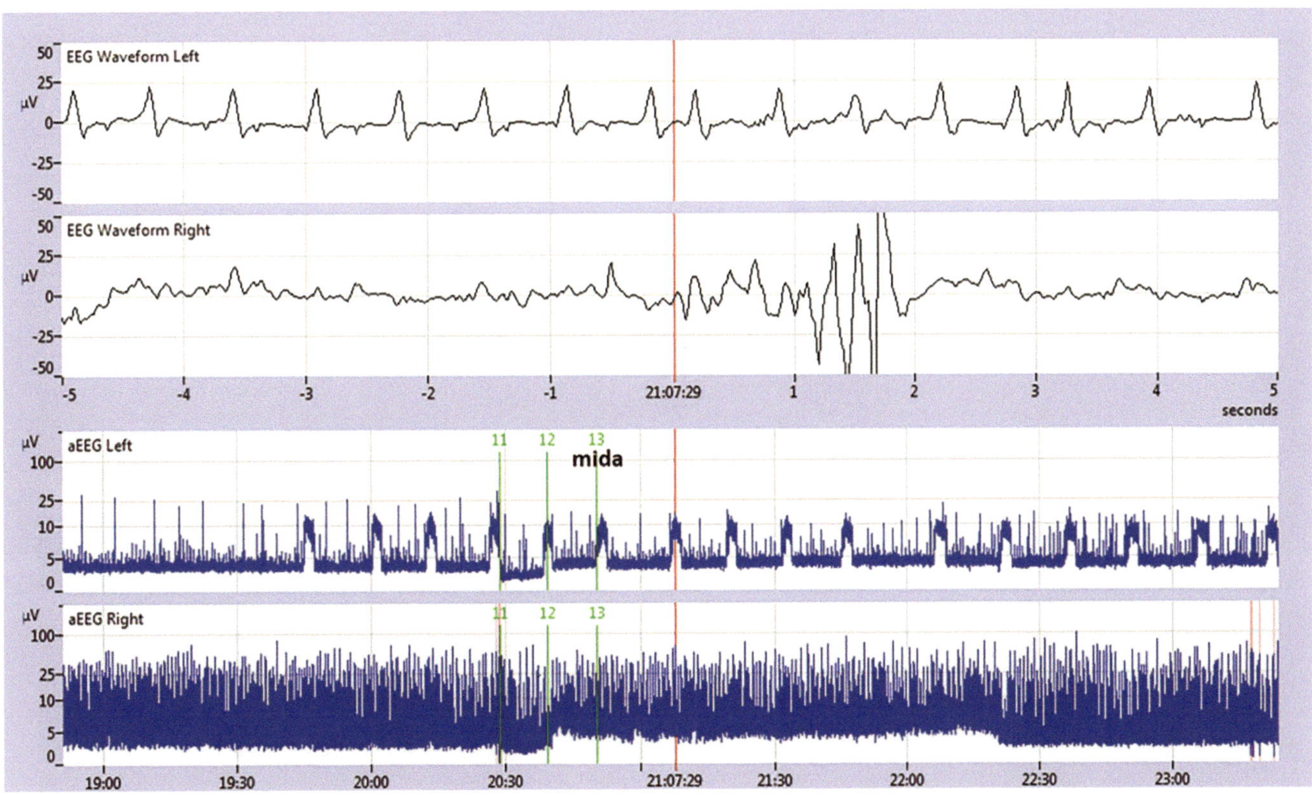

FIGURE 5.14C

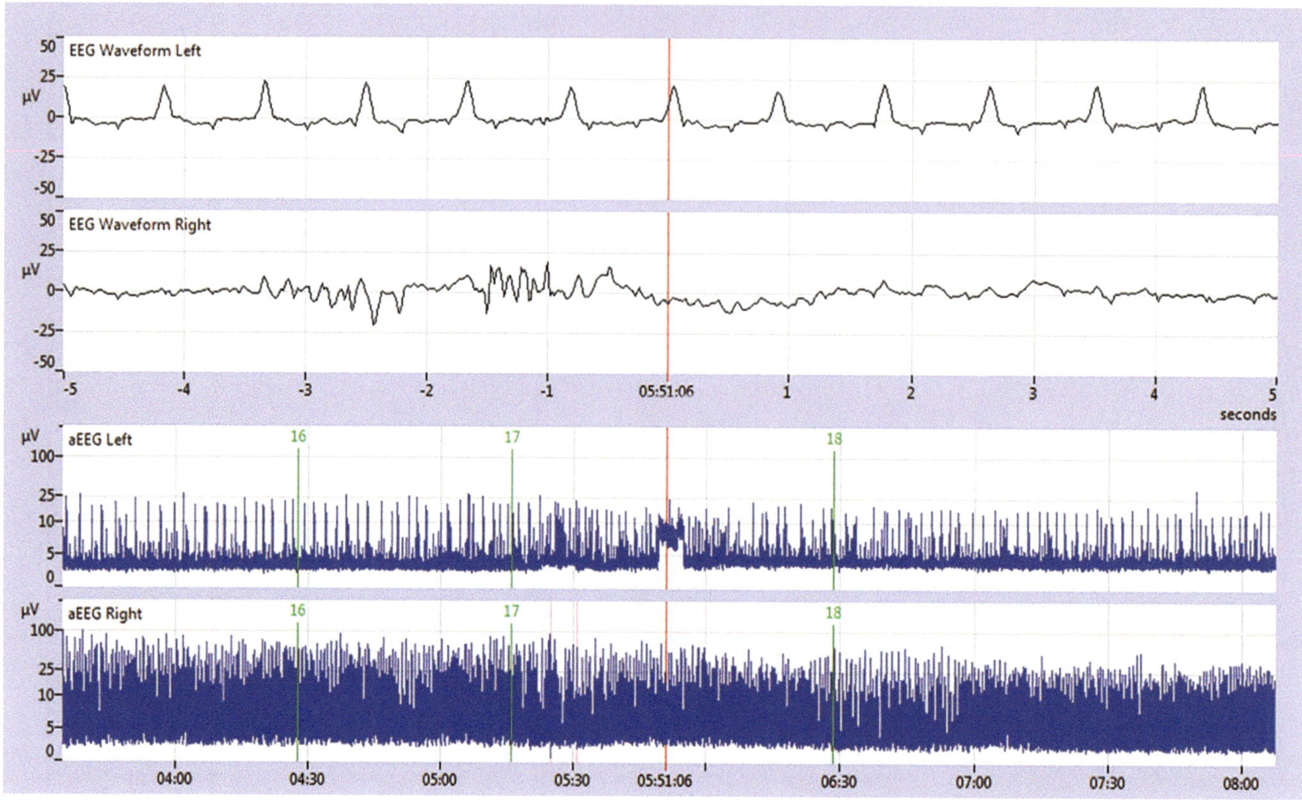

FIGURE 5.14D

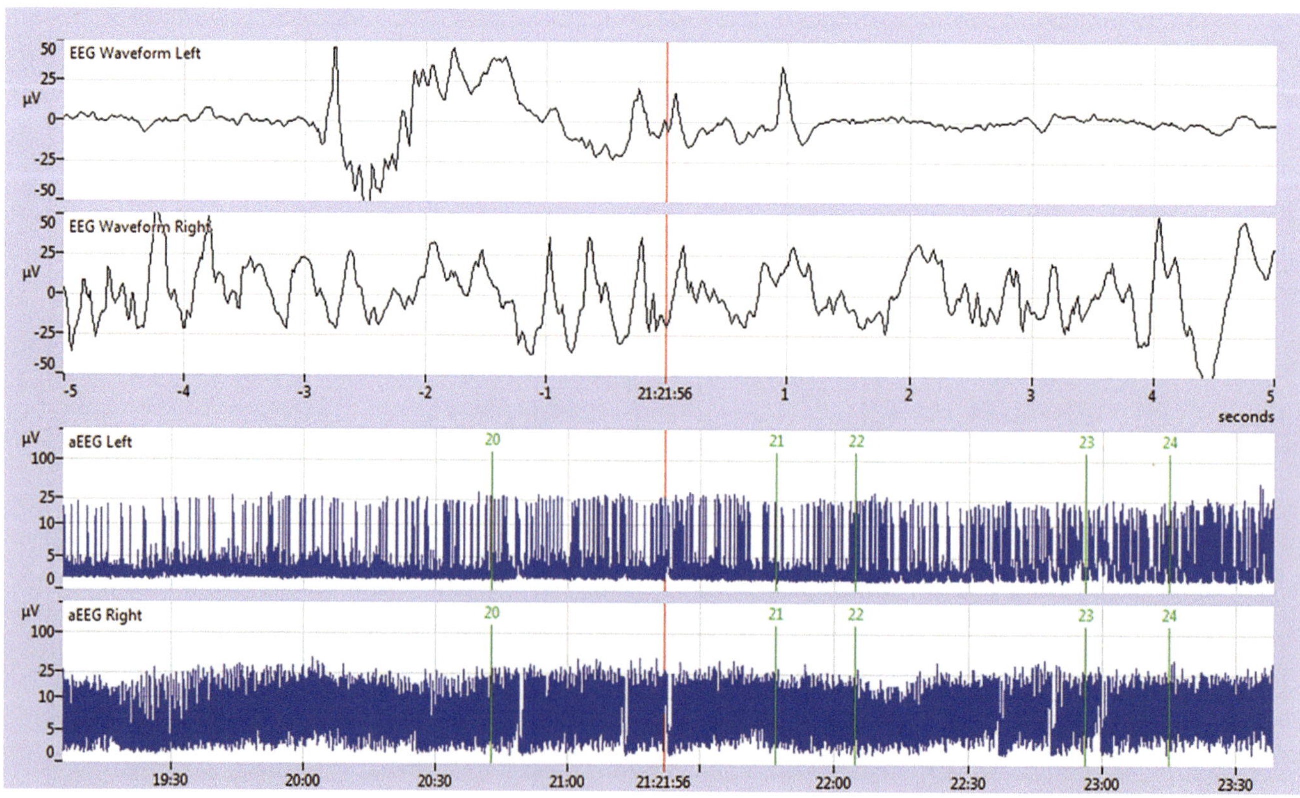

FIGURE 5.14E

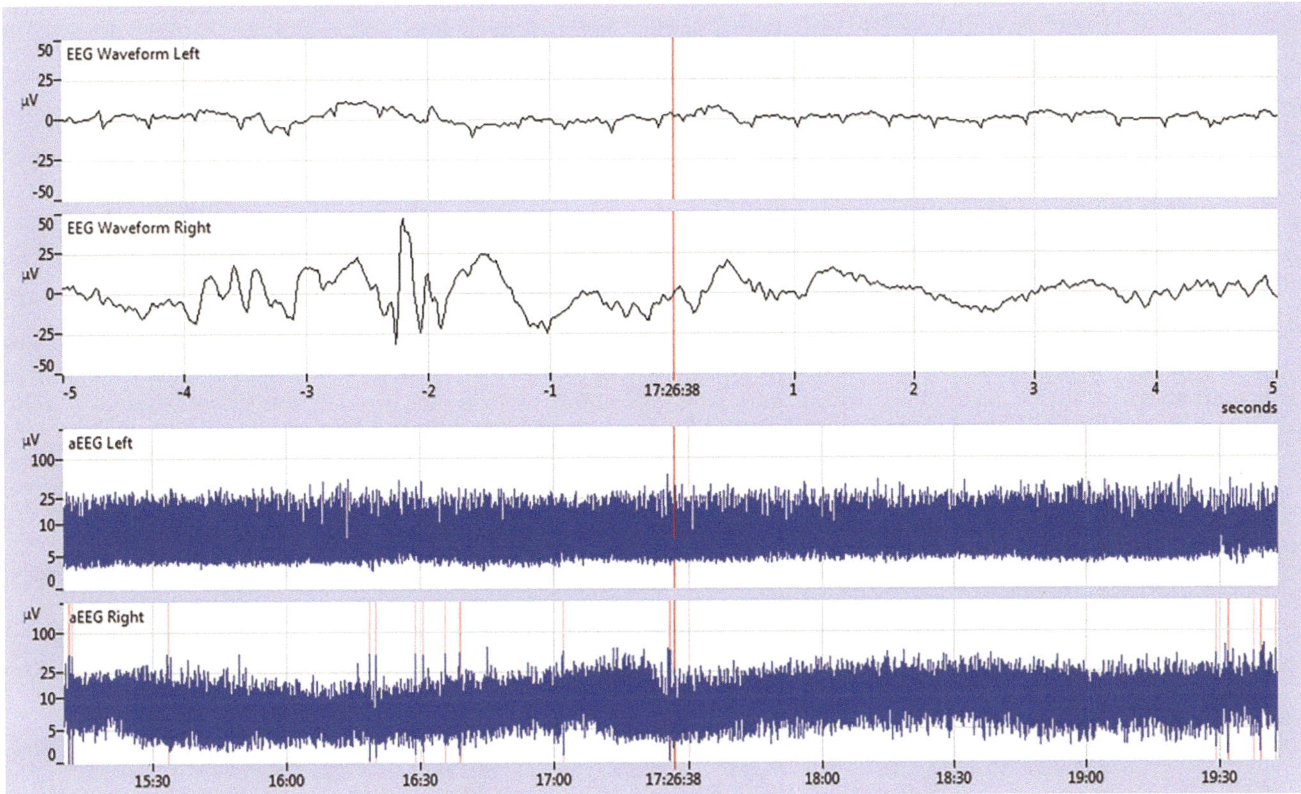

FIGURE 5.14F

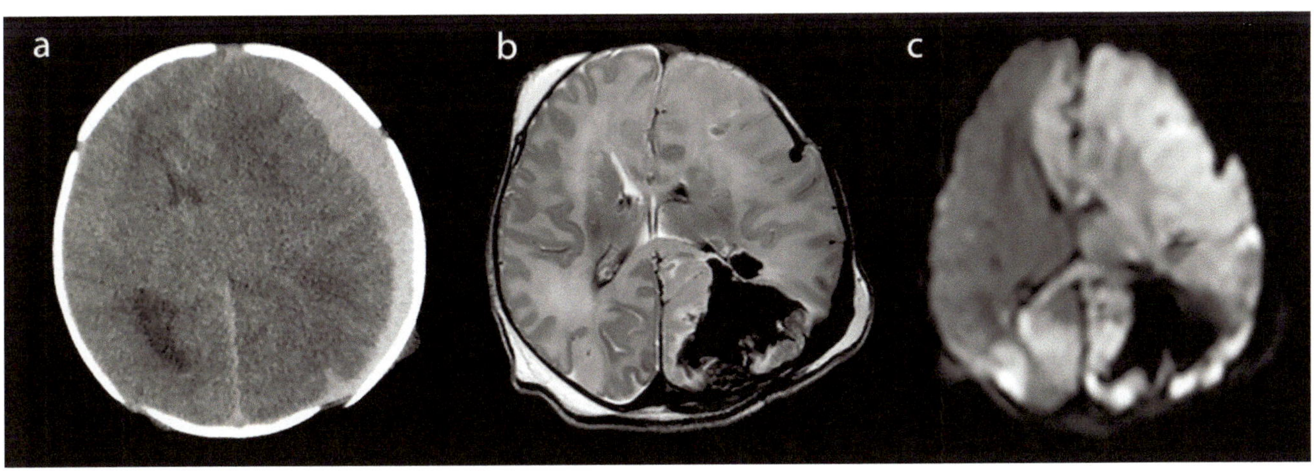

FIGURE 5.14G

Case 5.15 Full-Term Infant with Cortical Stroke

This term infant was born after an uneventful vaginal delivery and was doing well at home. The infant was admitted on day 11 with clonic movements of the left hand and arm. CPAP was required for insufficient respiration after a loading dose of phenobarbital (40 mg/kg iv in two doses). Bacterial and viral cultures were all negative. A cardiac echo did not show any abnormalities, except for a persisting foramen ovale.

The *aEEG* showed repetitive seizures originating in the right hemisphere, lasting up to 9 minutes at the arrow. Two additional doses of phenobarbital were given, each 10 mg/kg iv. There is asymmetry in background activity, and several periods of quiet sleep are seen (Figure 5.15A). Another very long seizure is seen in Figure 5.15B and Video 5.15, and the SWC present before this seizure is interrupted for several hours. No other anti-seizure medication (ASM) was given. In Figure 5.15C a very long seizure of 45 minutes is seen. Levetiracetam (20 mg/kg iv) was given during this seizure.

The Figure 5.15D shows the standard EEG. The SWC is recovering, and no further seizures occurred.

An *MRI* was performed 3 days after admission (Figure 5.15E) and showed a cortical branch MCA infarct, clearly seen on the T2 sequence (a) and DWI (b). Motor and cognitive scores were well within the normal range when seen at 2 years of age, with a composite cognitive score of 105 and combined motor score of 127. It remained unclear why this stroke developed at the end of the second week.

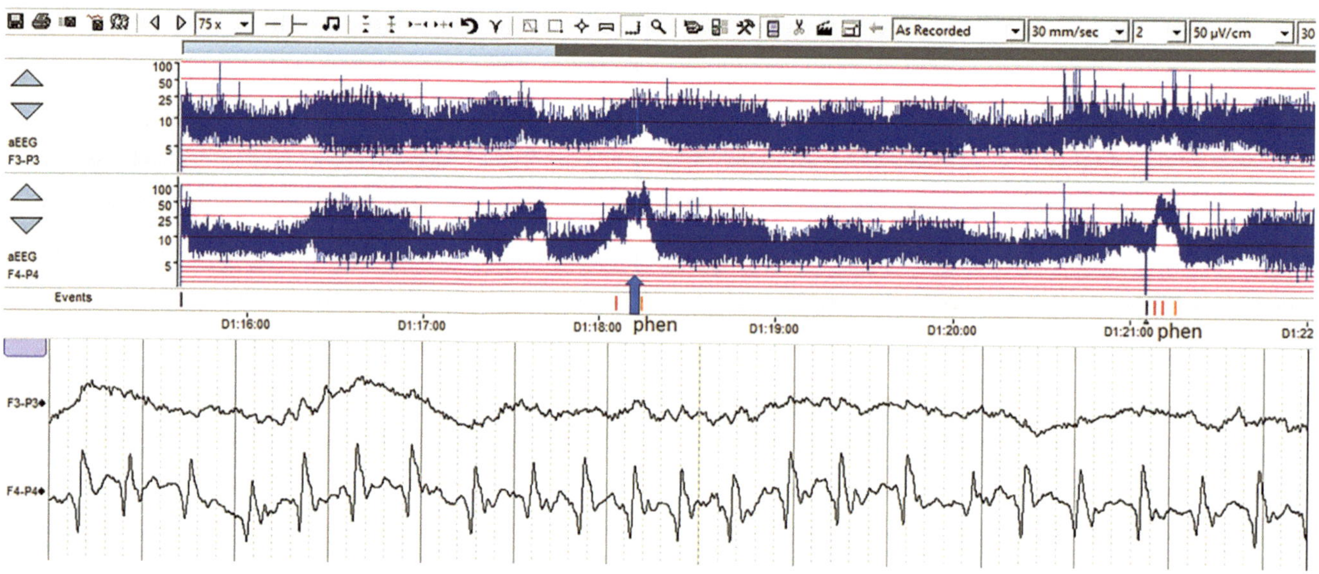

FIGURE 5.15A

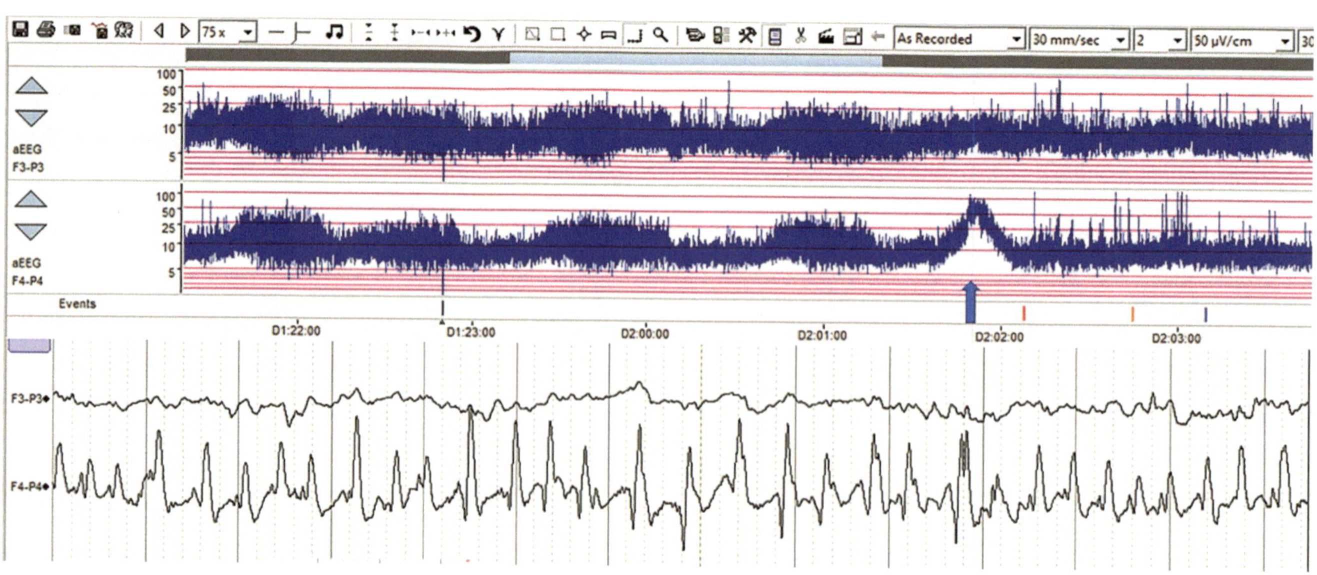

FIGURE 5.15B

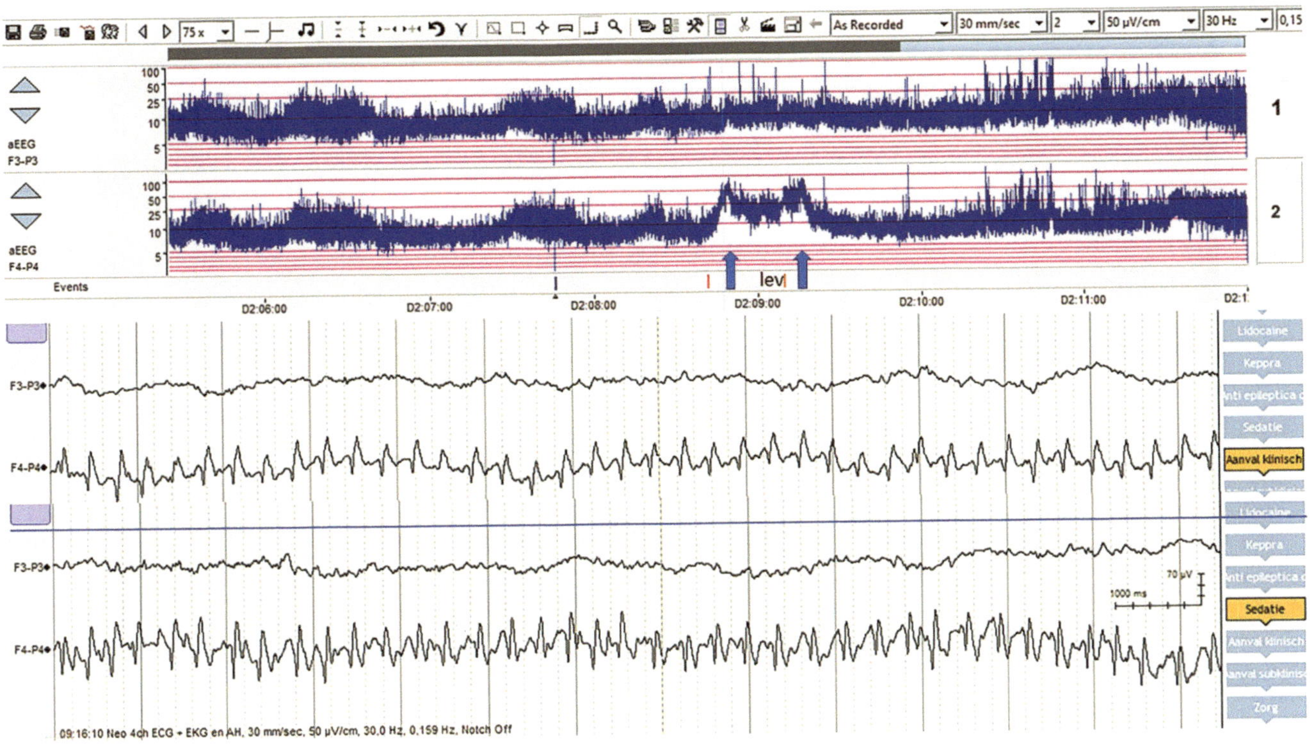

FIGURE 5.15C

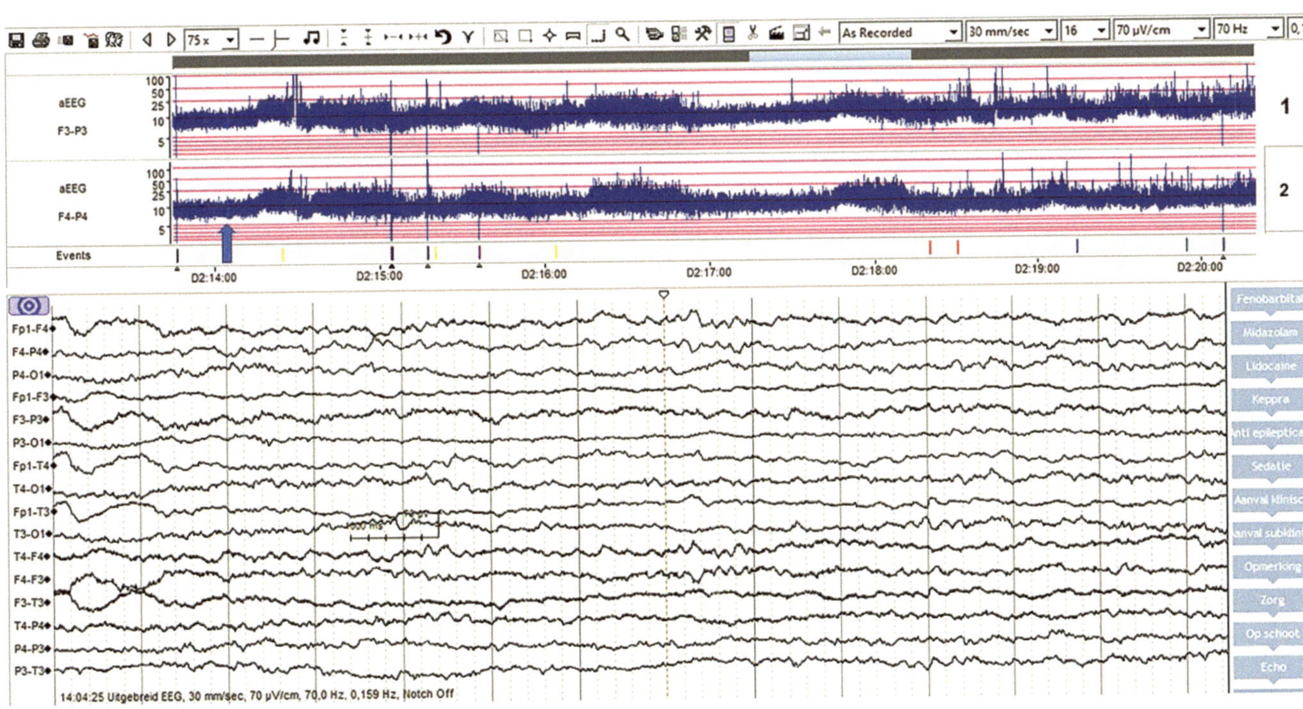

FIGURE 5.15D

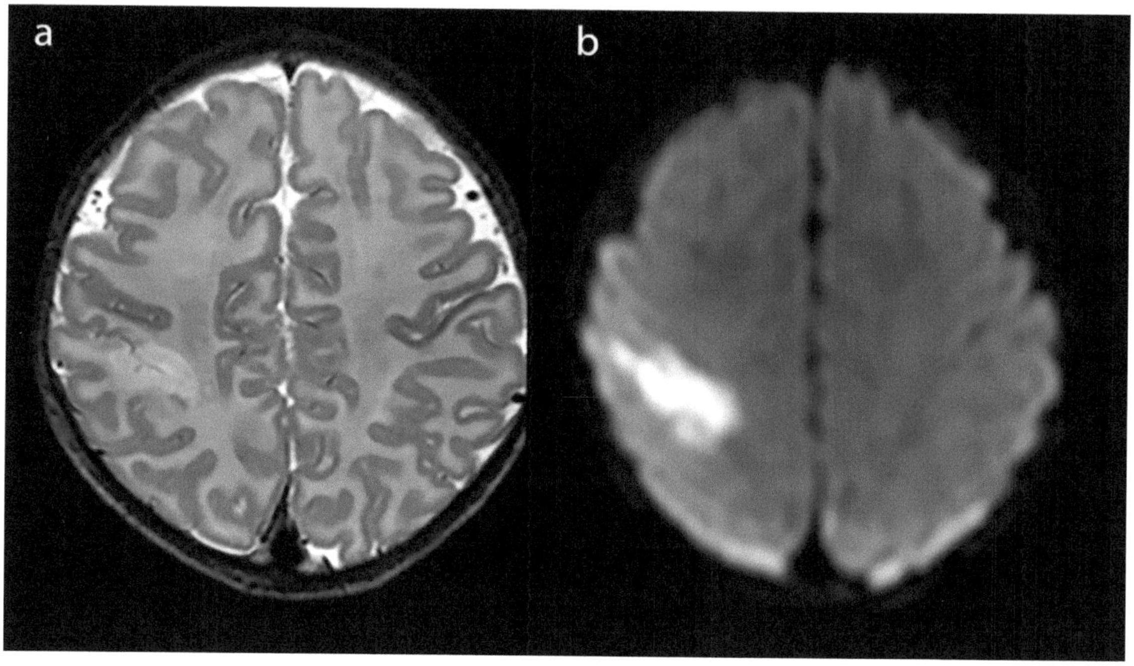

FIGURE 5.15E

Case 5.16 Full-Term Infant with Posterior Branch MCA

Term infant, born at 38 weeks' gestation, with a birthweight of 2510 grams. Confirmed feto-maternal transfusion with positive Kleihauer, requiring transfusion in the delivery room. Arterial umbilical pH was 7.27. Apgar scores were 1, 4 and 8 at 1 and 10 minutes, respectively. Transferred for respiratory problems. Thompson score was 7 on admission, but arrival was too late for hypothermia.

The *aEEG* showed ictal discharges almost immediately after starting the recording (Figure 5.16A) on a CNV pattern. Phenobarbital (20 mg/kg iv) was administered, and the background pattern changed to DNV. More discharges were seen, and a second dose of phenobarbital was given (10 mg/kg iv).

As seizures continued, midazolam was given (Figure 5.16B). This resulted in a further depression of the background activity (BS), but low-voltage seizures were still seen, and levetiracetam (20 m/kg iv) was given (Figure 5.16B). The seizures, however, evolved into a status epilepticus, and another dose of levetiracetam (20 mg/kg iv) was given. The status was stopped following administration of lidocaine (Figure 5.16C). At 48 hrs, a standard EEG was also performed showing a predominant BS pattern (Figure 5.16D). Recovery to a DNV and CNV pattern is seen at 60 hours of age (Figure 5.16E).

An *MRI* (Figure 5.16F, a, b) was performed on day 6 and showed increased signal intensity on T2-weighted sequence in the right posterior occipital lobe.

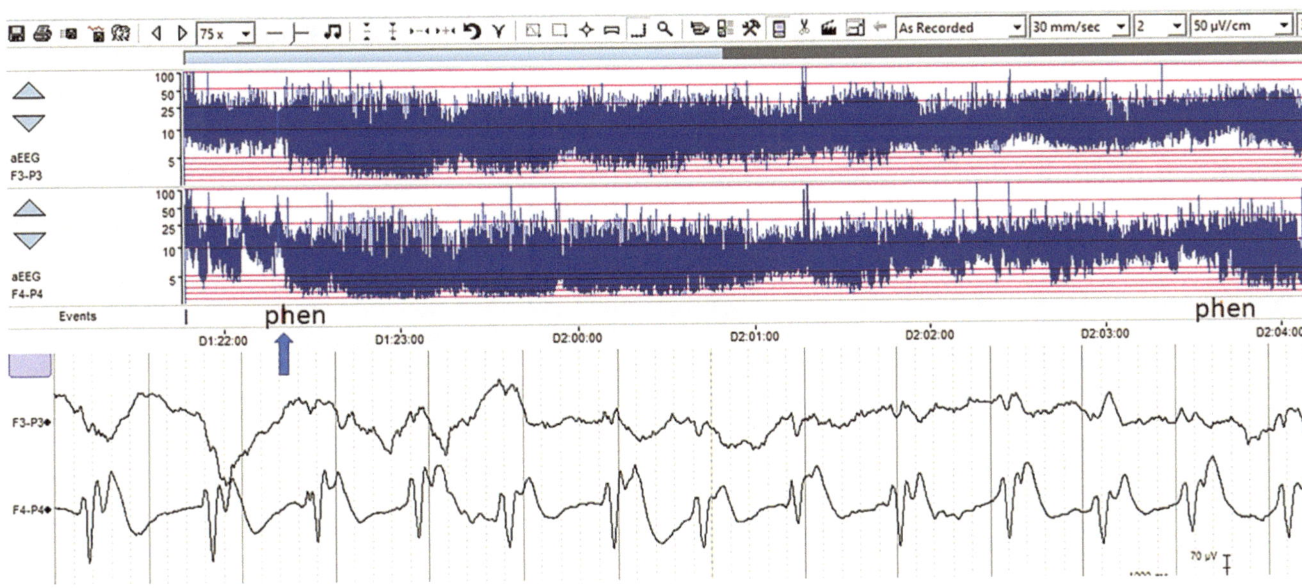

FIGURE 5.16A

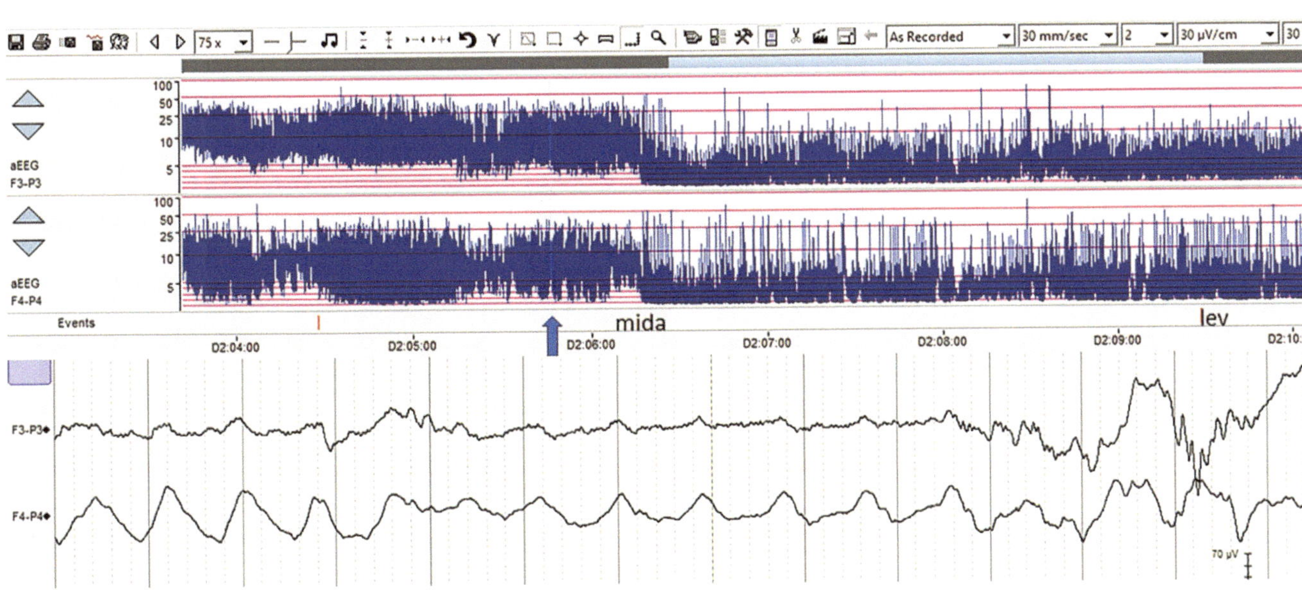

FIGURE 5.16B

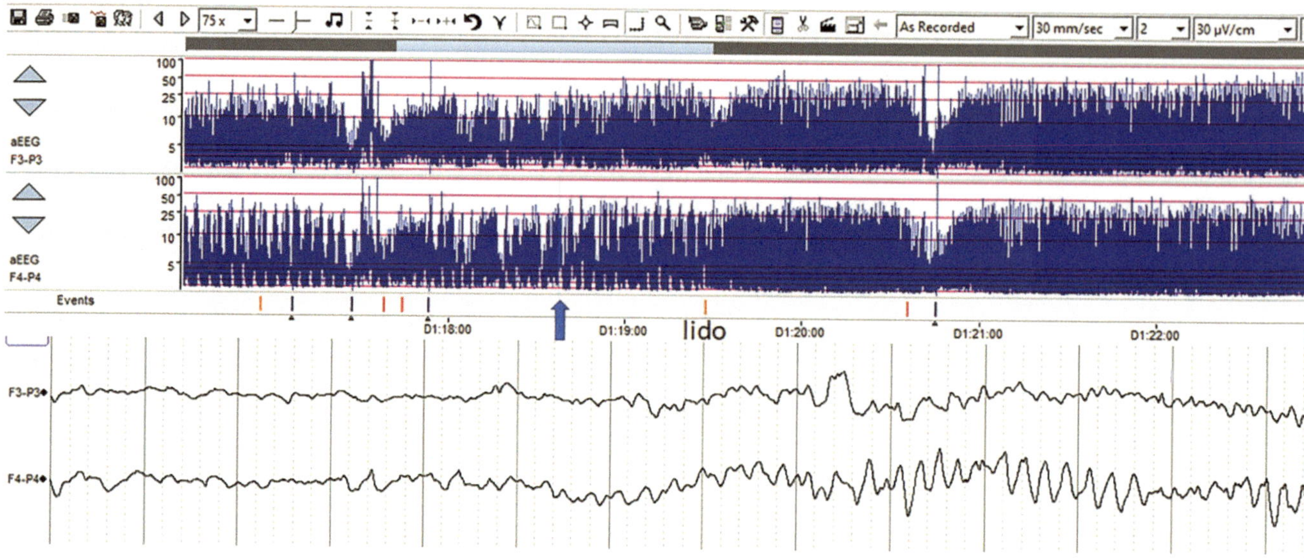

FIGURE 5.16C

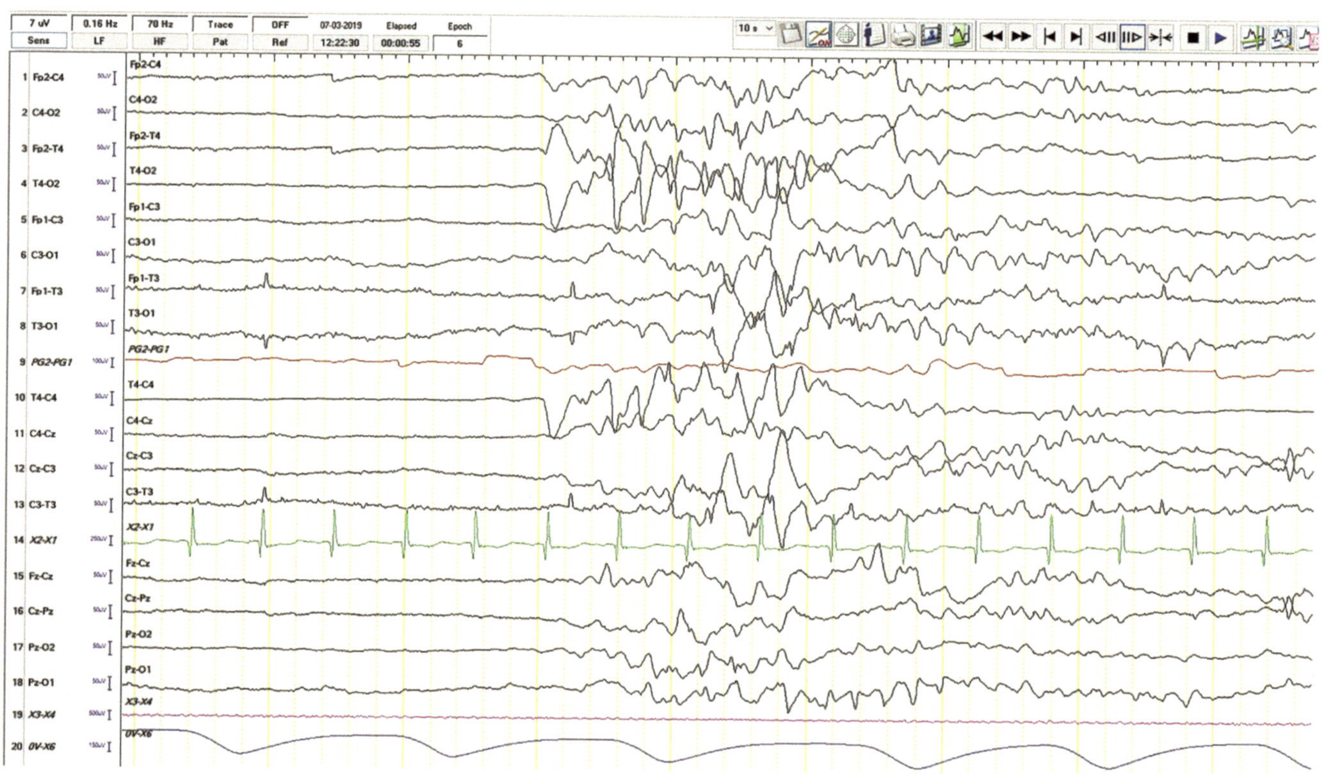

FIGURE 5.16D (Courtesy Selma Tromp, Department of Neurology, Leiden University Medical Center.)

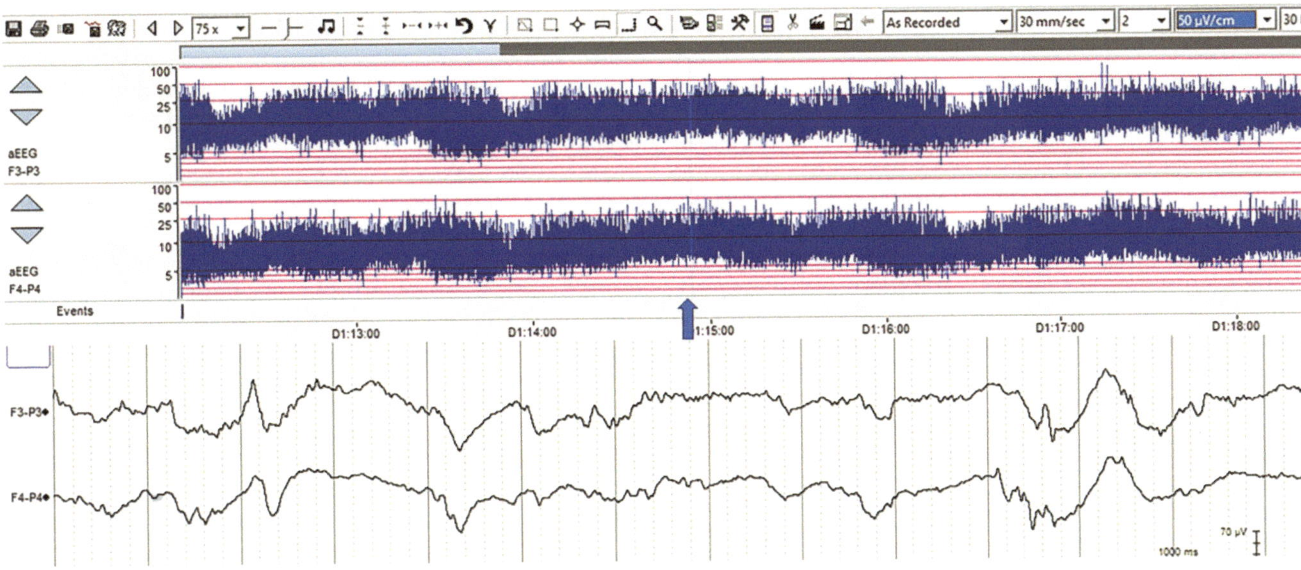

FIGURE 5.16E

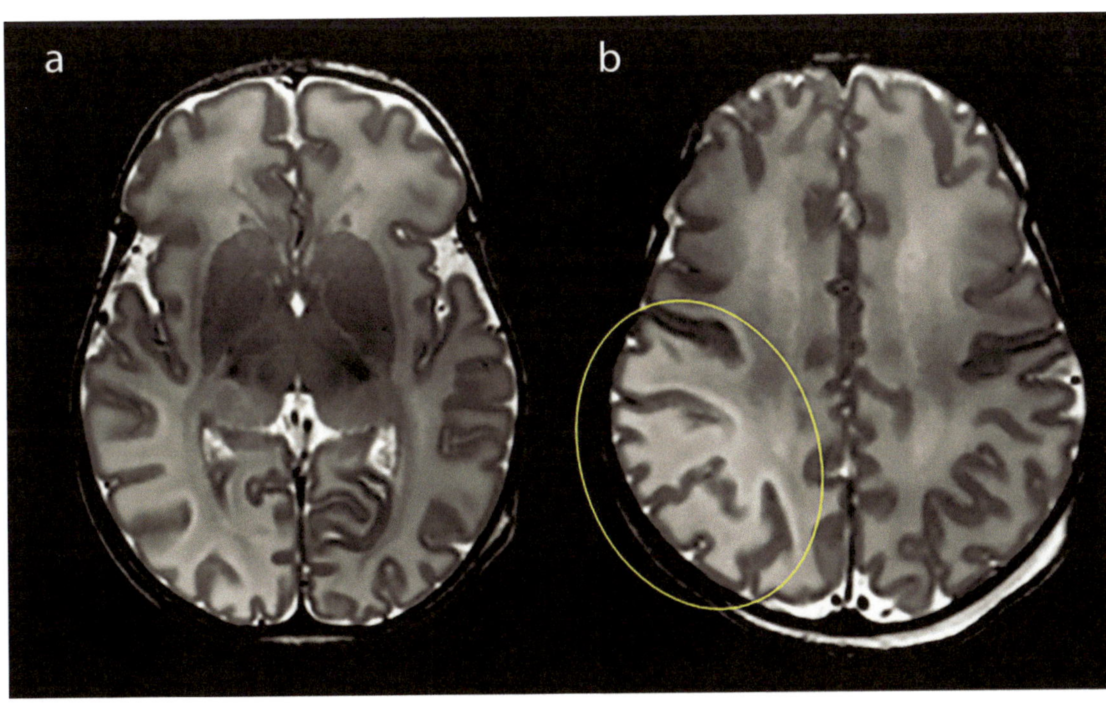

FIGURE 5.16F

Case 5.17 Full-Term Infant with MCA Stroke

This infant was born at 39 weeks' gestation by repeat caesarean section. Apgar scores were 8 and 8 at 1 and 5 minutes, respectively. The infant required CPAP for 10 min for respiratory distress and decreased O_2 saturation. The infant was observed in the triage for 2 hours, then admitted to the term nursery. At about 26 hours after birth and during routine nursery care, the infant was noted to have clonic jerks of the right leg and possible arm shaking. There was immediate transfer to the NICU, where another episode was noted with bilateral clonic jerks of the lower limbs but more on the right than left.

An *aEEG* was started, seizures, most prominent in the left hemisphere, were noted, and phenobarbital (20 mg/kg iv) was administered (not shown). As the seizures continued, another dose of phenobarbital (10 mg/kg iv) was given (Figure 5.17A), but repetitive seizures continued to occur. Some of the seizures are also recognized on the recording from the right hemisphere. The background pattern between the discharges is CNV with SWC noted on the less affected side. A loading dose of fosphenytoin (20 mg/kg iv) was given 4 hours later (Figure 5.17B), as the discharges were still not controlled. Soon after, no discharges were seen any more, and there is a CNV pattern with SWC on both sides.

An *MRI* (Figure 5.17C) was obtained the next day and showed a left-sided MCA stroke, clearly seen as high signal with loss of the cortical ribbon on the T2 sequence (a) and restricted diffusion (b).

It is of interest that this perinatal arterial ischemic stroke occurred following an elective caesarean section. It is also of interest that the background activity was not worse on the affected side and that SWC was noted on both sides immediately after the seizures were controlled. This case also shows that there is not always a negative effect of ASM on background activity and SWC.

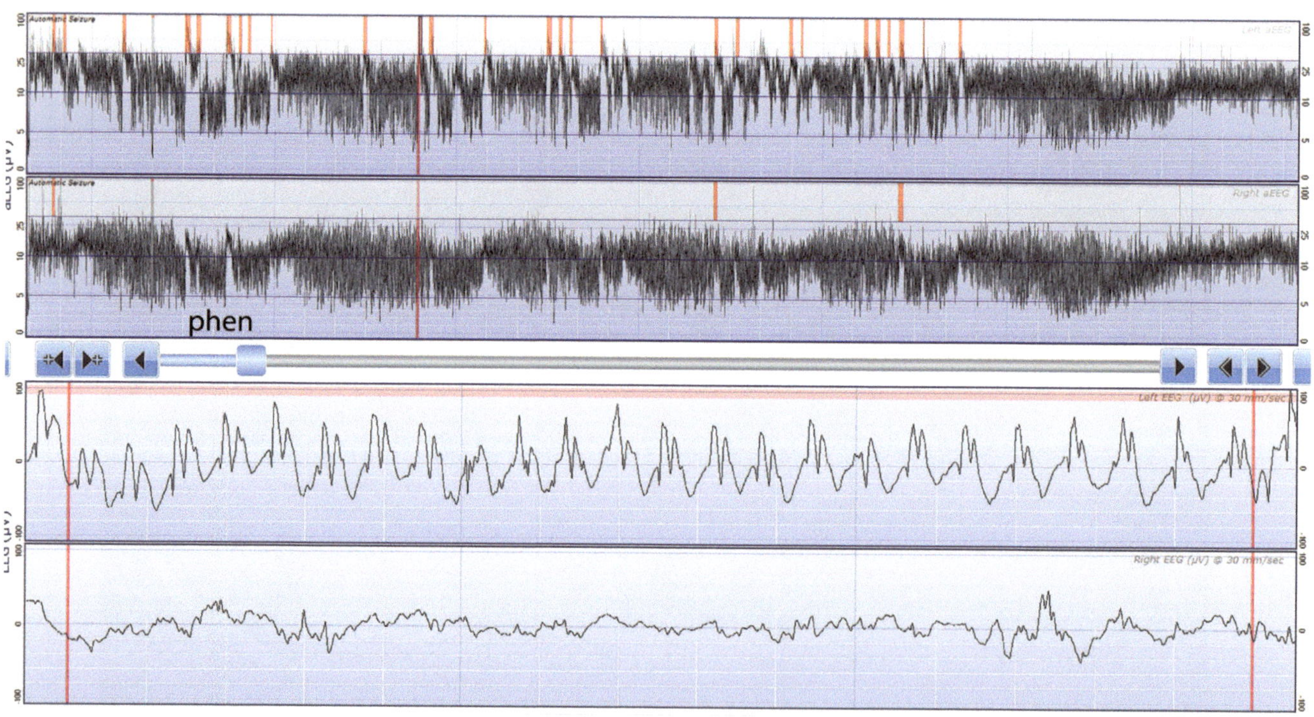

FIGURE 5.17A

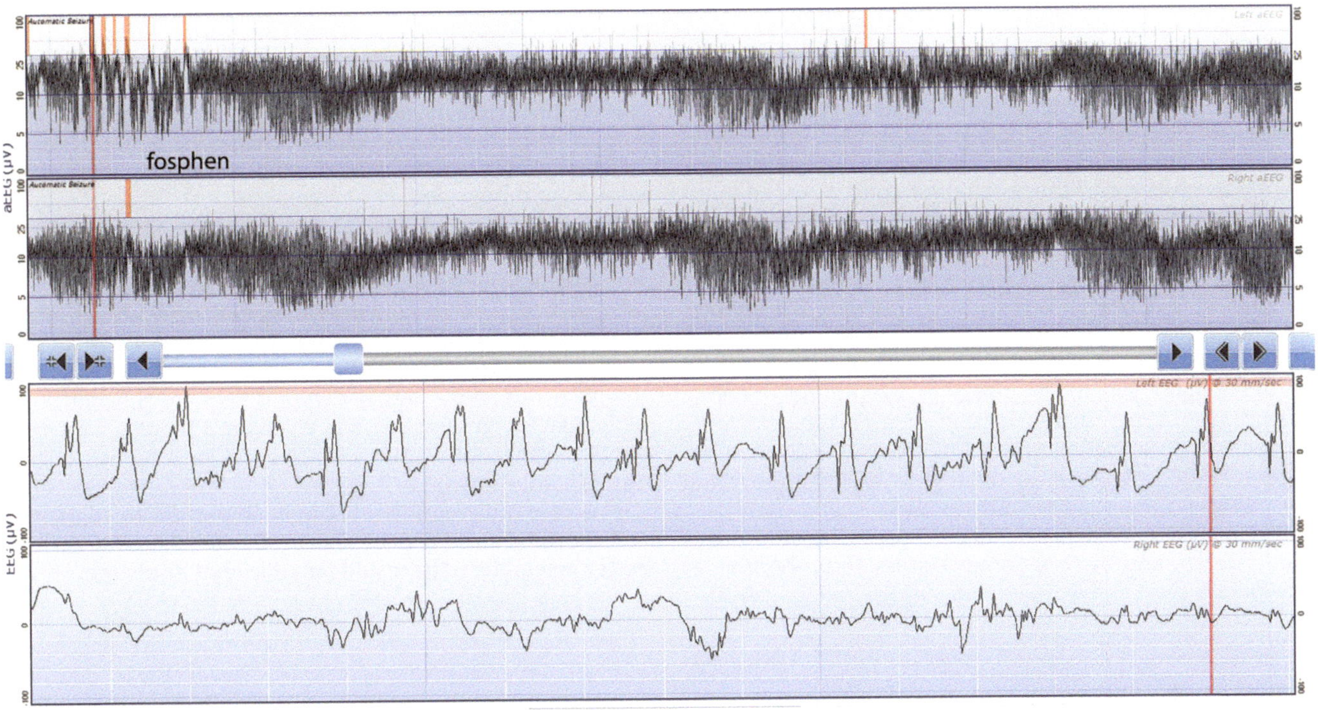

FIGURE 5.17B

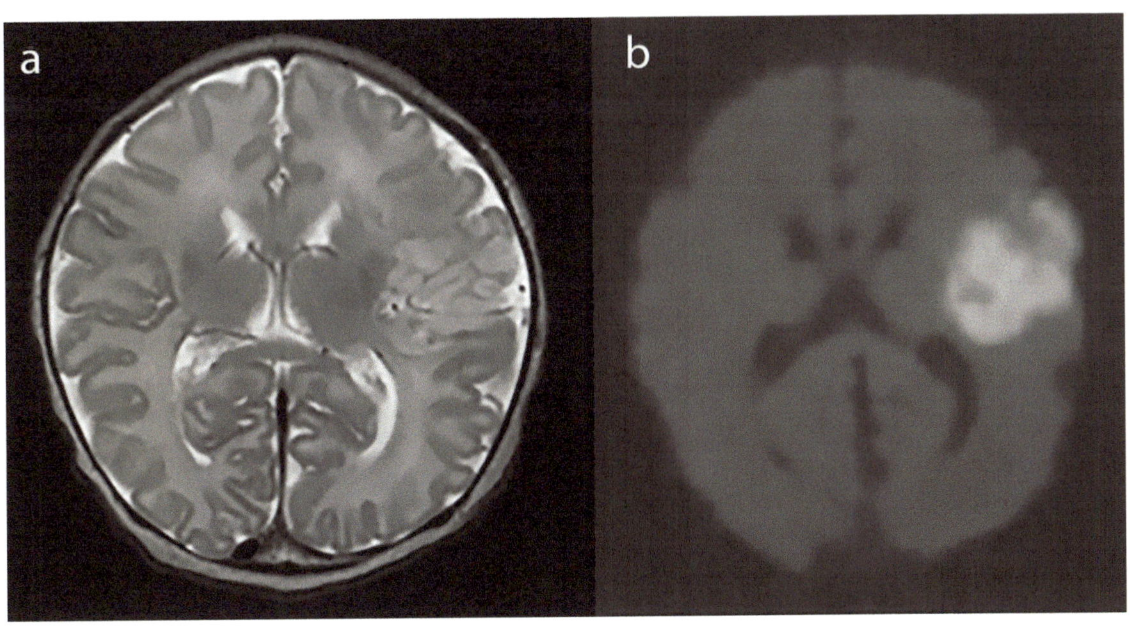

FIGURE 5.17C

Case 5.18 Full-Term Infant with Cerebral Sinovenous Thrombosis

This infant was born at 41 weeks' gestation with a birthweight of 4050 grams. Membranes had been ruptured for 48 hours. Delivery was by ventouse extraction. Apgar scores were 9, 10 and 10 at 1, 5 and 10 minutes, respectively. The infant was observed in the hospital for concern for an infection and was discharged home the next day. Clonic jerks were noted in the right leg and arm on day 3 on four occasions, the infant was readmitted, a septic workup was done, and antibiotics as well as acyclovir was started. Blood and CSF cultures were negative.

aEEG was started and immediately showed three short seizures (Figure 5.18A; see also Video 5.18) and one long seizure. The upper margin of the long seizure can only be seen after adjusting the scale from 100 to 200 µV (Figure 5.18B). After a loading dose of phenobarbital (20 mg/kg iv), no further seizures were seen. There is a small difference in the background activity before ASM is administered, and there is some depression on both sides following administration of phenobarbital. In Figure 5.18C, taken only 6 hours after admission, established SWC is present, especially in the second part of the panel. There is still a slight difference in bandwidth, especially outside the periods of quiet sleep.

An *MRI* (Figure 5.18D) was performed the next day showing diffusion restriction in the distribution of the medullary veins, as well as the CC and thalamus in the left hemisphere (a). Susceptibility weighted imaging (SWI) (b) shows small hemorrhages in the medullary vein network. Magnetic resonance venography (MRV) (c) showed occlusion of the straight sinus and internal cerebral vein on the left. Low molecular weight heparin was given for 3 months, and only partial recanalization of the sinuses was seen on the follow-up MRI (not shown).

This case illustrates that it can be important to adjust the scale of the recording to be able to see the upper margin and better assess the pattern and possible ictal discharge.

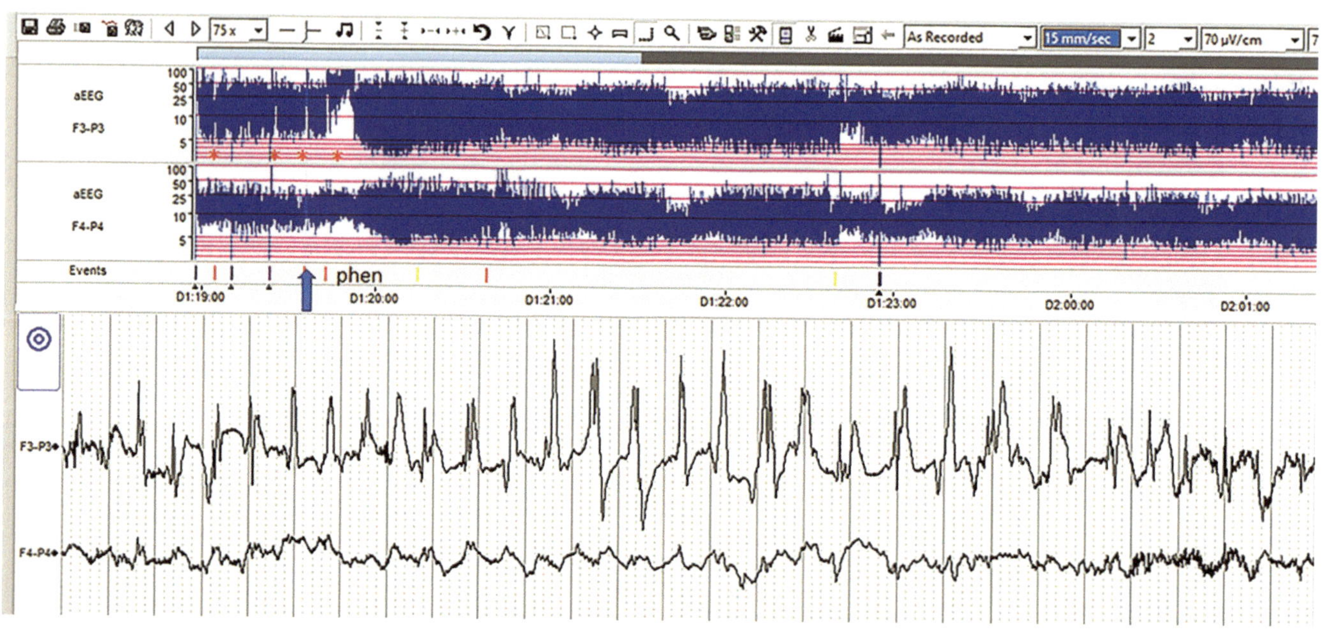

FIGURE 5.18A

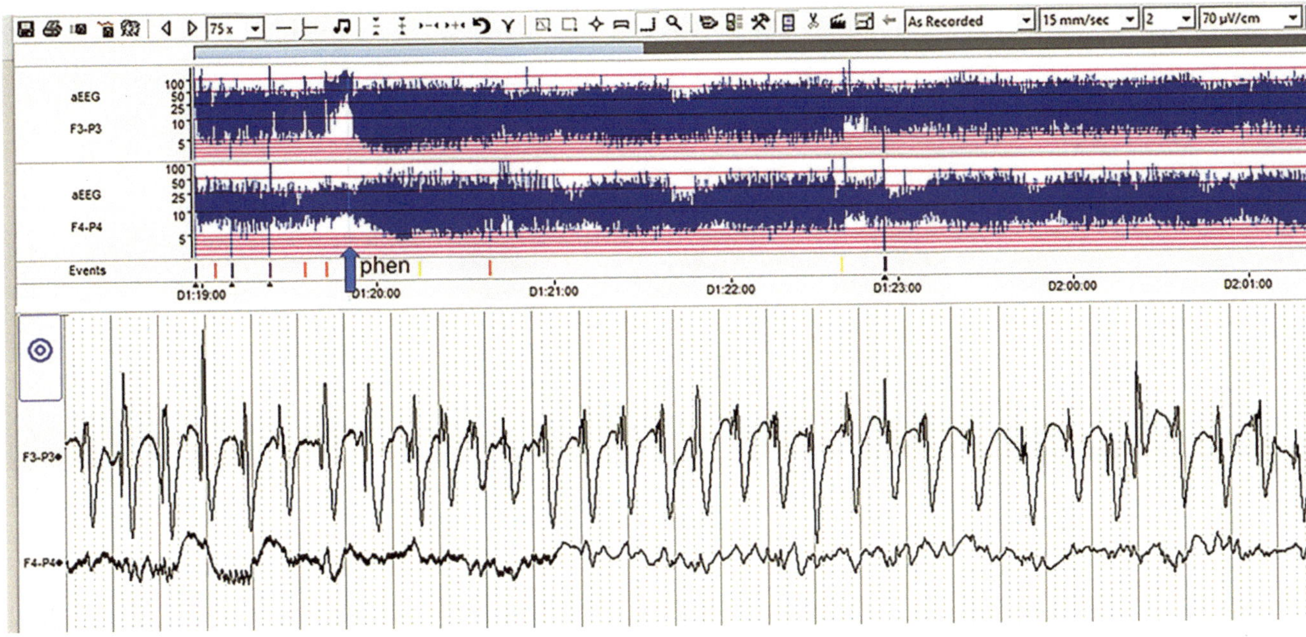

FIGURE 5.18B

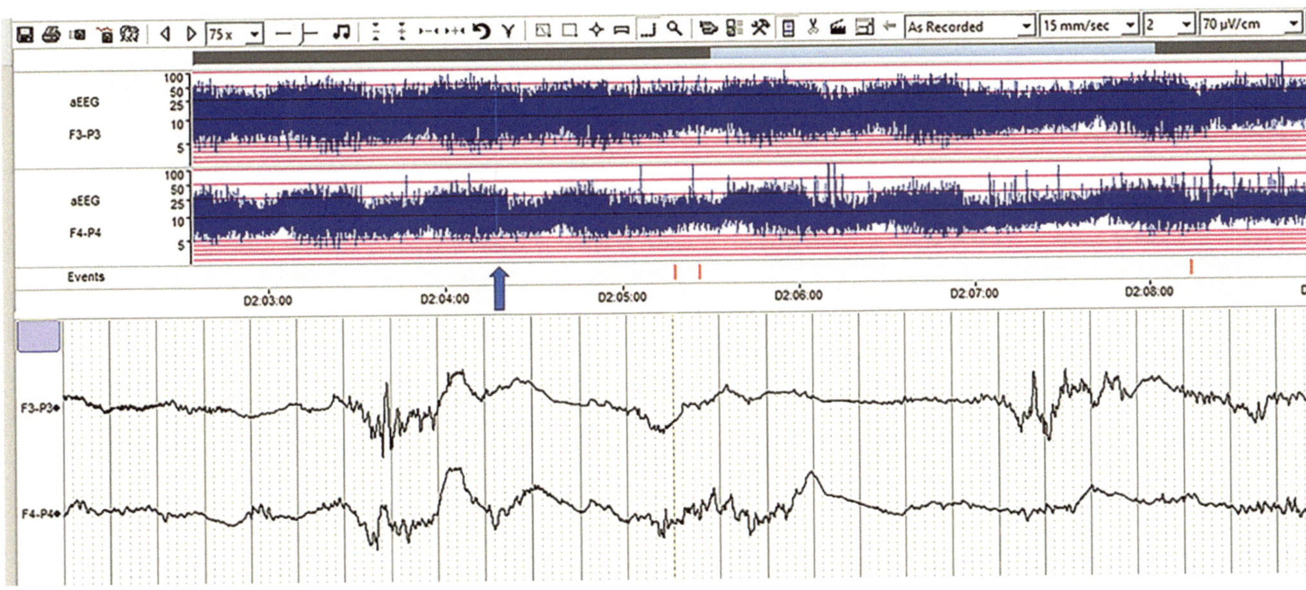

FIGURE 5.18C

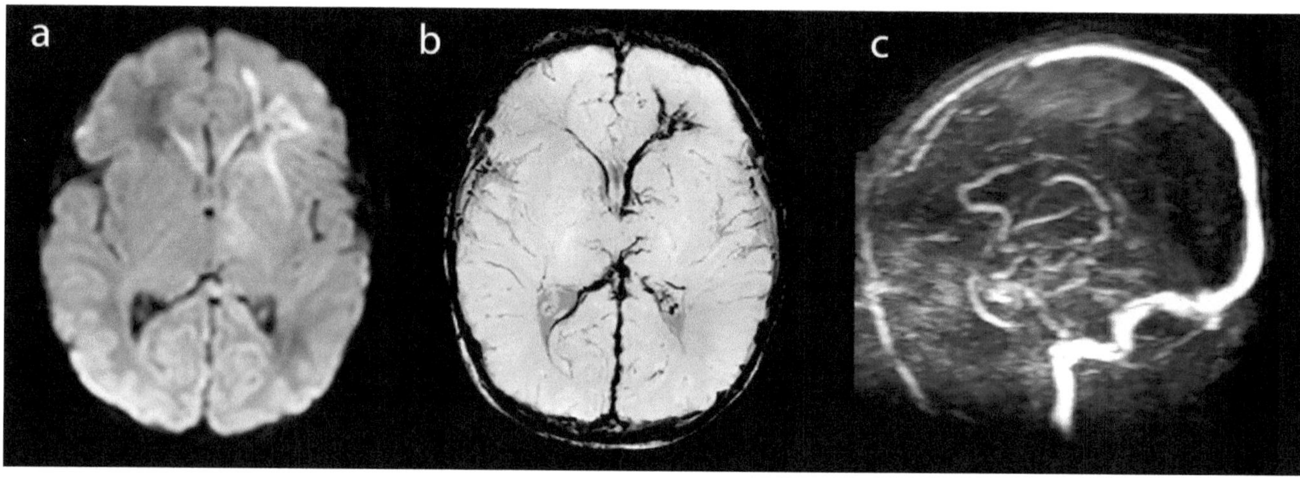

FIGURE 5.18D

6 NEONATAL ENCEPHALOPATHY DUE TO INFECTIONS, METABOLIC DISORDERS AND GENETIC CAUSES

Linda S de Vries and Sonia L Bonifacio

SUMMARY

- Most aEEG/EEG changes due to metabolic diseases, CNS infections or malformations are non-specific.
- The most common aEEG findings include overall background depression, lack of sleep-wake cycling and the presence of seizures.
- A burst-suppression background pattern is often present in non-ketotic hyperglycinemia.
- Channelopathies present with a typical aEEG pattern and a sodium channel blocker should be tried following recognition.
- A standard EEG should be recorded early in all infants with cerebral symptoms due to metabolic disturbances, including hypoglycemia, infections and cerebral malformations.

Neonatal encephalopathy (NE) is seen in a variety of disorders where newborns present with an altered level of consciousness, seizures, poor tone and inability to initiate or maintain sufficient respiration. The use of aEEG monitoring has been reported to be useful in these infants to assess the background activity as well the presence of seizures. A selection of aEEG examples with corresponding EEG traces from newborn infants with various causes of NE are provided. Infections and hypoglycemia are common in newborn infants, while metabolic diseases and cerebral malformations are rare. Most EEG changes in these conditions are non-specific and include acute stage background abnormalities such as electrocortical background depression and seizures. Bedside EEG measures in infants with NE are related to the severity of brain injury seen on a neonatal MRI. A minimum amplitude of < 4 μV appears useful in predicting outcome.

The aEEG examples in this chapter cannot cover all rare conditions but show how the aEEG can be used to give continuous information on brain function and its evolution during the clinical course in these infants.

6.1 Hypoglycemia

Hypoglycemia is probably the most common metabolic cause of acute cerebral dysfunction in newborn infants. Very little is known about evolution of EEG changes during hypoglycemic episodes in newborns, but adult studies indicate an increase in slow EEG activity that is not seen in the aEEG trend. Mild hypoglycemia may link to changes seen in the aEEG trends, while more severe hypoglycemia will lead to general cerebral depression and/or seizures, with accompanying depression in the aEEG background patterns (see Chapter 2). Severe hyperglycemia may also cause worsening of aEEG background scores, reduced sleep-wake cycling and even electrographic seizures.

6.2 Metabolic Diseases

Changes in cortical activity due to metabolic problems are unspecific, and they relate to the overall level of cerebral depression or likelihood of seizures: Hyperammonemia and organic/amino acidopathies often show marked electrocortical background depression with seizure activity. Peroxisomal disorders do not show major background abnormalities, but seizures can be seen. Molybdenum cofactor deficiency and sulphite oxidase deficiency may cause hard-to-treat seizures on a depressed aEEG background from the first hours of life. Non-ketotic hyperglycinemia is often characterized by a burst-suppression pattern, which, however, is a common finding with severe encephalopathies. Pyridoxine dependent seizures are quite rare, but the incidence is probably underestimated. aEEG activity may show a sudden change in background activity, with a sudden control of seizures. Seizures occurring in lethal hypophosphatasia are also vitamin B6 dependent.

6.3 Hyperbilirubinaemia

High bilirubin levels may affect the aEEG, mainly with increased slow activity. It has been reported that there is no direct effect of a high bilirubin level on the electrocortical activity but rather, a delayed effect seen in the second week after birth as also with a delayed onset of SWC. The predictive value of aEEG findings was not as good as that of the auditory brainstem responses (ABR). Very high bilirubin levels may be associated with seizures that are detected in the temporal and/or occipital lobe which can be missed using a typical aEEG montage (see Chapter 3).

6.4 Central Nervous System Infections

In infants with a central nervous system infection, the EEG or aEEG abnormalities are mainly non-specific and include background depression and seizures. The presence of low-voltage background, absence of SWC and presence of seizures were associated with an adverse outcome. Changes in the EEG background, such as a multifocal periodic pattern, are associated with neonatal herpes simplex meningoencephalitis, but this will not always be detectable in the aEEG trend.

6.5 Neurocutaneous Syndromes and Brain Malformations

Abnormal brain function in infants with brain malformations are often associated with including background changes, asymmetries and epileptic seizure activity. In this chapter,

DOI: 10.1201/b22858-6

examples are shown for infants with hemimegalencephaly, tuberous sclerosis and incontinentia pigmenti.

Congenital brain tumors are rare but may show similar abnormalities in the aEEG and EEG as brain malformation. These infants may present with macrocephaly and therapy-resistant seizures.

6.6 Neonatal Epilepsy

Seizures in the newborn are mostly spontaneously resolving and provoked by an acute brain injury or other compromise described elsewhere in this atlas. However, out of the newborns with seizures, 10–15% will eventually be diagnosed with epilepsy, and 15–20% of them will have a channelopathy. The aEEG pattern may help in early recognition of channelopathies: The most common channelopathies (*KCNQ2, SCN2A* and *KCNQ3*) show a short increase in lower and upper margin, followed by a prolonged amplitude suppression. Recognizing this pattern may expedite treatment with a sodium channel blocker, such as carbamazepine. A distinction between acute provoked seizures and genetic epilepsy can be facilitated by seizure semiology: Newborns with genetic epilepsy typically show tonic or myoclonic seizures, whereas provoked seizures are often clonic. However, distinction of these semiologies needs expertise, and they are not diagnostic *per se* (see also Chapter 4).

Bibliography

Cornet M-C, Morabito V, Lederer D, et al. Neonatal presentation of genetic epilepsies: Early differentiation from acute provoked seizures. *Epilepsia*. 2021;62(8):1907–1920.

Falsaperla R, Sciuto L, La Spina L, et al. Neonatal seizures as onset of inborn errors of metabolism (IEMs): From diagnosis to treatment. A systematic review. *Metab Brain Dis*. 2021;36(8):2195–2203.

Gürses D, Kiliç I, Sahiner T. Effects of hyperbilirubinemia on cerebrocortical electrical activity in newborns. *Pediatr Res*. 2002; 52(1):125–130.

Harris DL, Weston PJ, Williams CE, et al. Cot-side electroencephalography monitoring is not clinically useful in the detection of mild neonatal hypoglycemia. *J Pediatr*. 2011;159(5):755–760.e1.

Hellström-Westas L, Blennow G, Rosén I. Amplitude-integrated encephalography in pyridoxine-dependent seizures and pyridoxine-responsive seizures. *Acta Paediatr*. 2002;91(8):977–980.

Ishiguro T, Sugiyama Y, Ueda K, et al. Findings of amplitude-integrated electroencephalogram recordings and serum vitamin B6 metabolites in perinatal lethal hypophosphatasia during enzyme replacement therapy *Brain Dev*. 2019;41(8):721–725.

Klinger G, Chin CN, Otsubo H, et al. Prognostic value of EEG in neonatal bacterial meningitis. *Pediatr Neurol*. 2001;24(1):28–31.

Nabbout R, Soufflet C, Plouin P, Dulac O. Pyridoxine dependent epilepsy: A suggestive electroclinical pattern. *Arch Dis Child Fetal Neonatal Ed*. 1999;81(2):F125–F129.

Ohtsuka Y, Ohno S, Oka E. Electroclinical characteristics of hemimegalencephaly. *Pediatr Neurol*. 1999;20(5):390–393.

Olischar M, Shany E, Aygün C, et al. Amplitude-integrated electroencephalography in newborns with inborn errors of metabolism. *Neonatology*. 2012;102(3):203–211.

Pijpers JA, Au PYB, Weeke LC, et al. Early recognition of characteristic conventional and amplitude-integrated EEG patterns of seizures in SCN2A and KCNQ3-related epilepsy in neonates. *Seizure*. 2023;110:212–219.

Pinchefsky EF, Hahn CD, Kamino D, et al. Hyperglycemia and glucose variability are associated with worse brain function and seizures in neonatal encephalopathy: A prospective cohort study. *J Pediatr*. 2019;209:23–32.

Schmitt B, Baumgartner M, Mills PB, et al. Seizures and paroxysmal events: Symptoms pointing to the diagnosis of pyridoxine-dependent epilepsy and pyridoxine phosphate oxidase deficiency. *Dev Med Child Neurol*. 2010;52(7):e133–e142.

Shah DK, Lavery S, Doyle LW, et al. Use of 2-channel bedside electroencephalogram monitoring in term-born encephalopathic infants related to cerebral injury defined by magnetic resonance imaging. *Pediatrics*. 2006;118(1):47–55.

Shellhaas RA, Wusthoff CJ, Tsuchida TN, et al.; Neonatal Seizure Registry. Profile of neonatal epilepsies: Characteristics of a prospective US cohort. *Neurology*. 2017;89(9):893–899.

ter Horst HJ, Bos AF, Duijvendijk J, Hulzebos CV. Moderate unconjugated hyperbilirubinemia causes a transient but delayed suppression of amplitude-integrated electroencephalographic activity in preterm infants. *Neonatology*. 2012;102(2):120–125.

ter Horst HJ, van Olffen M, Remmelts HJ, et al. The prognostic value of amplitude integrated EEG in neonatal sepsis and/or meningitis. *Acta Paediatr*. 2010;99(2):194–200.

Vilan A, Mendes Ribeiro J, et al. A distinctive ictal amplitude-integrated electroencephalography pattern in newborns with neonatal epilepsy associated with KCNQ2 mutations. *Neonatology*. 2017;112(4):387–393.

Wilson MP, Plecko B, Mills PB, Clayton PT. Disorders affecting vitamin B_6 metabolism. *J Inherit Metab Dis*. 2019;42(4): 629–646.

Yuan X, Song J, Gao L, et al. Early aEEG predicts long-term outcomes in term and near-term newborns with severe hyperbilirubinemia. *Pediatr Neurol*. 2019;98:68–73.

Zhang L. Severe neonatal hyperbilirubinemia induces temporal and occipital lobe seizures. *PLoS One*. 2018;13(5):e0197113.

Zhang L, Zhou Y, Li X, Cheng T. Hyperbilirubinemia influences sleep-wake cycles of term newborns in a non-linear manner. *PLoS One*. 2017;12(1):e0169783.

Case 6.1 Full-Term Infant with Hypoglycemia Due to Insulinoma

This infant was born at home at 37 weeks' gestation; birthweight was 3700 g, and Apgar scores were 9 and 10 at 1 and 5 minutes, respectively. Breastfeeding was difficult, and the next morning, the infant was found to be hypothermic, sweaty and pale and was taken to the local hospital, where the first blood glucose was < 0.1 mmol/L. It was difficult to normalize the blood glucose levels, and she was intubated and transferred to the regional NICU for further treatment. The insulin level was increased (15 mIE/L). There was a gene defect encoding for the protein SUR1 of the pancreatic β cell K_{ATP} channel.

aEEG was initially recorded with an analogue machine, started soon after admission, and showed suspected repeated ictal discharges on a normal voltage pattern to start with (Figure 6.1A). Following administration of lidocaine, the background pattern became discontinuous with a BS pattern, even though the lower margin is around 5 μV (a). Several hours later, clinical as well as subclinical seizures were noted on a BS background. Midazolam was added to the medication, and the seizures were temporarily under control (Figure 6.1B).

The digital (NicoletOne, Natus) comparison confirms that these are brief ictal discharges with a very sudden onset and end of the discharge (Figure 6.1C). In Figure 6.1D, a BS is seen without ictal discharges. It is also clear in Figure 6.1 A-C, that there is an ECG artefact that lifts the baseline to 4-5 μV.

Cranial *ultrasound* showed extensive increased echogenicity throughout the thalami and the periventricular white matter (not shown). The *MRI* performed on day 4 showed extensive injury with loss of grey-white matter differentiation on the inversion recovery sequence in the occipital regions (Figure 6.1E) and more extensive abnormalities extending anteriorly involving the thalami on diffusion-weighted imaging (Figure 6.1F).

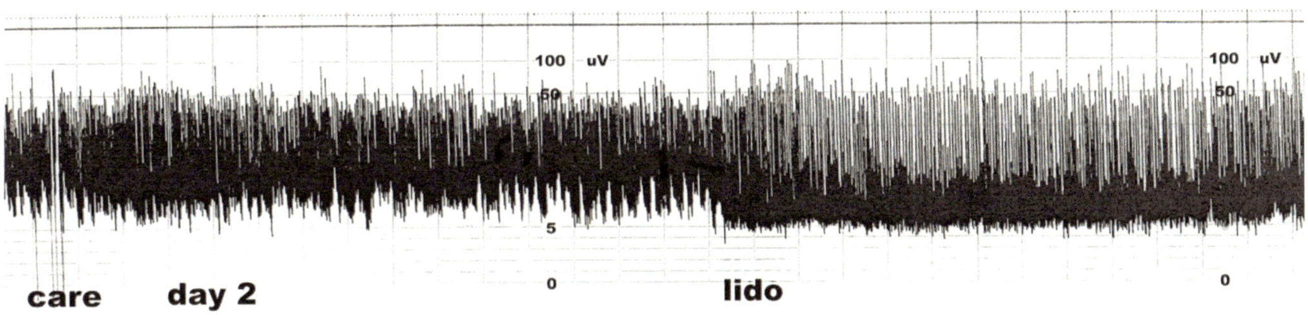

FIGURE 6.1A

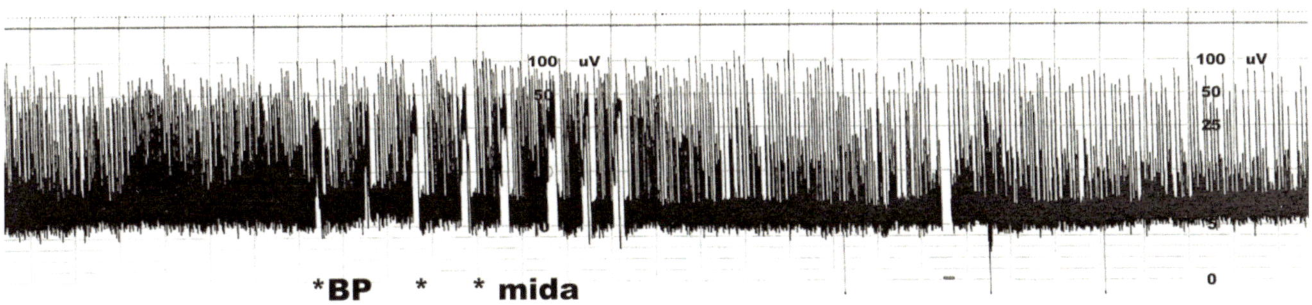

FIGURE 6.1B

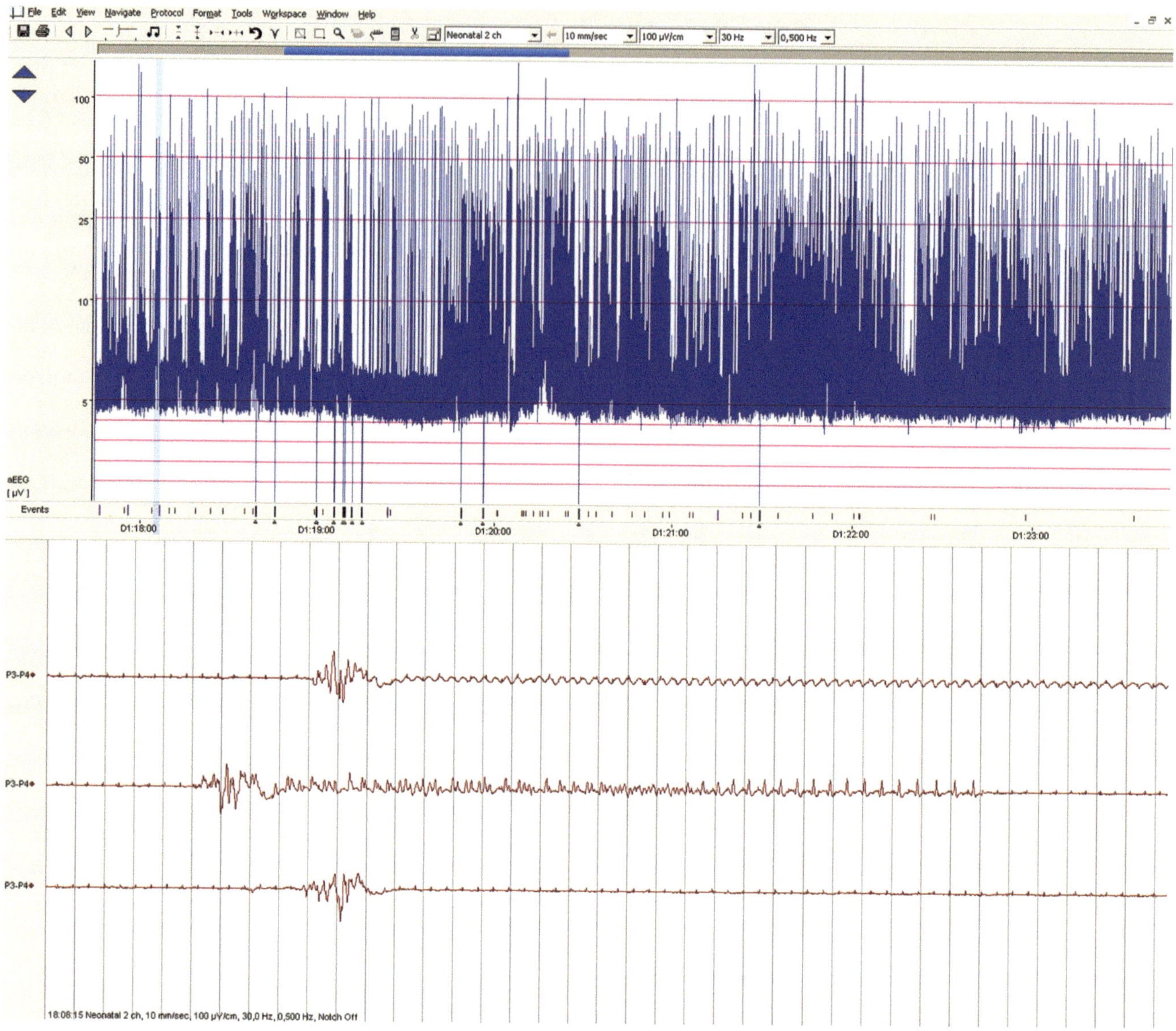

FIGURE 6.1C

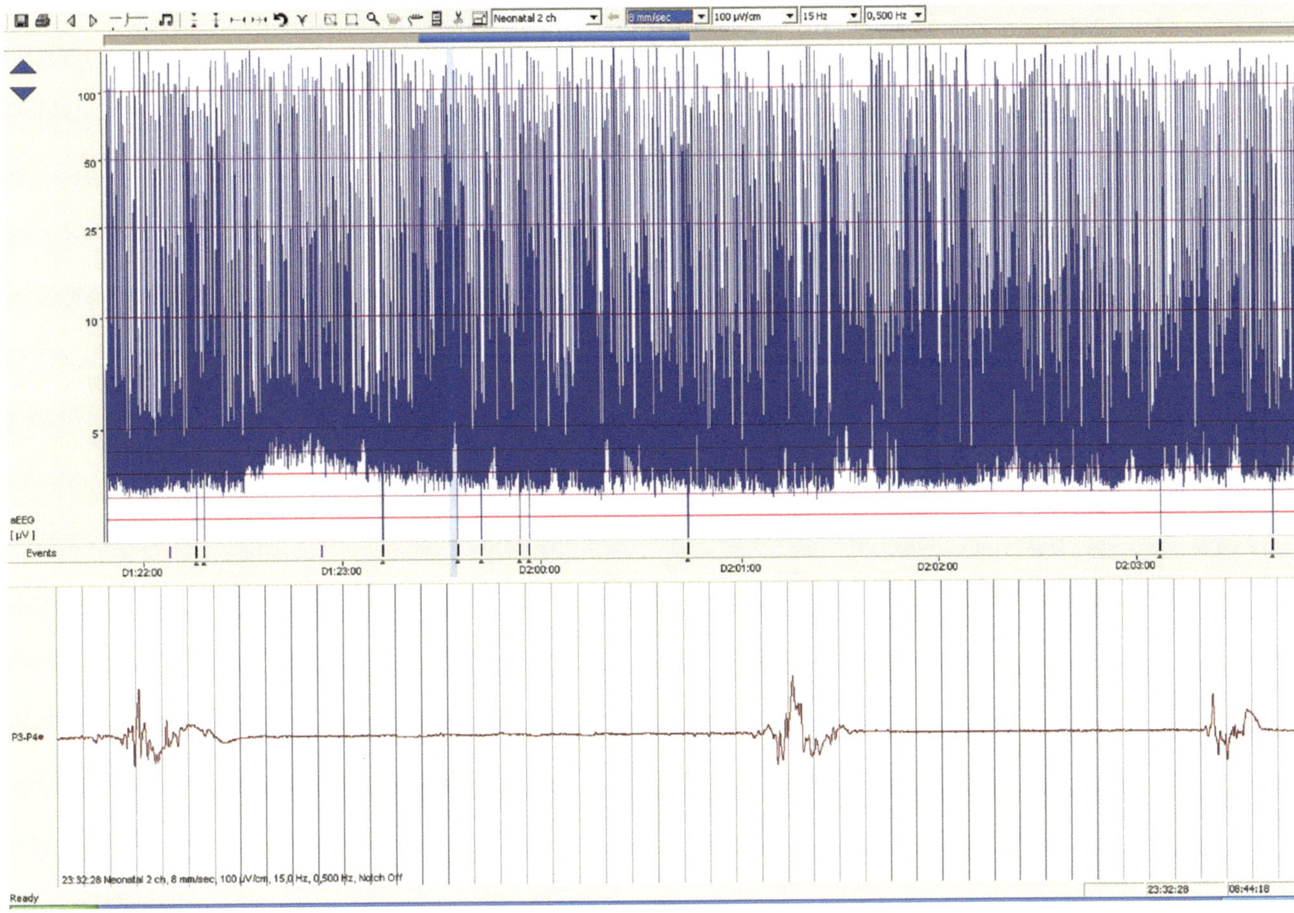

FIGURE 6.1D

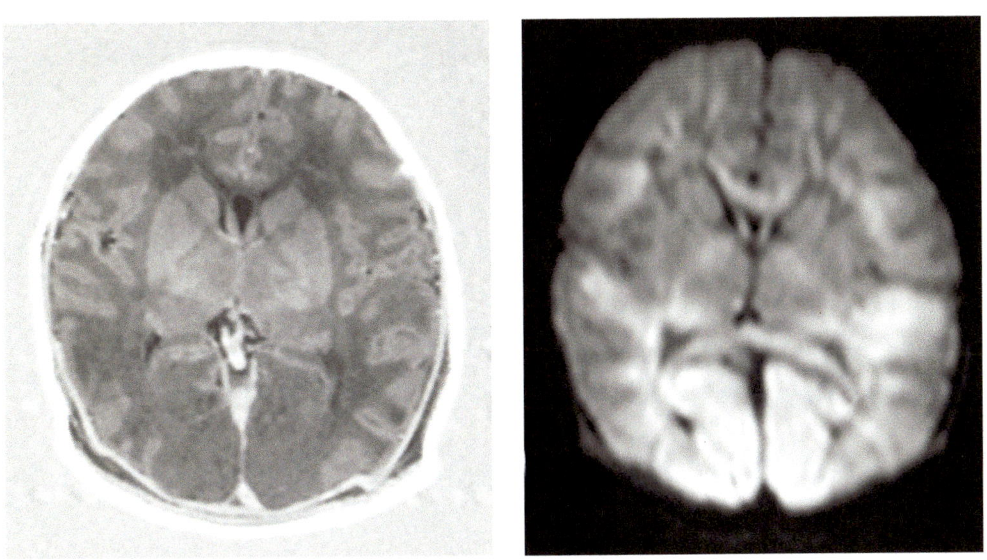

FIGURE 6.1E AND F

Case 6.2 Full-Term Infant with Hypoglycemia

This term infant was born by a caesarean section because of a suboptimal CTG at 41 weeks' gestation and a birthweight of 3770 g. Arterial umbilical pH was 7.17, with a BE of 14 mmol/L. Apgar scores were 7, 9 and 9 at 1, 5 and 10 minutes, respectively. At 12 hrs of age, the infant developed apneas. The plasma-glucose was 1.4 mmol/L, and the next one was 1.9 mmol/L. There were four seizures noted in the level-two hospital, with staring and nystagmus, but no medication was given. The infant was transferred to a level-three unit for further care and neuromonitoring. On admission, the glucose was 1.3 mmol/L, and an arterial lactate was 4 mmol/L. There was mild polycythaemia, with a level of 0.61 L/L.

The *aEEG* was started 46 hrs after birth and showed a continuous background pattern with some cycling. However, there are repetitive seizures predominantly from the left hemisphere (Figure 6.2A). The seizures could easily be missed without access to the raw EEG, as they were not as sharp on the aEEG as we tend to see. The infant had received phenobarbital (20 mg/kg iv) before start of the aEEG recording. Repetitive subclinical seizures continued for another 12 hours after admission, and an additional dose of phenobarbital (10 mg/kg iv) was administered. Figures 6.2A and B show repeated seizures that were not adequately recognized and treated during the night. Seizures are marked *. The cEEG (Figure 6.2C) obtained at 72 hrs after birth showed no abnormalities.

An *MRI* (Figure 6.2D) performed on day 3 shows typical changes seen in infants with symptomatic hypoglycemia. The DWI sequence (a, b) shows loss of grey-white matter differentiation (cortical ribbon) in the occipital lobes, as well as diffusion restriction in the optic radiation and pulvinar. The MRI was repeated 5 weeks later, and the T1-weighted sequence shows gliosis and some volume loss, especially in the right occipital lobe (c, d). Myelination of the PLIC was within the normal range.

At 2 years, cognitive outcome was just within the normal range (composite score 87), and the combined motor score was 89. There was a strabismus and the infant was referred for assessment of cerebral visual impairment.

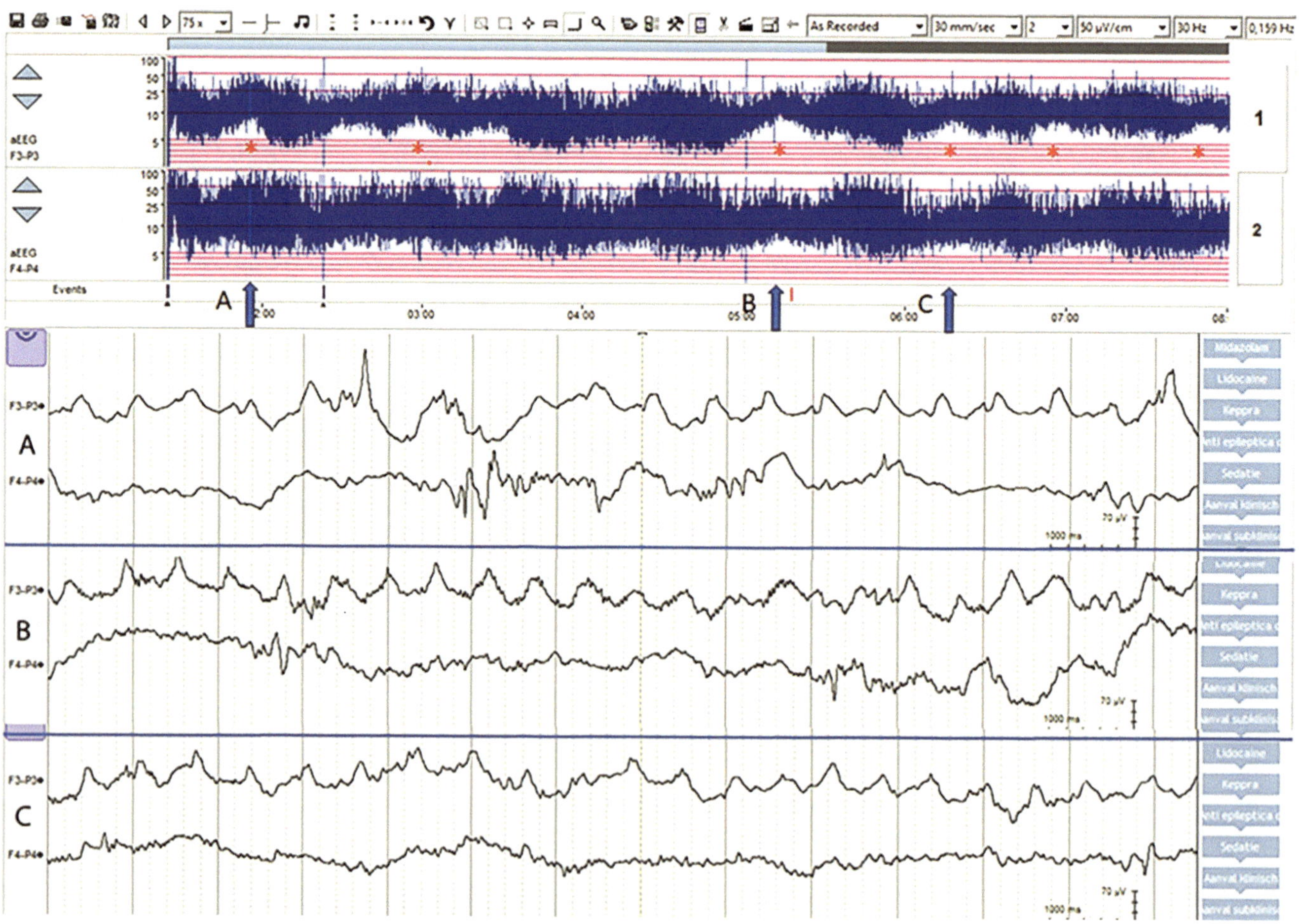

FIGURE 6.2A

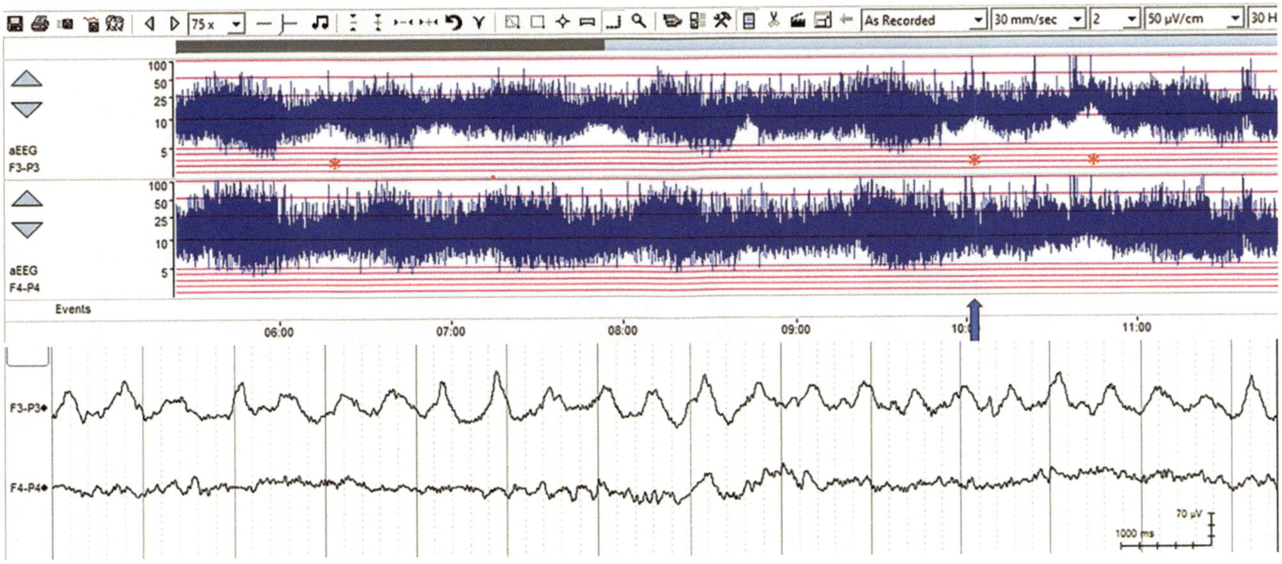

FIGURE 6.2B

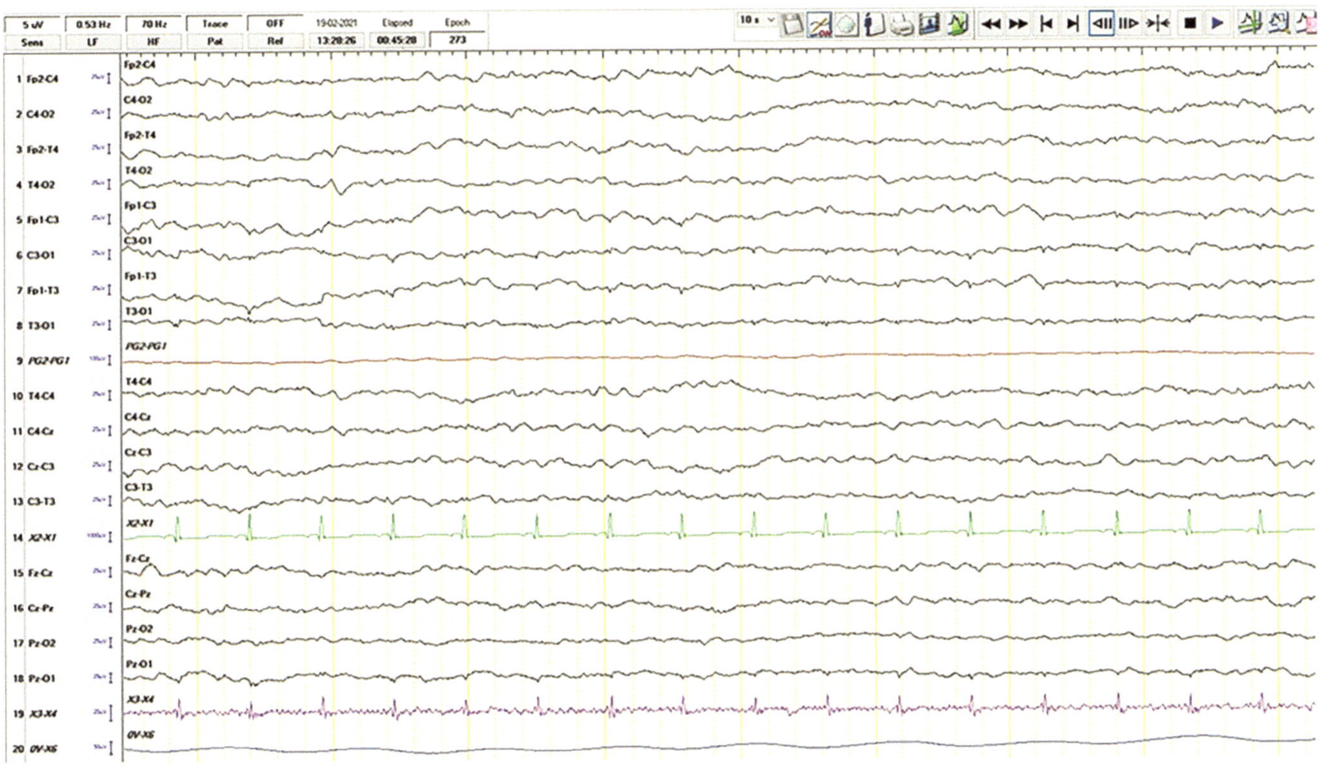

FIGURE 6.2C (Courtesy Selma Tromp, Department of Neurology, Leiden University Medical Center.)

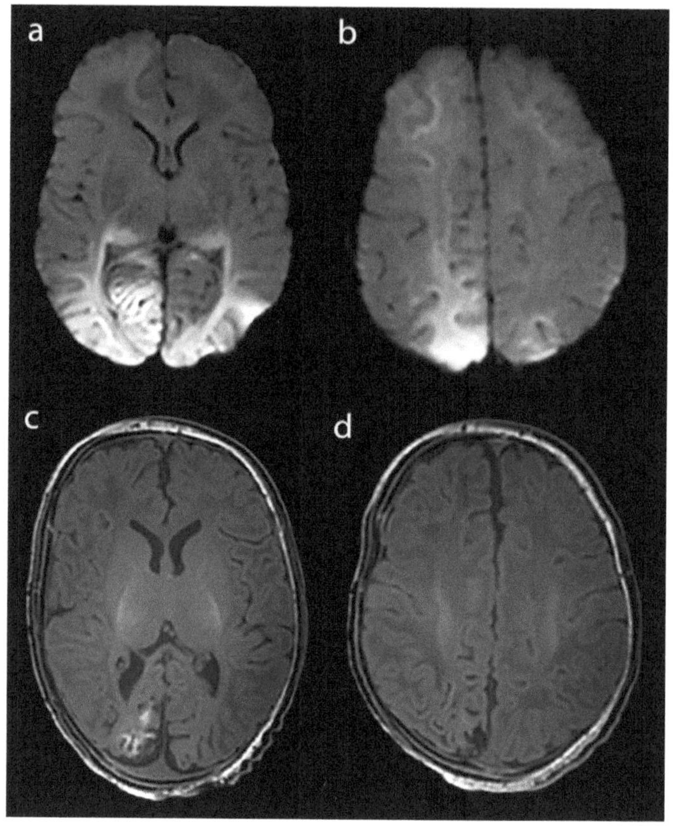

FIGURE 6.2D

Case 6.3 Full-Term Neonate with Molybdenum Cofactor Deficiency

This infant was born at 41 weeks, with a birthweight of 3600 g following a vaginal planned home delivery. The pregnancy was uneventful, and the infant had Apgar scores of 9 and 10 at 1 and 5 minutes, respectively. There was no consanguinity. Tremors developed, feeding was difficult, and the infant was admitted at 24 hours with suspected septicemia. CRP was 194 mg / L, and the infant was treated with broad spectrum antibiotics as well as acyclovir, but blood and CSF cultures and PCR for herpes remained negative. Seizures developed at 30 hrs of age and were hard to control and persisted in spite of administration of phenobarbital, midazolam, lidocaine and levetiracetam. The uric acid was very low (< 0.10 mmol/L). This suggested molybdenum cofactor deficiency, which was confirmed with a mutation in MOCS 1 gene. In view of the severe MRI abnormalities and ongoing seizures, intensive care was discontinued.

aEEG was started on admission and showed repetitive seizures (Figure 6.3A). Phenobarbital was given (green marker 2) and resulted in background depression and fewer, but longer, seizures. A bit later (Figure 6.3B), midazolam was started, and the background activity changed to a flat trace. Thirty-six hours after admission, lidocaine was started, and seizures still continued on a very depressed background (Figure 6.3C). Seventy-two hours after admission (Figure 6.3D), the background activity had recovered to a burst-suppression pattern, but brief seizures were still present.

Cranial ultrasound (Figure 6.3E, a) showed diffuse increase in echogenicity and brain swelling, and an *MRI* (Figure 6.3E, b) showed extensive diffusion restriction of the white matter, including the cerebral peduncles but sparing the cerebellum.

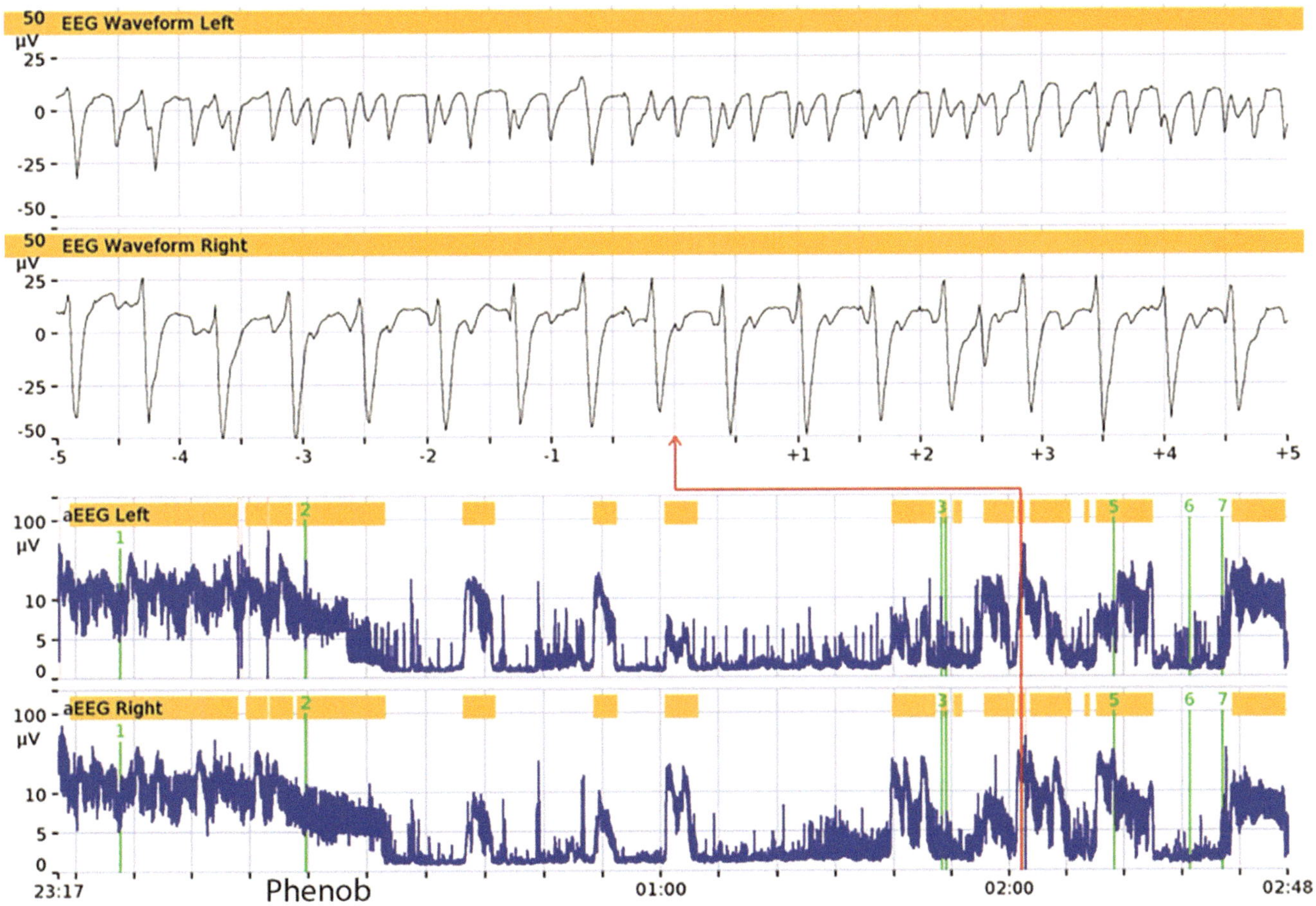

FIGURE 6.3A

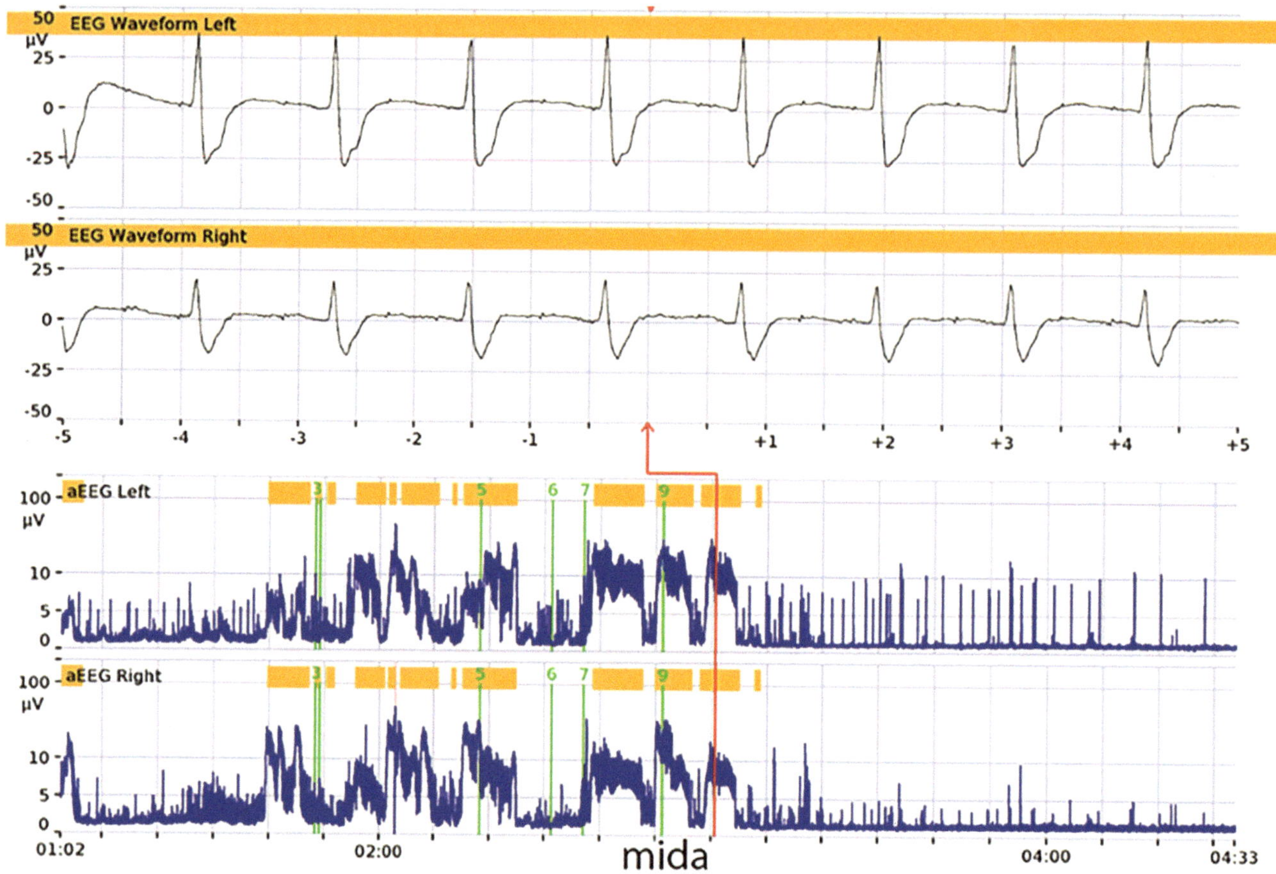
EEG Waveform Left
EEG Waveform Right
aEEG Left
aEEG Right
mida
01:02
02:00
04:00
04:33

FIGURE 6.3B

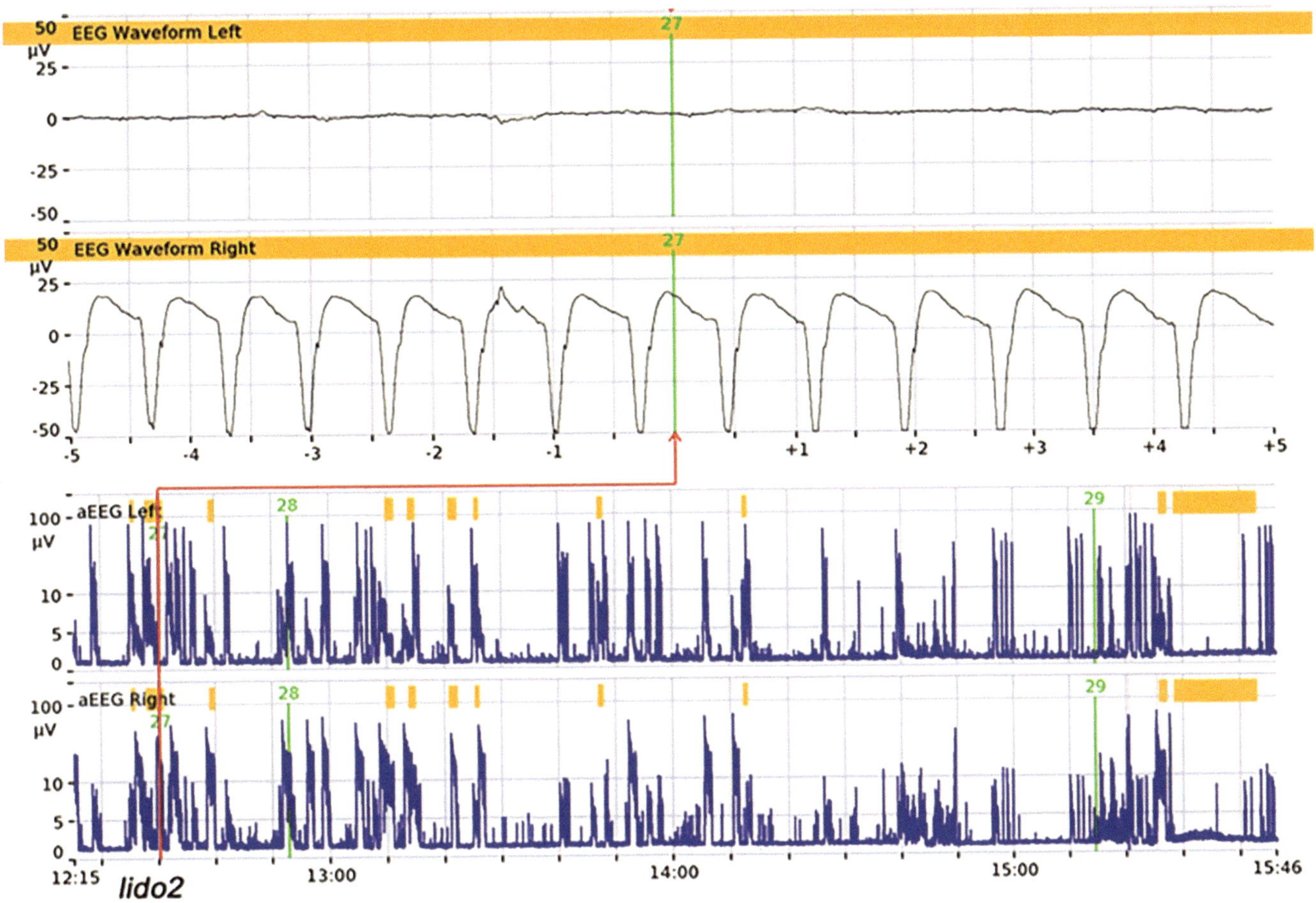
EEG Waveform Left
EEG Waveform Right
aEEG Left
aEEG Right
µV
27
28
29
12:15
13:00
14:00
15:00
15:46
lido2

FIGURE 6.3C

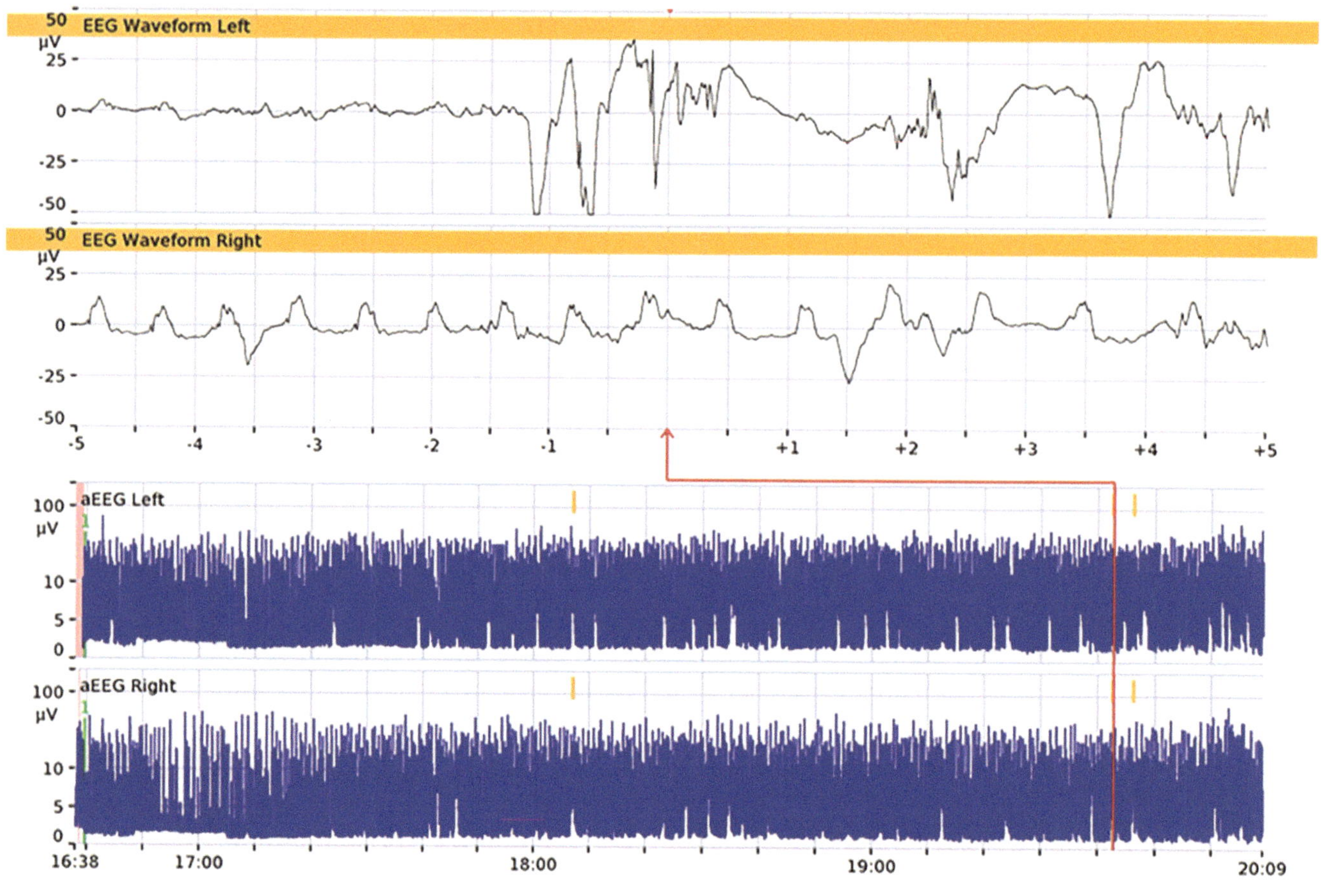

FIGURE 6.3D

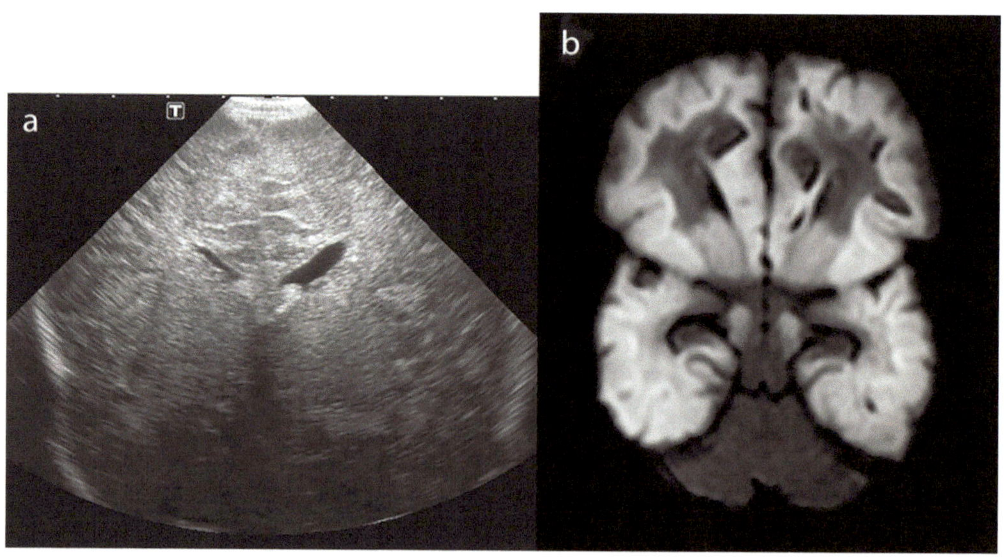

FIGURE 6.3E

Case 6.4 Ornithine Transcarbamylase (OTC) Deficiency

This infant was born as the third male infant to non-related parents. The pregnancy was normal as was the delivery at 40 weeks' gestational age. Birthweight was 4020 g, and Apgar scores were 9 and 10 at 1 and 5 minutes, respectively. Vomiting started at 24 h, and the infant became lethargic and tachypneic. Suspected clinical seizures, resembling hiccups, were noted. On arrival at the regional NICU at 4 days of age, the infant was comatose and unresponsive and had severe hyperammonemia (930 µmol/l). Dialysis was initiated within a few hours. The diagnosis of OTC deficiency was later established. The infant survived the neonatal period but died within some months.

The *aEEG* was started 3 hours after arrival and showed continuously ongoing subclinical status epilepticus (Figure 6.4A). At this time point, the infant was very unstable and needed inotrope support to maintain blood pressure. There was a transient drop in amplitude at time 02:30, but there are no explanatory notes. However, it is possible that this drop could have been caused by hypotension. Figure 6.4B began 8 hours later, when the infant was on dialysis, and showed a continuous subclinical status epilepticus.

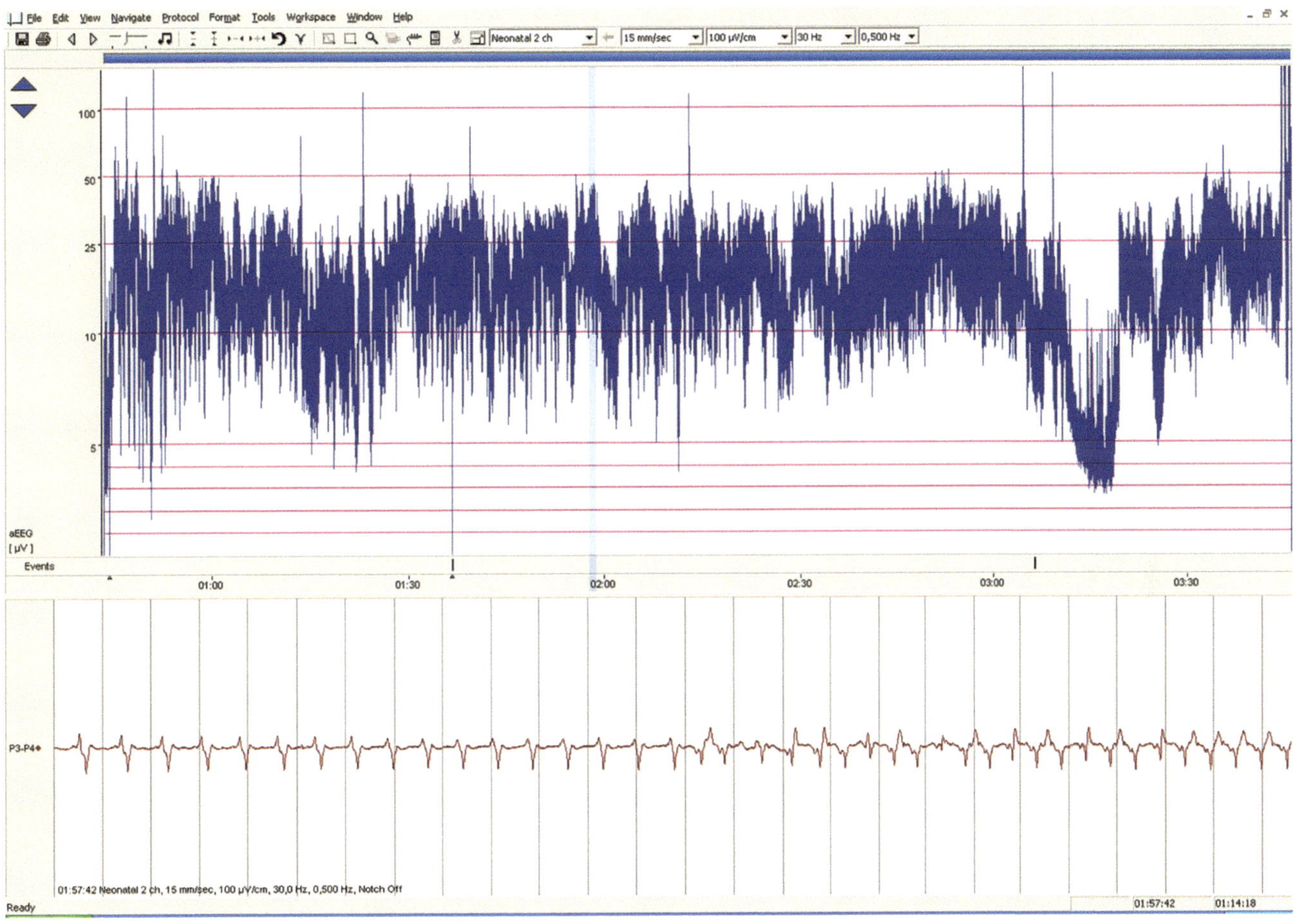

FIGURE 6.4A

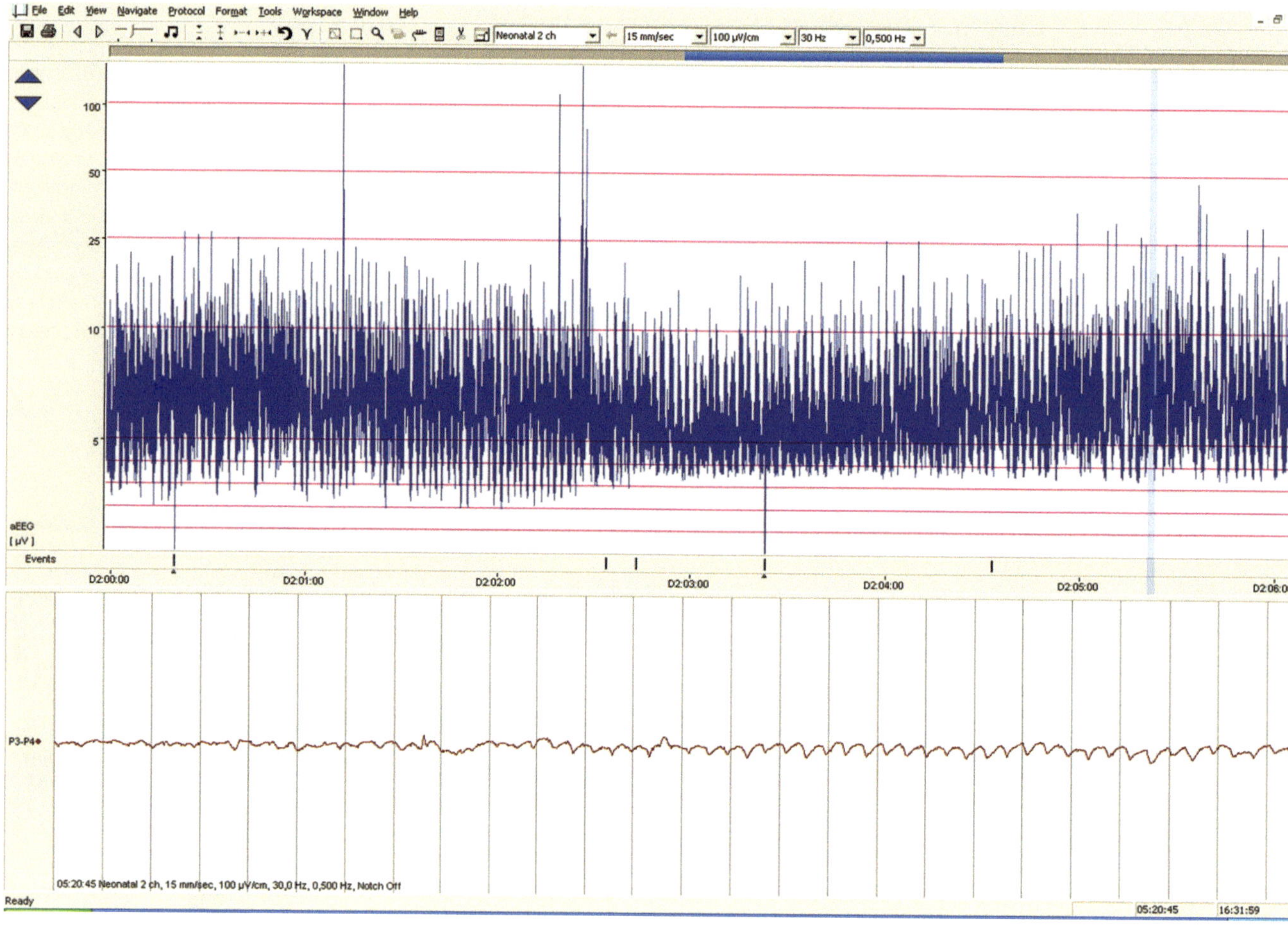
File Edit View Navigate Protocol Format Tools Workspace Window Help
Neonatal 2 ch
15 mm/sec
100 µV/cm
30 Hz
0,500 Hz
100
50
25
10
5
aEEG
[µV]
Events
D2:00:00
D2:01:00
D2:02:00
D2:03:00
D2:04:00
D2:05:00
D2:06:00
P3-P4
05:20:45 Neonatal 2 ch, 15 mm/sec, 100 µV/cm, 30,0 Hz, 0,500 Hz, Notch Off
Ready
05:20:45
16:31:59

FIGURE 6.4B

Case 6.5 Full-Term Infant with Non-Ketotic Hyperglycinemia

This infant was born by an uneventful vaginal delivery at 37 weeks. Apgar scores were 9, 10 and 10 at 1, 5 and 10 minutes, respectively. The birthweight was 2550 g. From birth onwards, feeding was difficult. The infant was hypotonic, became encephalopathic on the second day, and was transferred for further investigation.

A diagnosis of non-ketotic hyperglycinemia was considered likely on the basis of the clinical history, the dysplastic corpus callosum seen on cranial ultrasound performed after admission and subsequently on MRI and the burst-suppression pattern on the aEEG.

The plasma glycine was raised to 1669 (upper limit of normal being 689 μmol/L). The cerebrospinal fluid (CSF) glycine was 404 (upper limit of normal being 8 μmol/L). The CSF-to-plasma-glycine ratio was 0.24 (normal < 0.06). She was found to have two heterozygous mutations in the GLDC gene.

The *aEEG* shows a burst-suppression background pattern (Figure 6.5A) with a single seizure (Figure 6.5B). An interburst interval of 24 seconds was noted on the cEEG (Figure 6.5C).

Cranial ultrasound (not shown) showed changes compatible with a dysplastic corpus callosum, the 'bull-horn sign' on the coronal view. The *MRI* (Figure 6.5D) confirmed the dysplastic corpus callosum on the midsagittal view (a) and also showed lack of myelination of the PLIC on the axial T1-weighted image (b). A rather diffuse increase in signal intensity of the white matter on the T_2SE is noted; there is also a small bilateral IVH (c). A glycine peak was noted on proton-*MRS* at 3.5 ppm (not shown).

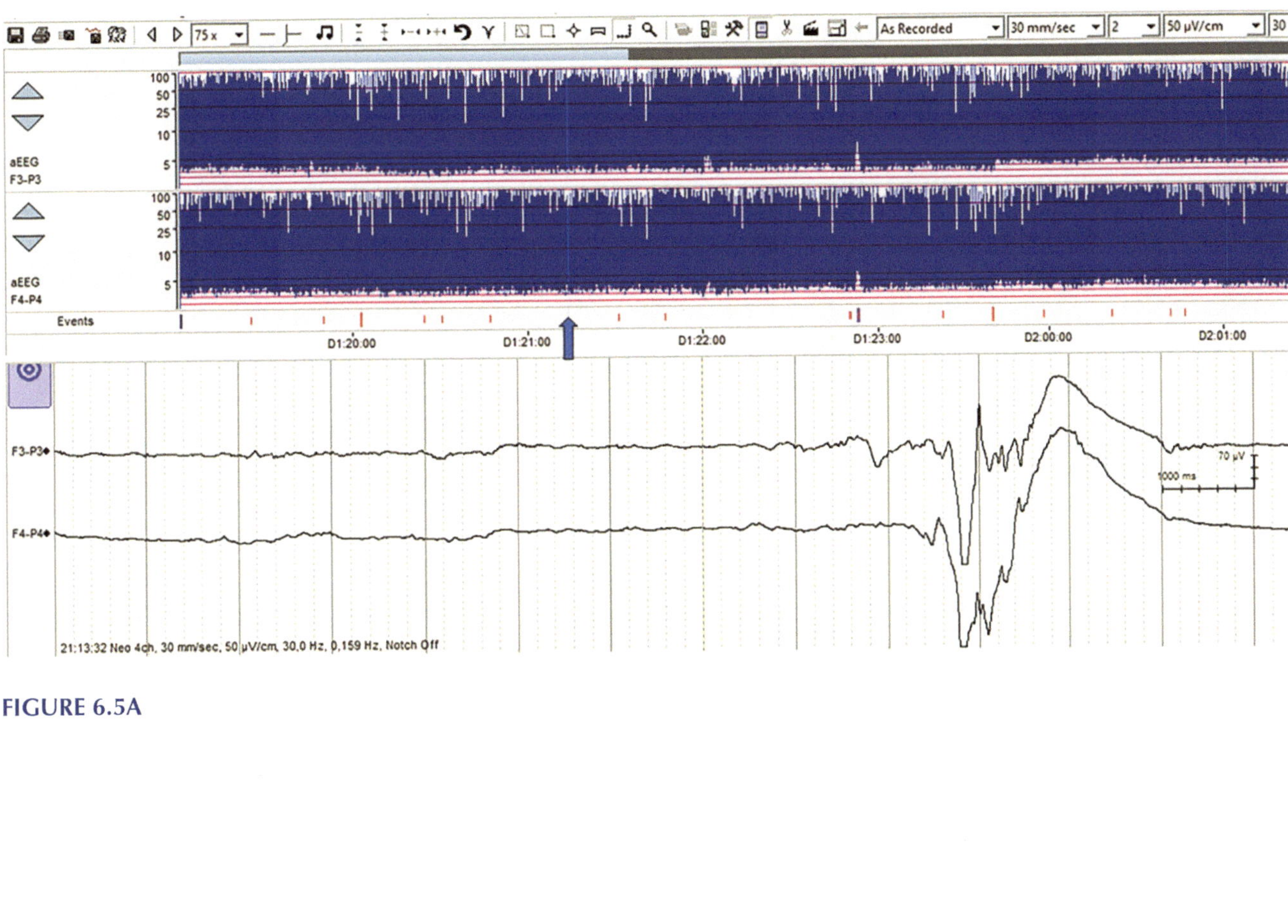

FIGURE 6.5A

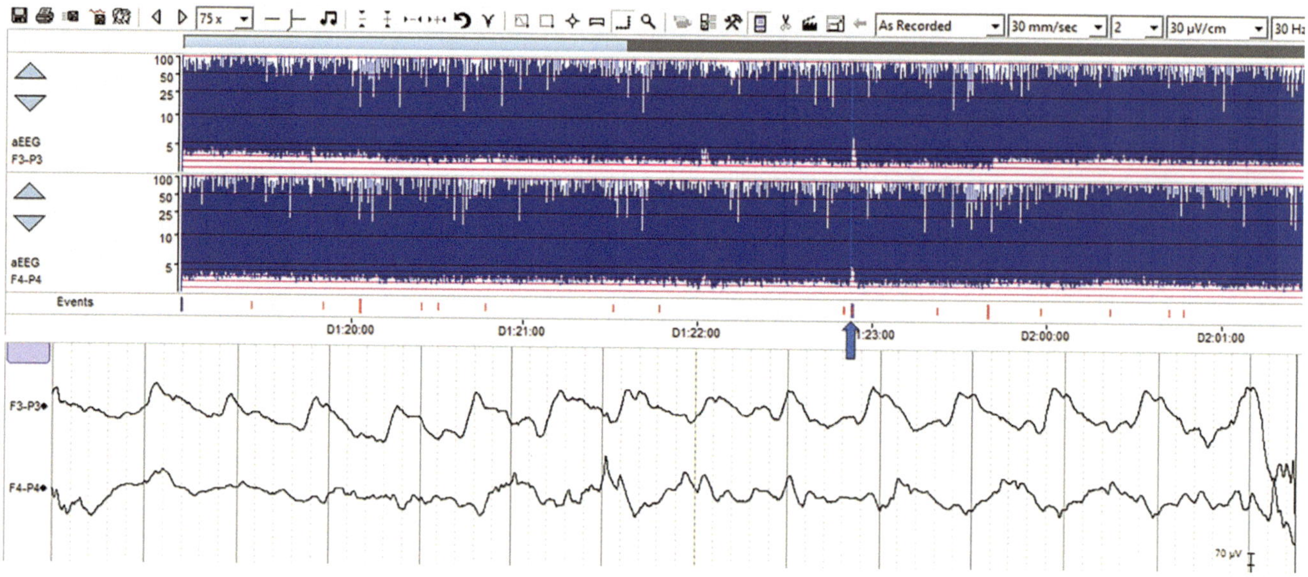

FIGURE 6.5B

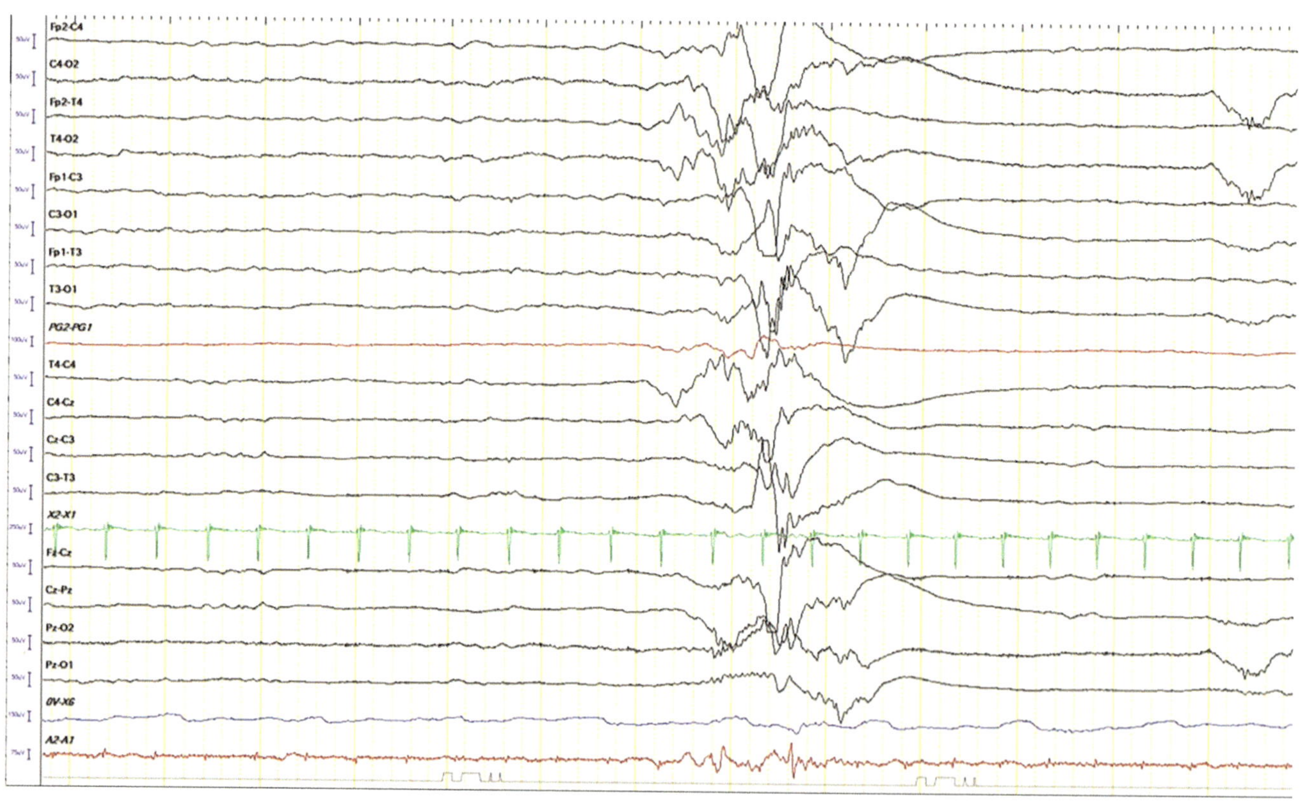

FIGURE 6.5C (Courtesy Selma Tromp, Department of Neurology, Leiden University Medical Center.)

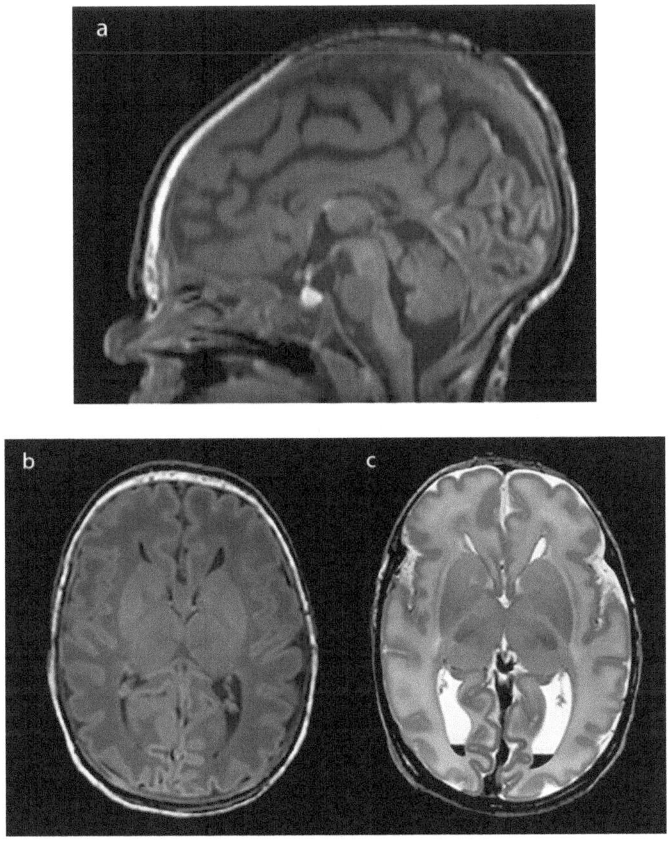

FIGURE 6.5D

Case 6.6 Pyridoxine-Responsive and Pyridoxine-Dependent Seizures

The two cases shown here illustrate (a) an infant with pyridoxine-responsive seizures and (b) an infant with pyridoxine-dependent seizures. The diagnosis of pyridoxine-dependent seizures is usually made when a child, after an initial response to pyridoxine, develops new seizures when pyridoxine treatment is temporarily discontinued. Since the child in (a) was never challenged, but probably has pyridoxine dependency, the diagnosis is still pyridoxine-responsive seizures.

INFANT A This full-term male infant was born after a normal pregnancy, with Apgar scores of 9, 9 and 10 at 1, 5 and 10 minutes, respectively, an umbilical artery pH of 7.21 and a meconium-stained amniotic fluid. He was admitted to the neonatal unit because he was irritable and had moderate metabolic acidosis. Myoclonic seizures started at 12 h and continued for several days in spite of treatment with diazepam, phenobarbitone, lidocaine and phenytoin. Two standard EEGs showed BS and normal activity, respectively. Seizures recurred later, and again, antiepileptic treatment with diazepam, phenobarbital, lidocaine and phenytoin was not effective. This time pyridoxine was given, with immediate effect on the seizure activity (see later). He remained on pyridoxine, and a decision to withdraw the pyridoxine was changed when very subtle episodes of arrested activity occurred with a corresponding left-sided rhythmic theta activity on the EEG. He has a moderate cognitive impairment.

The *aEEG* (Figure 6.6A) was recorded when the seizures recurred at 15 days. The recurrent electroclinical seizures can be seen as a 'sawtooth pattern' during the first 4 hours of the tracing. The seizures were totally abolished 15 min after 100 mg pyridoxine was given orally (at the arrow) through the nasogastric feeding tube (there was no iv pyridoxine available). After the administration of pyridoxine, the aEEG showed continuous background with a slightly periodic pattern (low minimum amplitude but normal maximum voltage) and cyclical fluctuations suggestive of sleep-wake cycling.

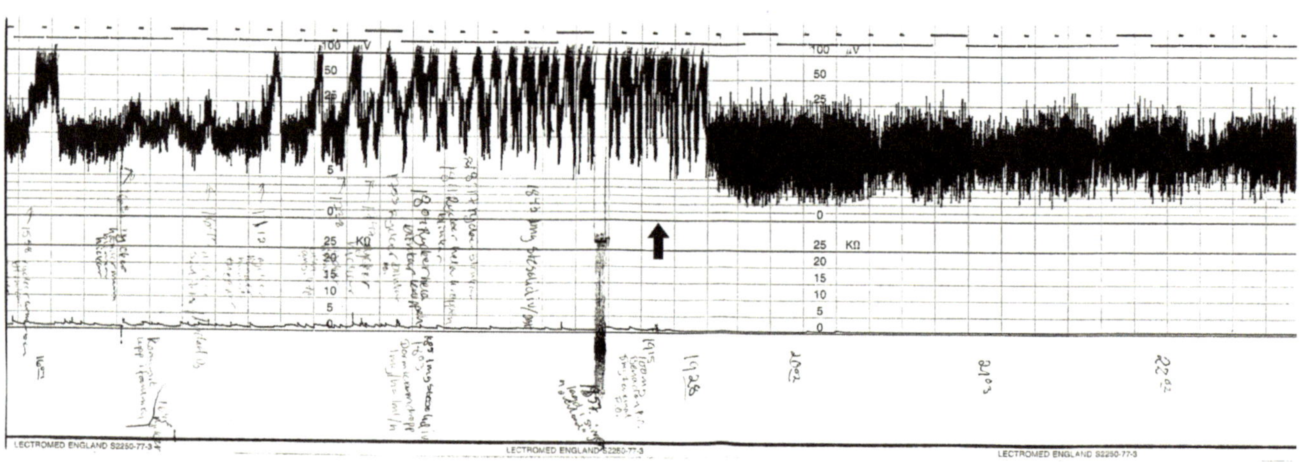

FIGURE 6.6A

INFANT B This female infant was born at 34 weeks' gestation with Apgar scores of 6, 8 and 9 at 1, 5 and 10 minutes, respectively, and a birthweight of 2240 g. The pregnancy was normal except for a routine ultrasound examination at 32 weeks' gestation that showed suspected bowel dilatation. Soon after birth, she became restless and irritable. Abdominal ultrasound and X-rays were normal. She had a metabolic acidosis with a pH of 7.08, a base excess of −21 mmol/L and a plasma lactate of 20 mmol/L. At 12 h, she needed sedation (with midazolam and morphine) and mechanical ventilation due to the irritability. On the third day of life, she developed multifocal myoclonic seizures. She received iv diazepam and lidocaine with no effect and was then given 100 mg pyridoxine iv. The seizures stopped within 2 minutes, and she became profoundly hypotonic. A standard EEG on the following day was discontinuous with bilateral epileptiform activity, but the EEG normalized within 3 days. She had no more seizures and was extubated after 5 days. A trial of pyridoxine withdrawal was done when she was 2.5 years old and resulted in recurrent seizures and continuing pyridoxine medication. Her development is slightly delayed.

The *aEEG* (Figure 6.6B) showed high-amplitude recurrent, almost continuous, electrographic seizure activity concomitant with the clinical seizures. After pyridoxine administration (at the arrow), the aEEG changed dramatically, the electrographic seizure activity ceased almost immediately, and the background amplitude became extremely low in voltage. The aEEG background recovered slowly during the following 8–10 h.

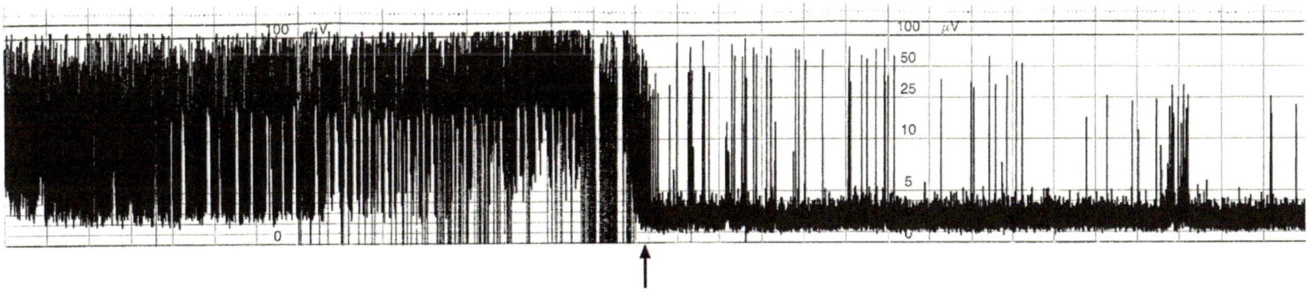

FIGURE 6.6B

Also see Chapter 4, Figure 4.6 for comparison.

Bibliography

Hellström-Westas L, Blennow G, Rosén I. Amplitude-integrated encephalography in pyridoxine-dependent seizures and pyridoxine-responsive seizures. *Acta Paediatr*. 2002;91(8):977–980.

Case 6.7 Full-Term Infant with a Peroxisomal Disorder

INFANT A The infant was born at 40 weeks with a birthweight of 3285 g. The vaginal delivery was uncomplicated. Apgar scores were 5, 6 and 9 and 1, 5 and 10 minutes. Because of insufficient respiration, the infant was intubated and ventilated. At 2 hours of age, a glucose of 0.9 mmol/L was measured. There was hypotonia with facial dysmorphisms (low-set ears), and the anterior fontanelle was enlarged. Fetal ultrasonography had shown ventriculomegaly.

aEEG was started 12 hrs after birth, showing repetitive seizures on a DNV pattern (Figure 6.7A; see also Video 6.7). The discharges at (a) and (b) were recognized by the seizure-detection algorithm (yellow markers), but the seizure at (c) was not detected by the algorithm. The seizures had an onset in either the left or right hemisphere. Phenobarbital was given twice, at green markers 1 (20 mg/kg iv) and 2 (10 mg/kg iv). A single seizure was seen at 24 hrs of age, and another dose of phenobarbital was given (10 mg/kg iv) (Figure 6.7B).

Postnatal *cranial ultrasound* (coronal view, Figure 6.7C, a) confirmed the enlarged ventricles and also showed germinolytic cysts, lenticulostriate vasculopathy and a poorly folded sylvian fissure, all suggestive of Zellweger syndrome. An *MRI* (Figure 6.7C, b) was obtained the next day, and an axial T2 sequence clearly showed extensive perisylvian polymicrogyria. A mutation in the PEX2 gene was found.

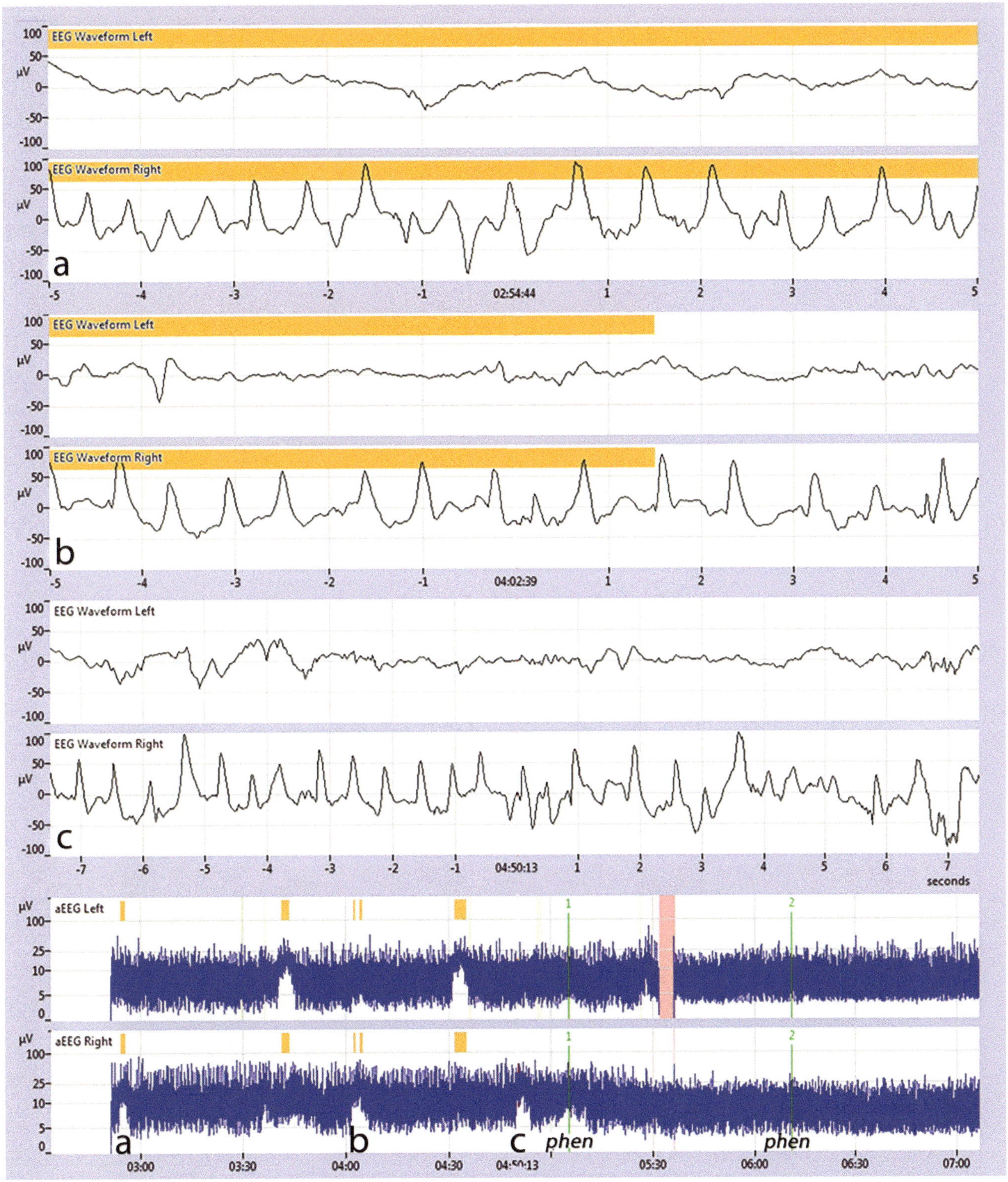
EEG Waveform Left
EEG Waveform Right
a
02:54:44
b
04:02:39
c
04:50:13
seconds
aEEG Left
aEEG Right
phen
phen
03:00
03:30
04:00
04:30
05:30
06:00
06:30
07:00

FIGURE 6.7A

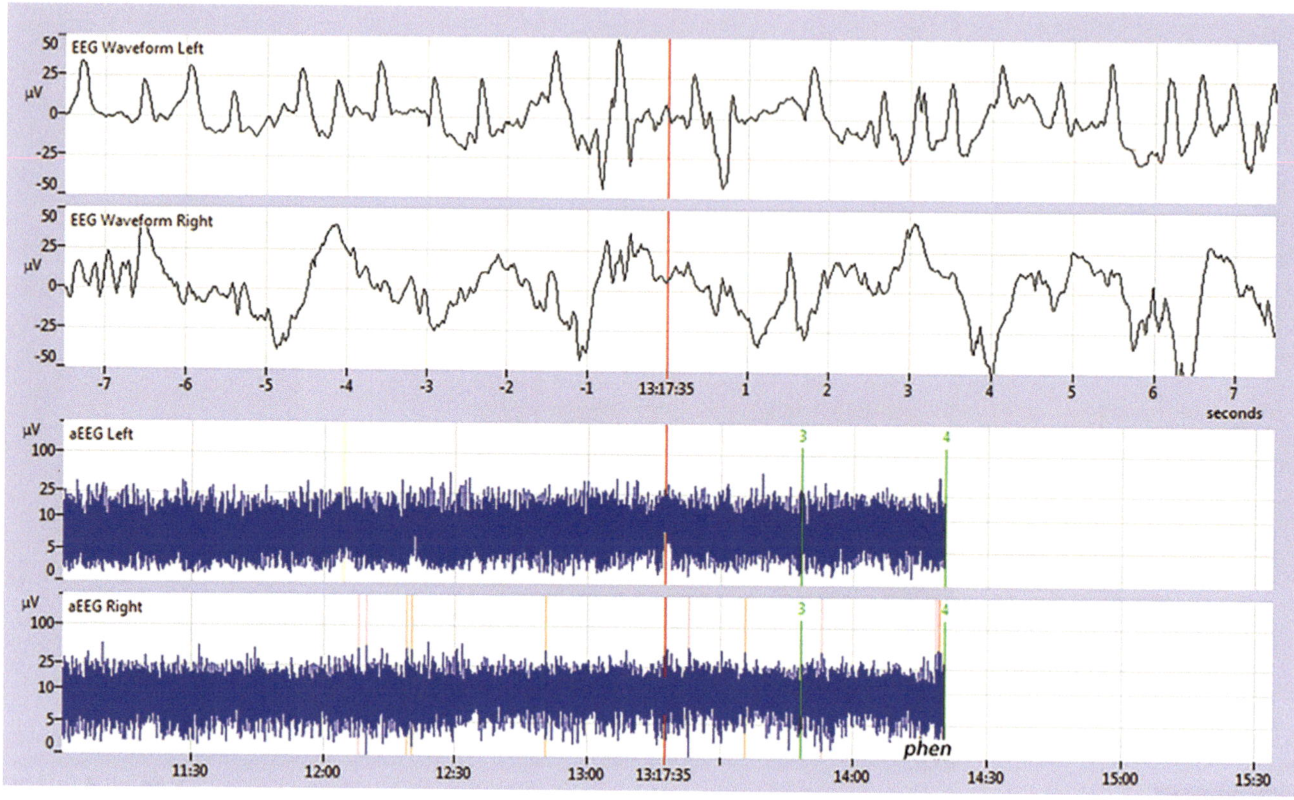

FIGURE 6.7B

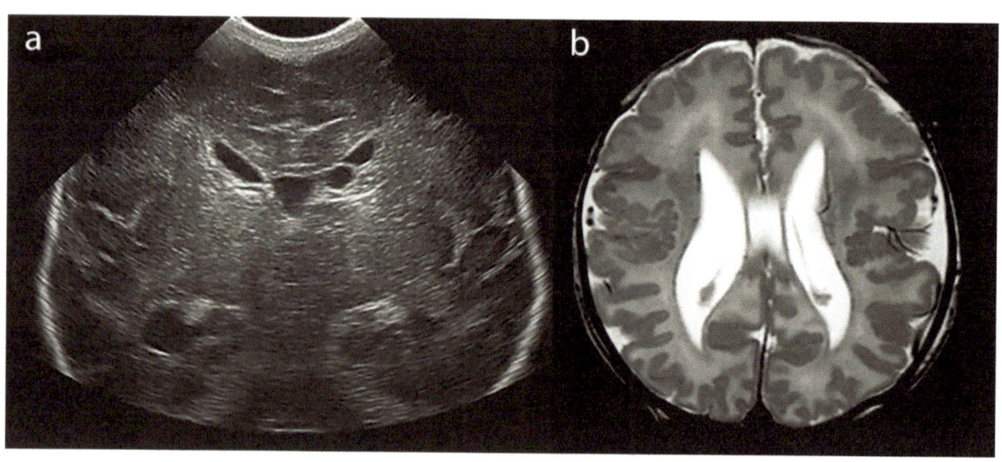

FIGURE 6.7C

INFANT B The infant was born at 41 weeks' gestation after a normal pregnancy and a normal delivery. The birthweight was 3700 g, and Apgar scores were 7, 7 and 7 at 1, 5 and 10 minutes, respectively. However, immediately after birth, the infant was hypotonic and rapidly developed respiratory insufficiency and required intubation at 10 minutes after the delivery. There was a large anterior fontanelle and wide sutures, a high forehead with a broad nasal ridge, low-set ears, adducted feet and hypospadias. *MRI* showed perisylvian polymicrogyria, ventricular dilatation and pachygyria. Zellweger syndrome was suspected and later confirmed. The infant died within a few weeks.

The *aEEG* from the second day of life shows a mainly continuous background without sleep-wake cycling during the 6-hour recording (Figure 6.7D). Four brief seizures are present in the recording (marked *); at A, there is a clinical note 'sleeping'. (B) shows a representative sample of the EEG background.

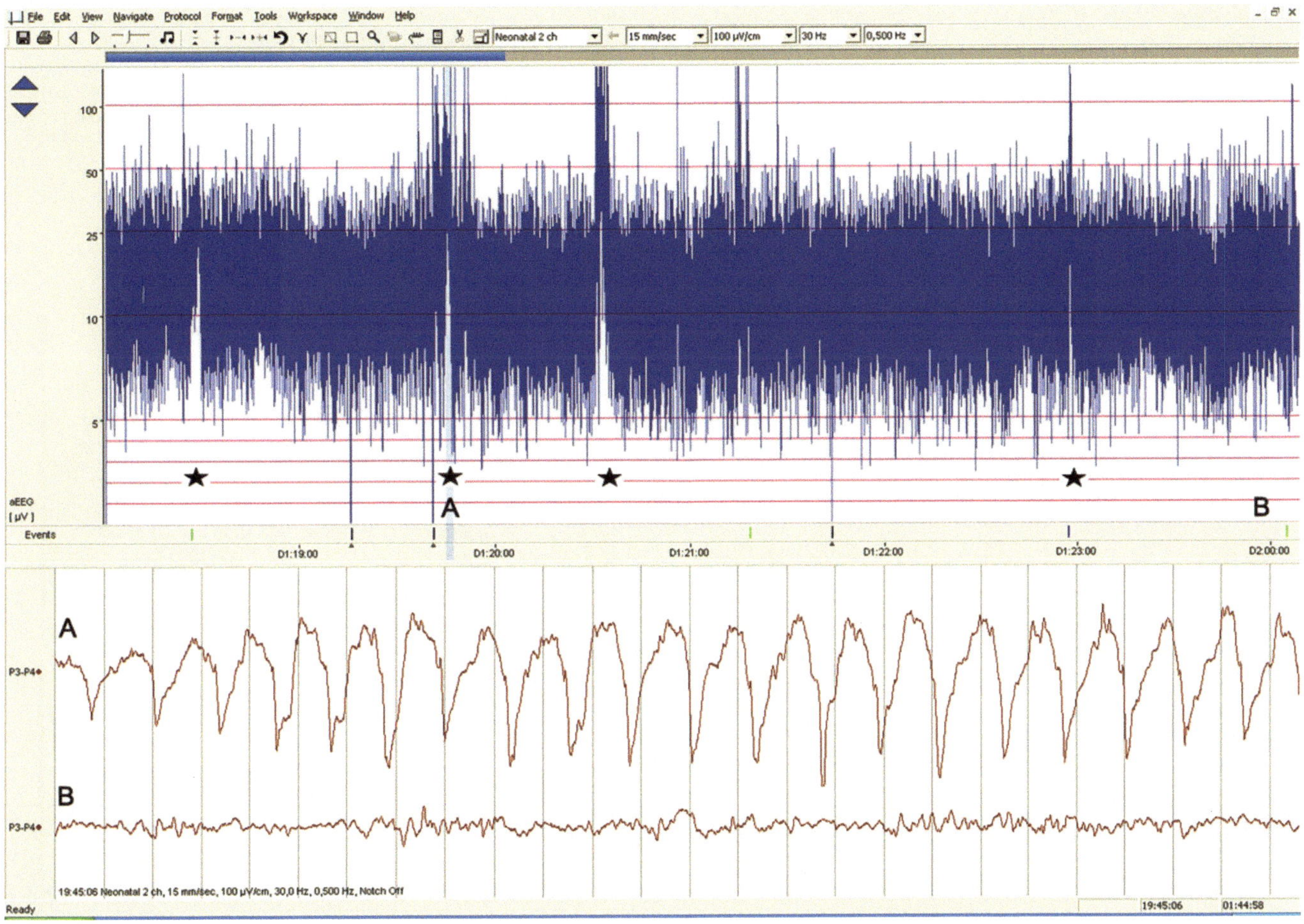

FIGURE 6.7D

Case 6.8 Full-Term Infant with Acute Bilirubin Encephalopathy

This infant was born at 37 weeks' gestation by vaginal delivery. Apgar scores were 9 and 10 at 1 and 5 minutes, respectively. On day 4, the baby was admitted with jaundice and a very high plasma bilirubin of 588 µmol/L. An exchange transfusion was performed. During the exchange transfusion, apneas were noted.

An *aEEG* recording was started and showed status epilepticus. A loading dose of phenobarbital (20 mg/kg iv) was given at the vertical dotted line (Figure 6.8A). No further seizures were detected, a DNV pattern was seen several hours later (Figure 6.8B), and no additional antiseizure medication was administered. Recovery to a CNV background with SWC was seen the next day (Figure 6.8C). (Figures 6.8A, B, and C were reproduced with permission from *Neurology; Neonatology Questions and Controversies*, 3rd edition, Weeke et al; aEEG and its potential role in augmenting management within the NICU, 235–255, Elsevier 2018.)

An *MRI* (Figure 6.8D) was performed on day 7, and the axial T1-weighted sequence showed increased signal intensity bilaterally in the globus pallidus, suggestive of kernicterus.

The infant was diagnosed to have glucose-6-phosphate dehydrogenase deficiency (G6PD). No motor or cognitive impairments developed, but there was an auditive neuropathy requiring hearing aids.

Reference

Weeke LC, Toet MC, de Vries LS. aEEG and its potential role in augmenting management within the NICU, *Neurology: Neonatology questions and controversies*, third edition, Elsevier, 2018, 235–255.

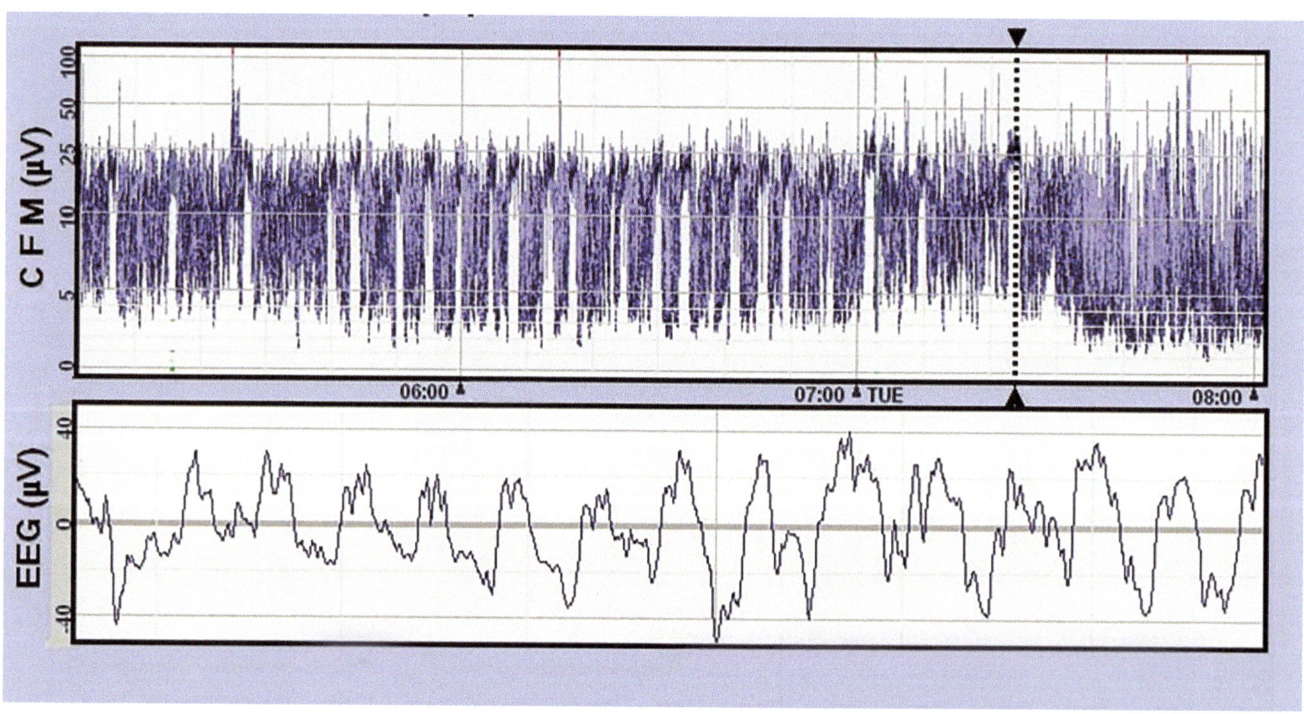

FIGURE 6.8A

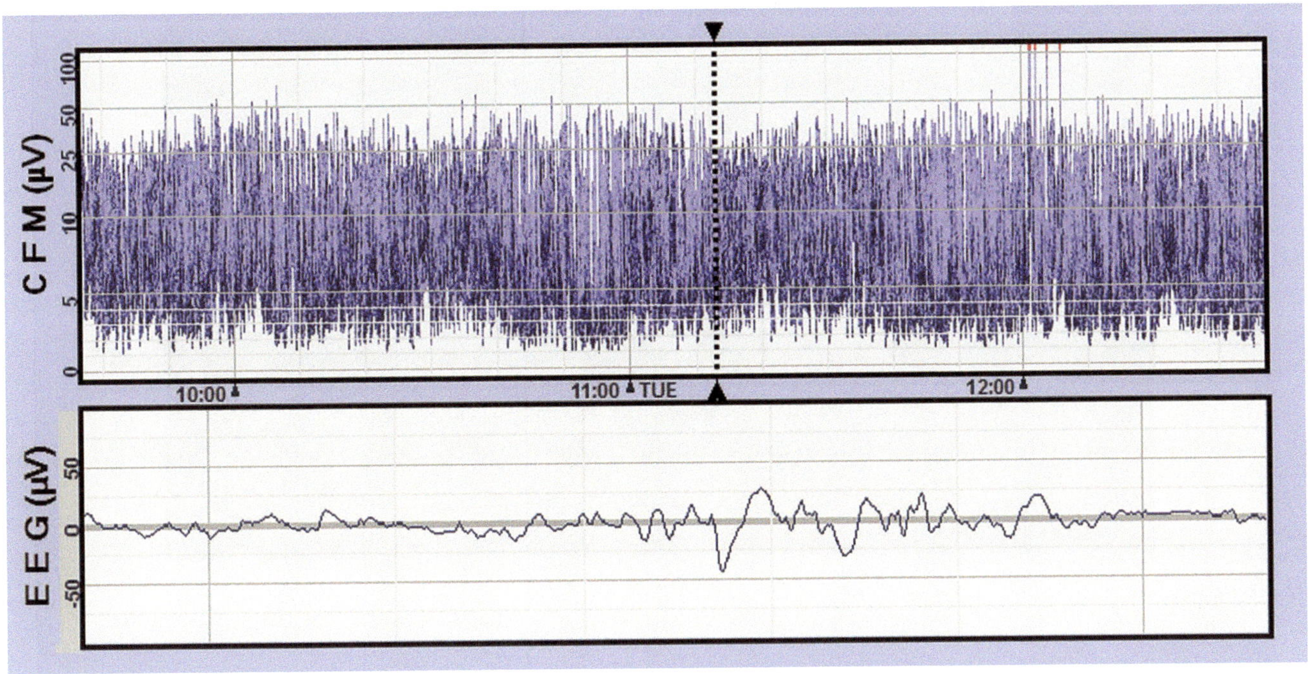

FIGURE 6.8B

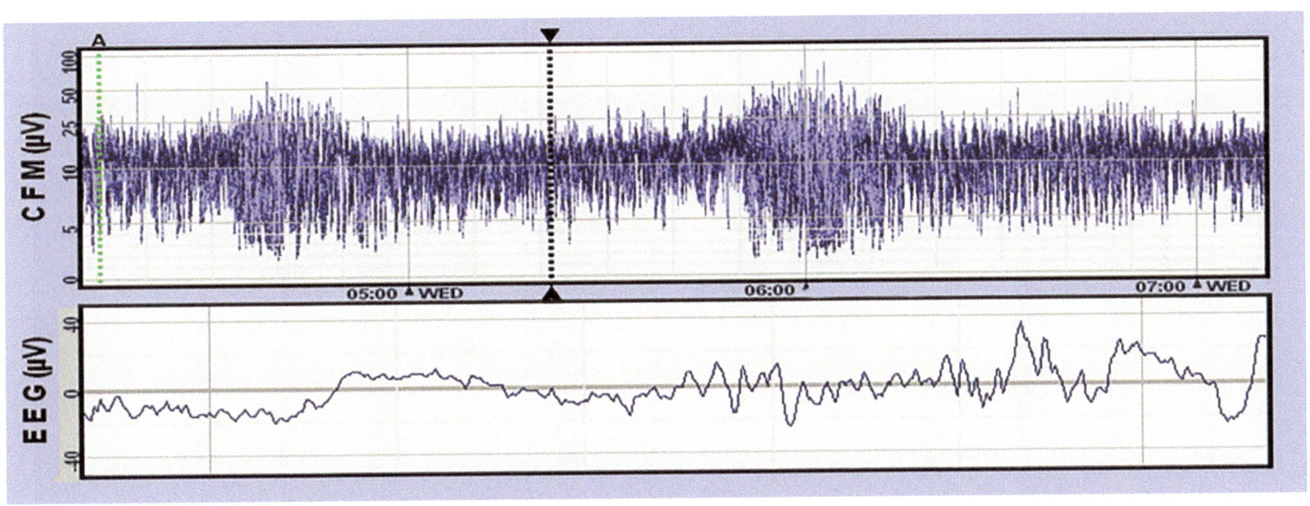

FIGURE 6.8C (From *Toet and de Vries 2012, with permission.*)

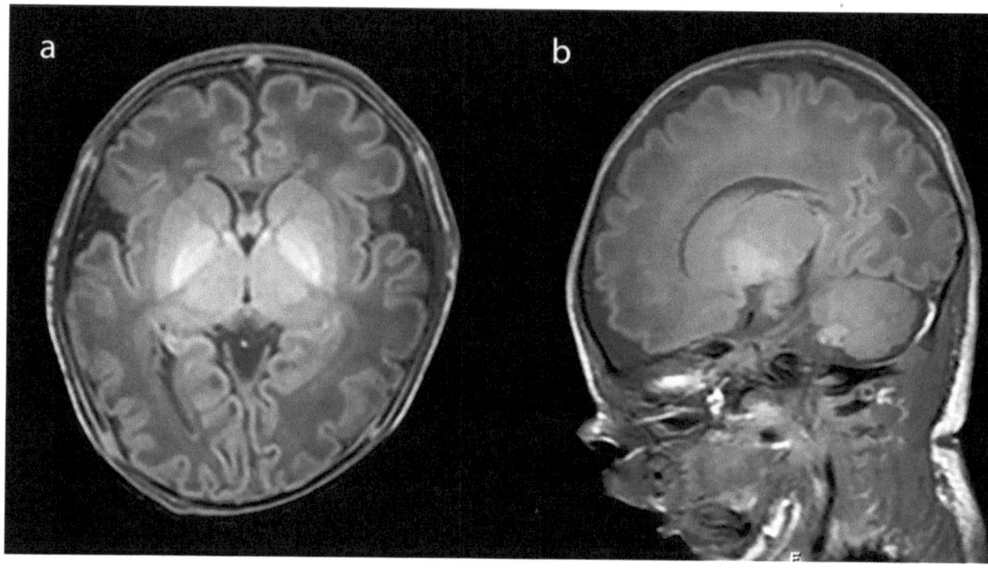

FIGURE 6.8D

Case 6.9 Full-Term Infant with Group B Streptococcus Meningitis

This infant was born at 39 weeks' gestation with a birthweight of 2910 grams. The delivery was by ventouse extraction. Apgar scores were 9, 10 and 10 at 1, 5 and 10 minutes, respectively.

The infant was admitted from home at 24 hrs, with grunting and an opisthotonic posture. Blood and CSF cultures were positive for Group B streptococci (GBS). Ventilation was required, along with inotropes for hypotension. Seizures developed within 24 hrs after admission, and phenobarbital (40 mg/kg iv), midazolam, levetiracetam (60 mg/kg iv) and lidocaine were administered in order to control the seizures.

Almost immediately after starting the *aEEG* recording, left-sided seizures (*) were noted on a predominantly burst-suppression background (Figure 6.9A). The seizures were temporarily stopped by two doses of levetiracetam (both 20 mg/kg iv) but recurred later (Figure 6.9B). After administration of lidocaine, a discontinuous pattern developed (Figure 6.9C). No further seizures were seen, and the next day, the aEEG background activity improved further and became CNV with SWC (Figure 6.9D).

Cranial ultrasound and *MRI* (Figure 6.9E) showed abnormalities in the deep grey matter, known as a typical pattern in GBS meningitis and perforator strokes. Increased echogenicity was seen on cUS (a), while MRI showed increased signal intensity on the T2-weighted sequence (b) and diffusion restriction (c).

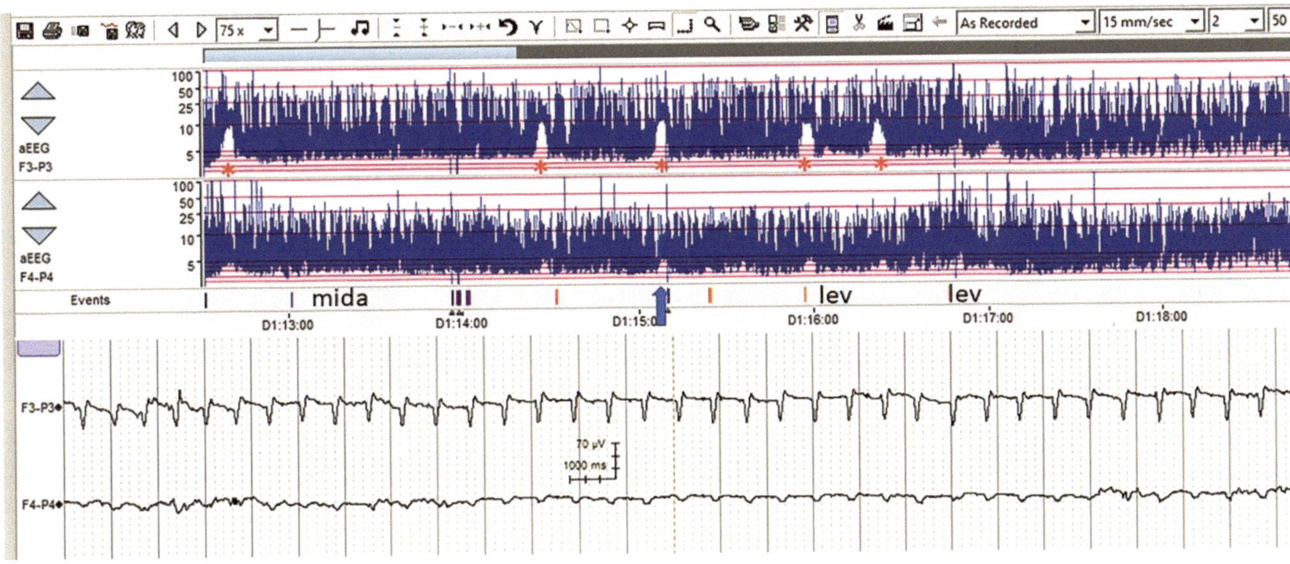

FIGURE 6.9A

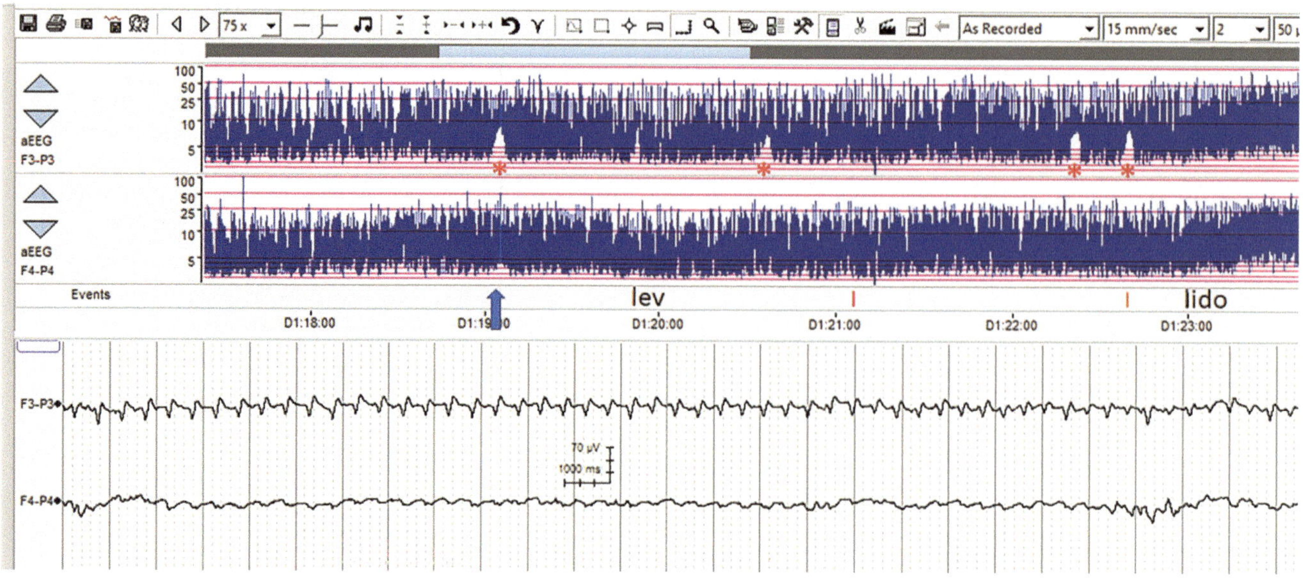

FIGURE 6.9B

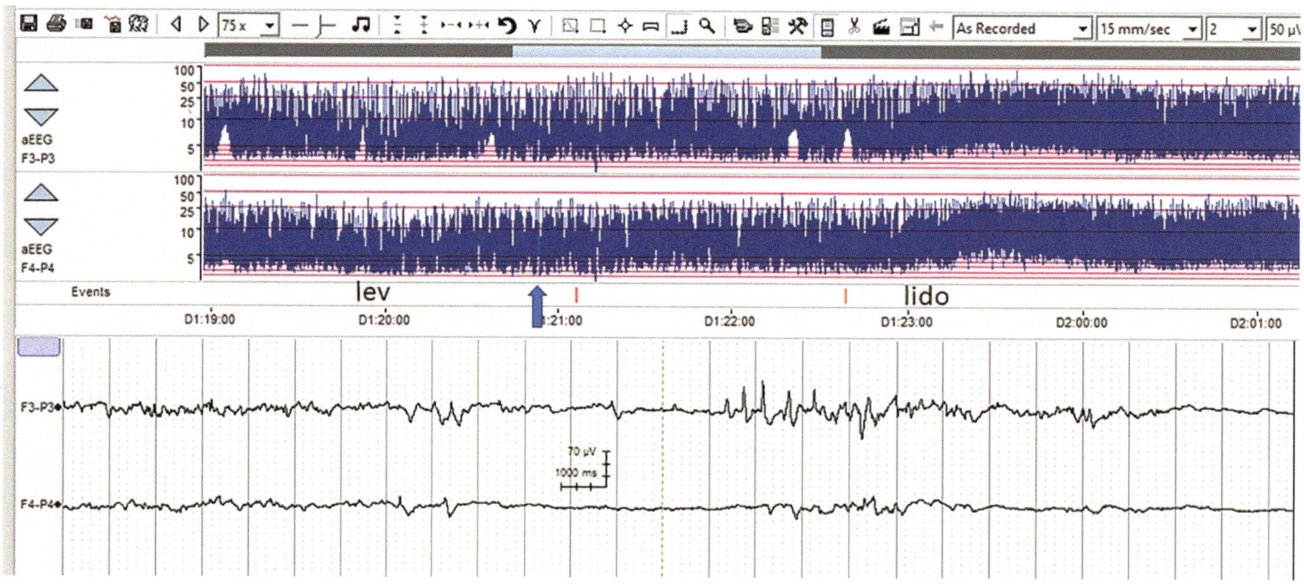

FIGURE 6.9C

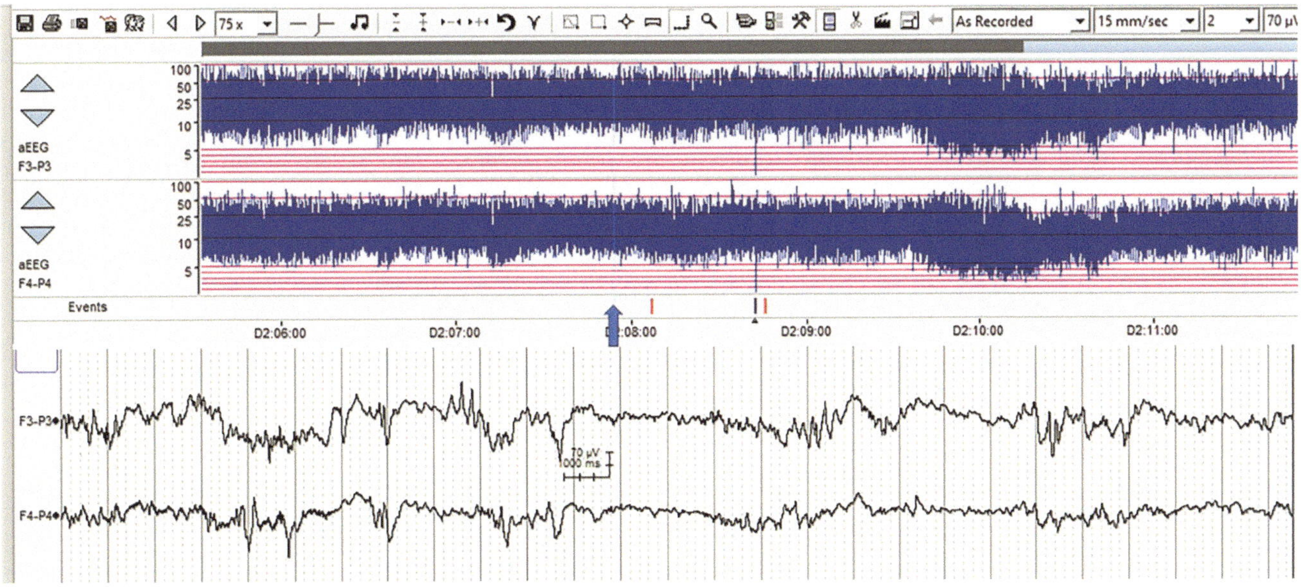

FIGURE 6.9D

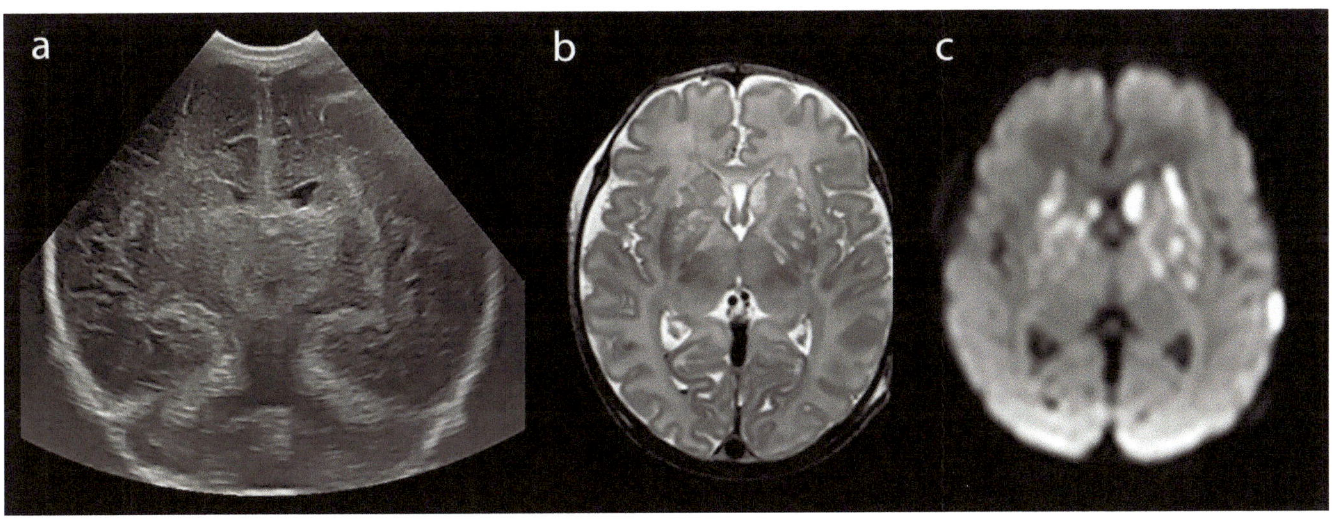

FIGURE 6.9E

Case 6.10 Full-Term Infant with HSV Meningoencephalitis

This was a term infant with an uncomplicated perinatal history who was discharged home after birth. On the seventh day after birth, the mother noted sleepiness and reported poor feeding. On day 8, the infant was brought to the emergency room for lethargy. On admission, there was encephalopathy with low tone. The baby underwent evaluation for sepsis and meningitis, and *aEEG* monitoring was initiated (Figure 6.10A).

The infant was also noted to be jaundiced, had elevated inflammatory markers and liver enzymes, and was started on antibiotics and antiviral medication.

On the *aEEG*, there were numerous areas that were interrogated and confirmed to be seizures shown with *. In between the seizures, there was a CNV background pattern. Figure 6.10B shows seven seizures and the response to phenobarbital. After phenobarbital was administered, resolution of the seizures was seen, and the background pattern became discontinuous. A lumbar puncture was performed, and PCR on the CSF was positive for herpes simplex virus.

An *MRI* (Figure 6.10C) was performed which demonstrated extensive multifocal injury. Due to significant multi-organ dysfunction and severe brain injury, care was redirected.

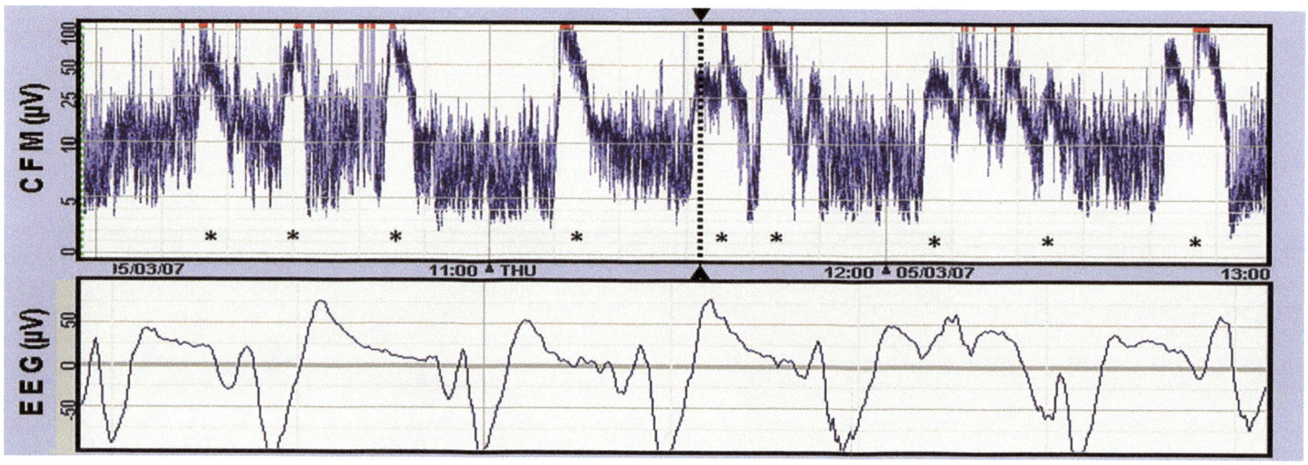

FIGURE 6.10A

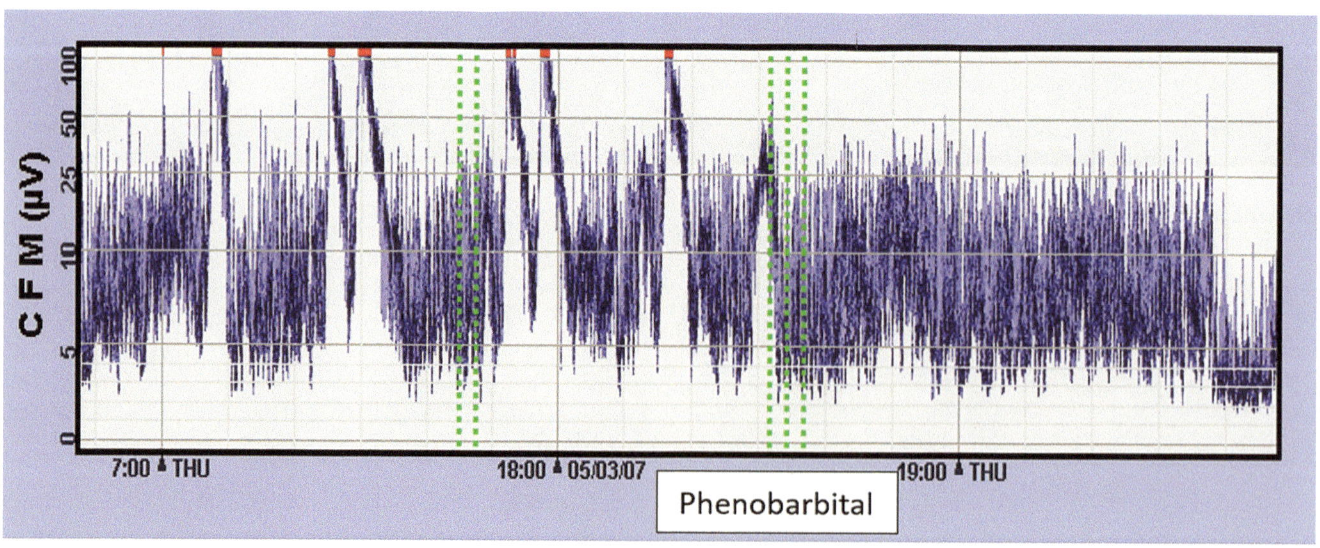

FIGURE 6.10B

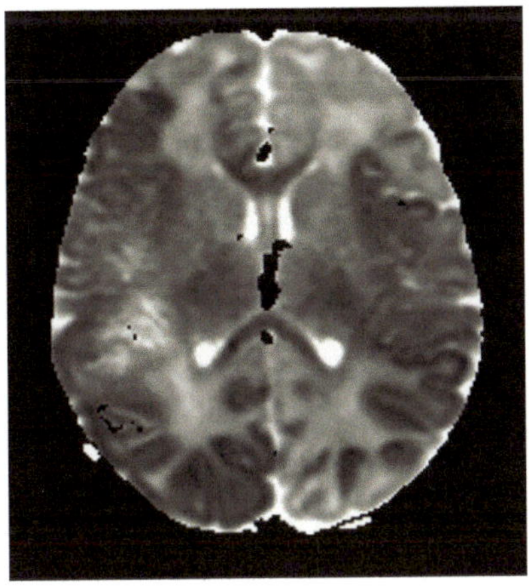

FIGURE 6.10C

Case 6.11 Late Preterm Infant with Rotavirus-Associated Encephalitis

This infant was born at 35 weeks' gestation by uneventful vaginal delivery. Birthweight was 2620 grams. The infant was discharged home after 7 days. On day 16, the infant was readmitted with drowsiness and seizures, but no fever and no diarrhea. Bacterial cultures, including CSF, were obtained, and antibiotics and acyclovir were started. Following the development of clinical and aEEG-suspected seizures, confirmed by the raw EEG trace, 20 mg/kg of phenobarbital iv was administered. Rotavirus was cultured from the stools.

aEEG was started on admission and immediately showed repetitive seizures, verified by the raw EEG, on a DNV pattern as indicated by the red asterisks. Phenobarbital was administered (20 mg/kg iv) and was able to stop the seizures (Figure 6.11A; see also Video 6.11). The next day, there was recovery of the background pattern with superimposed SWC (Figure 6.11B).

cUS (Figure 6.11C) on admission showed increased echogenicity in the periventricular white matter (a, b), and an *MRI* performed the next day (Figure 6.11D) showed high signal intensity of the white matter (a), scattered areas of restricted diffusion in the white matter, the corpus callosum (not shown), optic radiation and the pulvinar (b). A repeat MRI 6 weeks later showed cystic evolution (c). When last seen at 6 years, the movement ABC was below the 5th centile, and there were some concerns about her learning abilities.

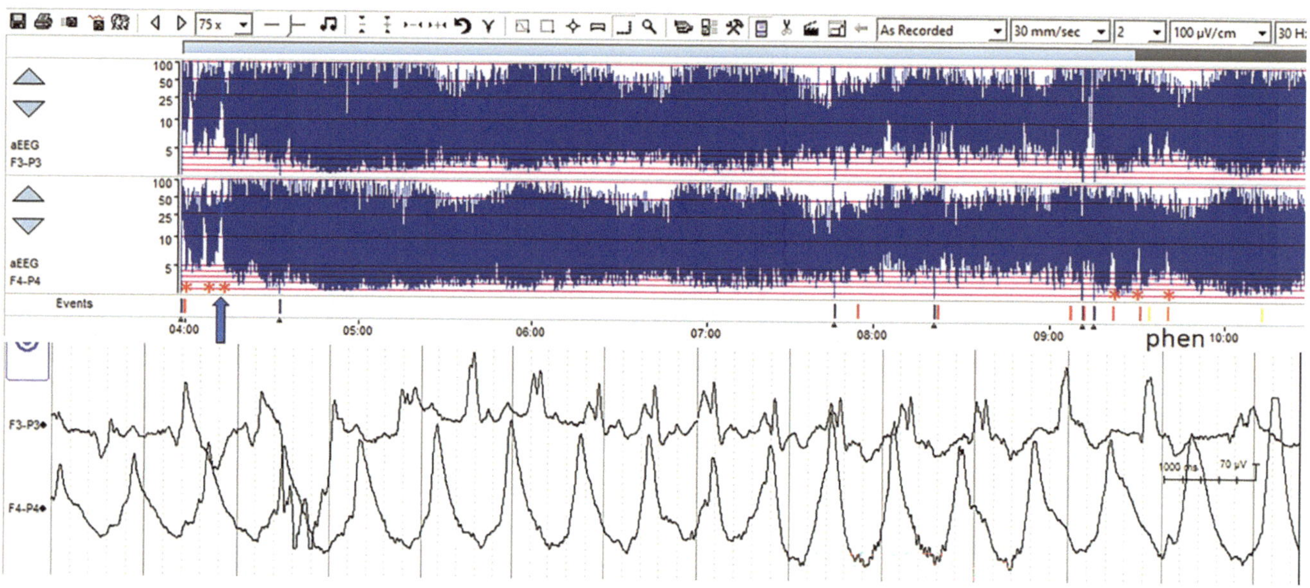

FIGURE 6.11A

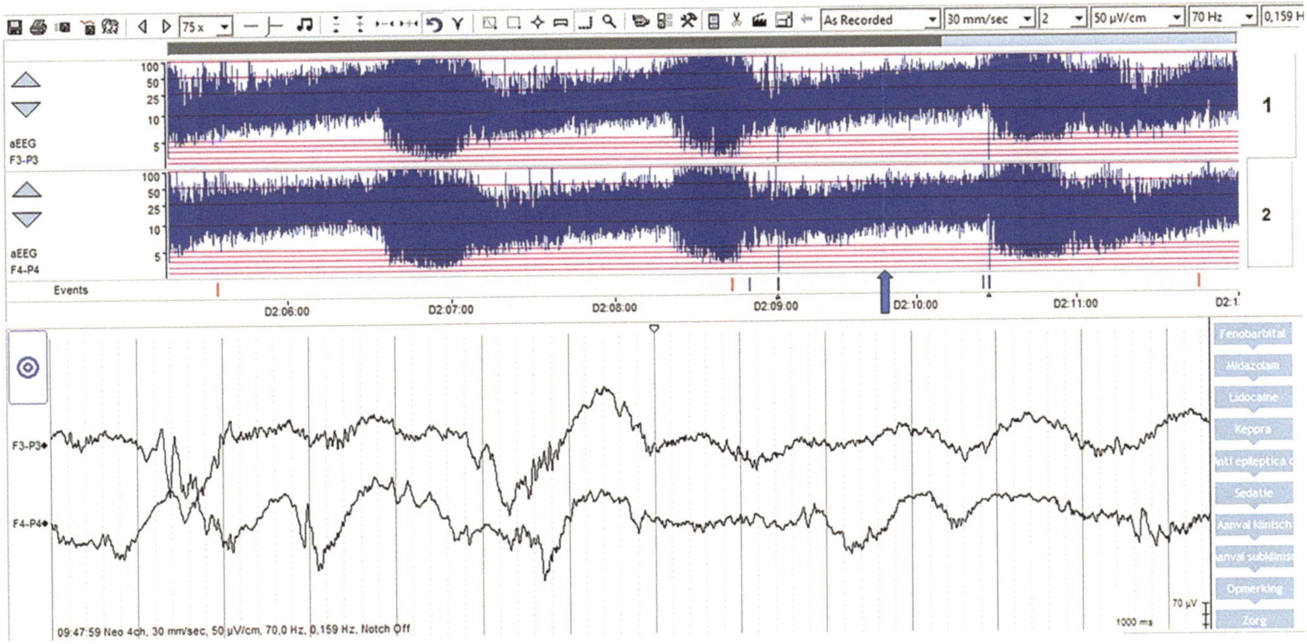

FIGURE 6.11B

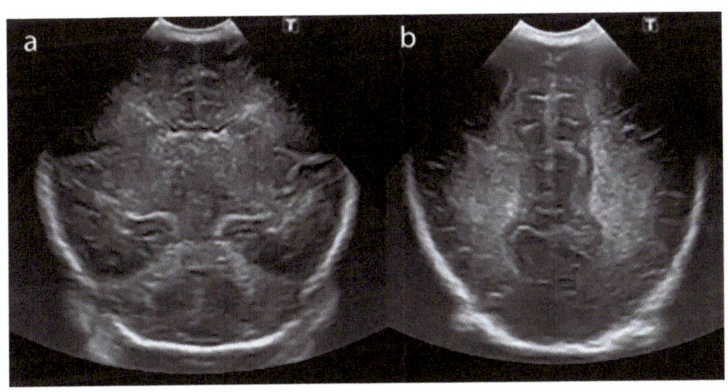

FIGURE 6.11C

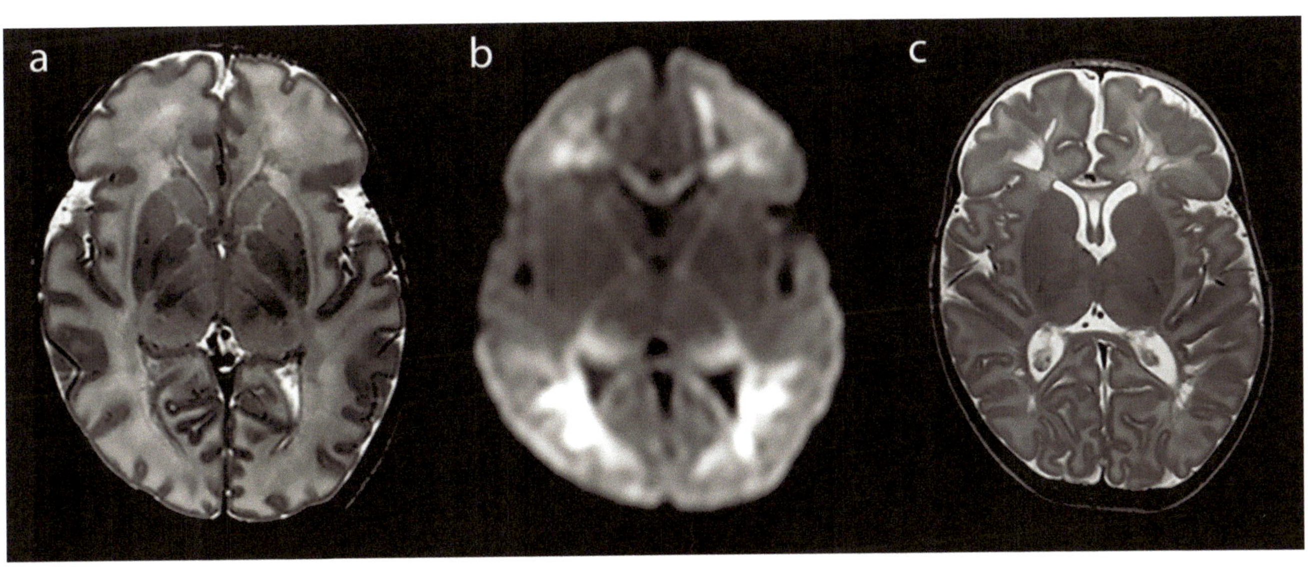

FIGURE 6.11D

Case 6.12 Full-Term Infant with Incontinentia Pigmenti

This infant was born at 39 weeks' gestation with a birthweight of 3260 grams and a head circumference of 33.5 cm. Pregnancy and delivery were uncomplicated. Apgar scores were 9 and 10 at 1 and 5 minutes, respectively.

From day 3, the infant had poor feeding, was difficult and was lethargic. The parents had noted a rash on the limbs the previous day. There also were problems keeping the temperature, and the infant was admitted to the hospital. On admission, there was a low muscular tone and a fixed posture of the head to the right, with nystagmus to the right as well. The infant developed apneas and was referred to the NICU for neuromonitoring.

The *aEEG* showed repetitive seizures on a CNV background (Figure 6.12A). The 12 seconds of EEG, below the aEEG, shows a right-sided seizure at time 10:04 (marked by a thick vertical line in the aEEG). The seizures were stopped after a loading dose of lidocaine (Figure 6.12B). The seizure shown occurred just before the administration of lidocaine. After which, the aEEG pattern became discontinuous, and no seizures were noted.

cUS showed inhomogeneous echogenicity, and the *MRI* performed the next day (Figure 6.12C) showed increased signal intensity on the T2 sequence (a) and DWI (b). A few cysts were seen in the left frontal lobe. The skin lesions following the lines of Blaschko were seen on the lower limb.

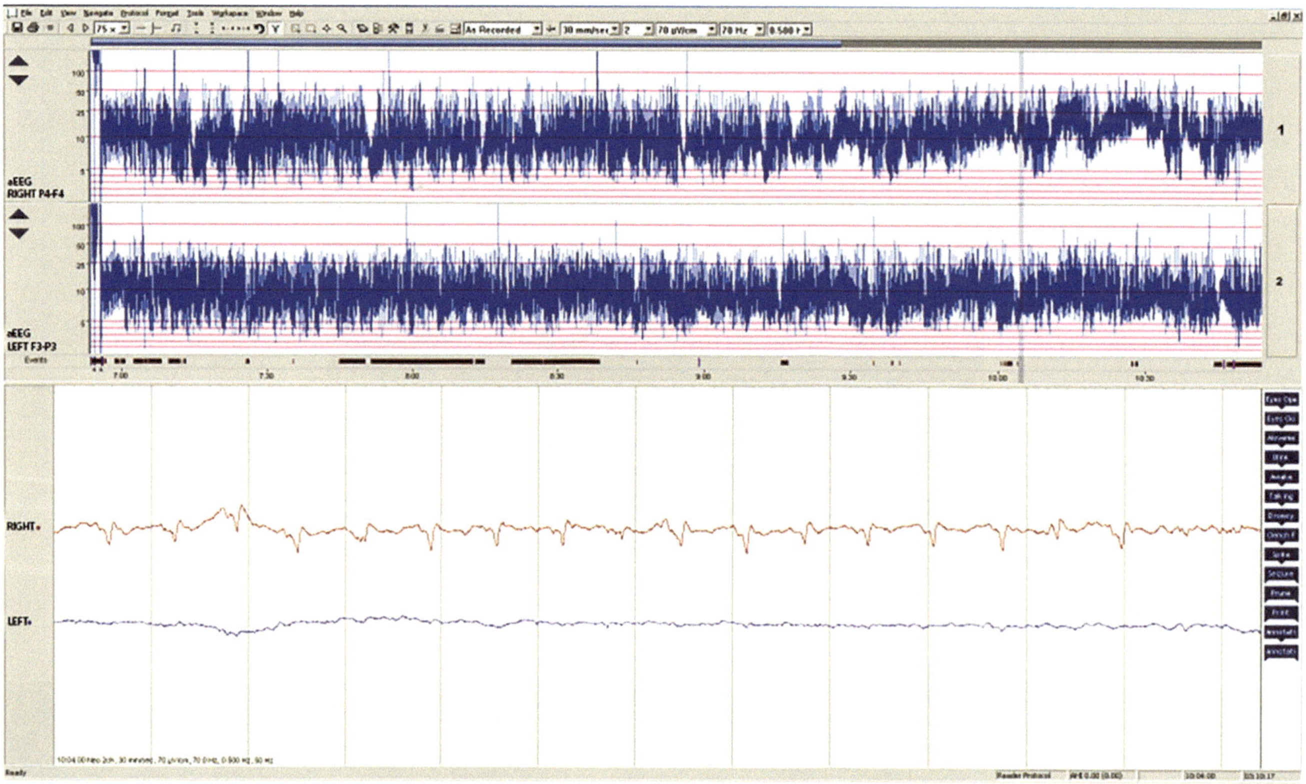

FIGURE 6.12A

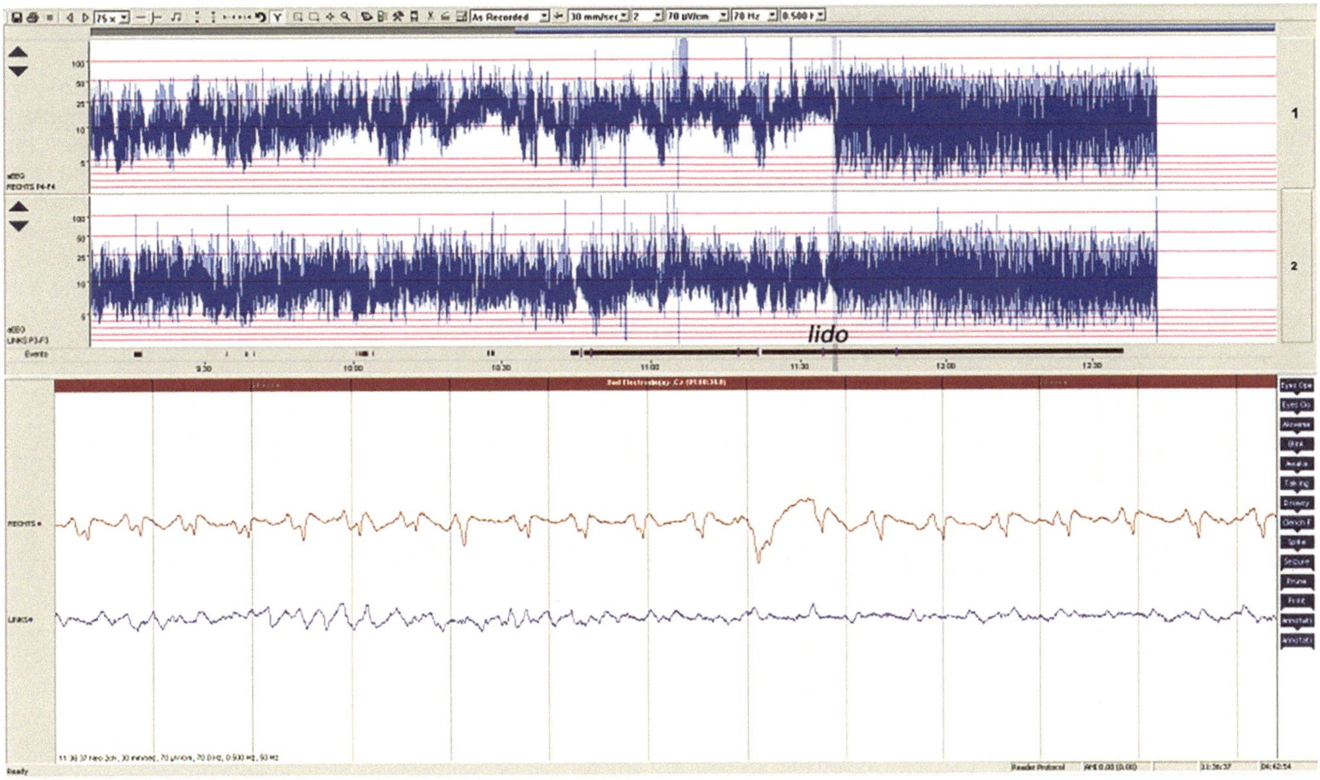

FIGURE 6.12B

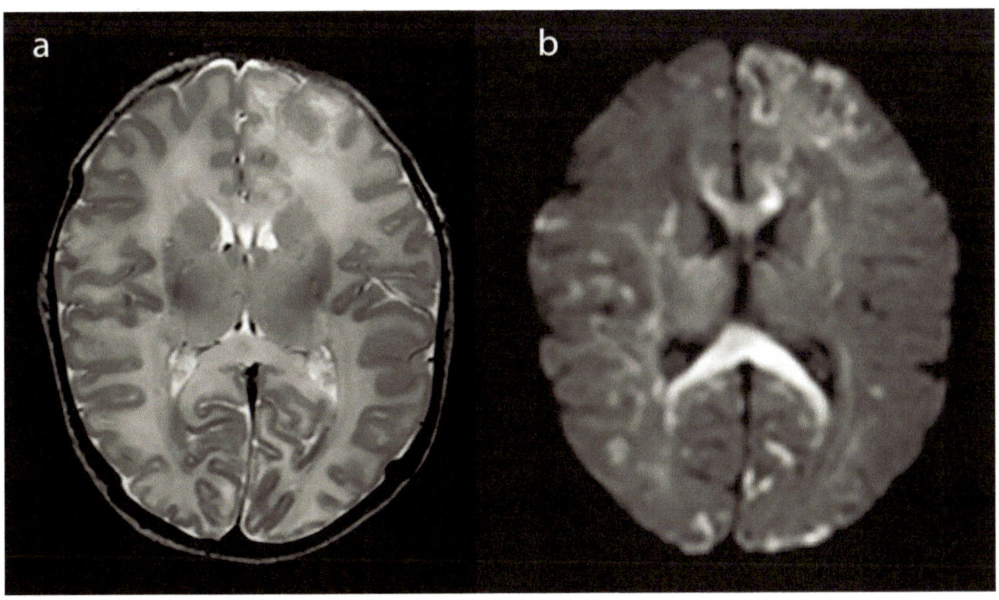

FIGURE 6.12C

Case 6.13 Full-Term Infant with Hemimegalencephaly

This term infant was born with an uncomplicated vaginal delivery and good Apgar scores of 7 and 9 at 1 and 5 minutes. Clinical seizures developed at one hour after birth and the infant was referred to the NICU for neuromonitoring.

Soon after starting the *aEEG*, suspected seizures were seen on aEEG and confirmed on the raw EEG. There was an asymmetry in amplitude, being higher on the affected side. The seizures lasted around 60 seconds and were seen over both hemispheres with a very high voltage on the affected left side. Following two doses of phenobarbital (each 20 mg/kg iv) and midazolam, lidocaine was given with a temporary reduction of the seizures (Figure 6.13A; see also Video 6.13). In Figure 6.13B, however, seizures recurred, and levetiracetam (20 mg/kg iv three times) was given, without a clear effect.

An *MRI* (Figure 6.13C, a and b) T2-weighted sequence shows the enlarged left hemisphere, with abnormal migration and periventricular noduli. A mutation in the *TSC1* gene was found.

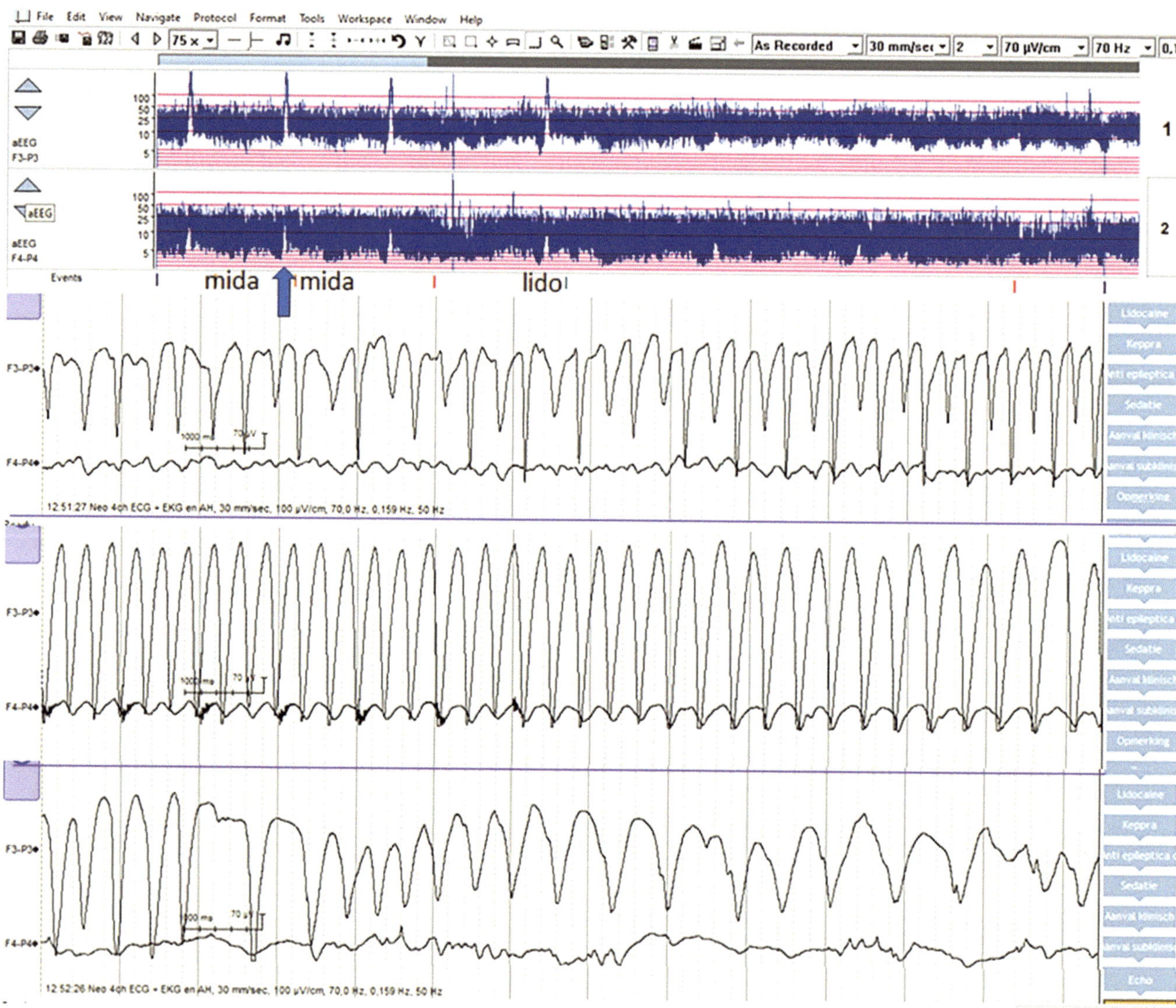

FIGURE 6.13A

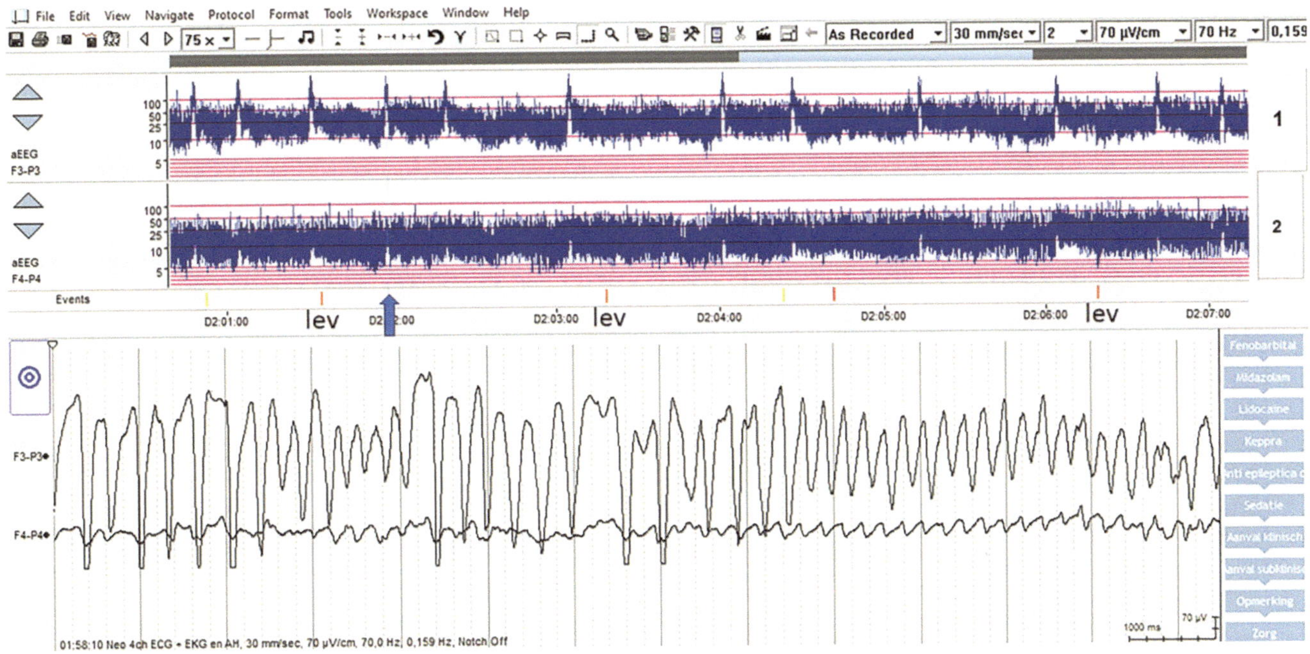

FIGURE 6.13B

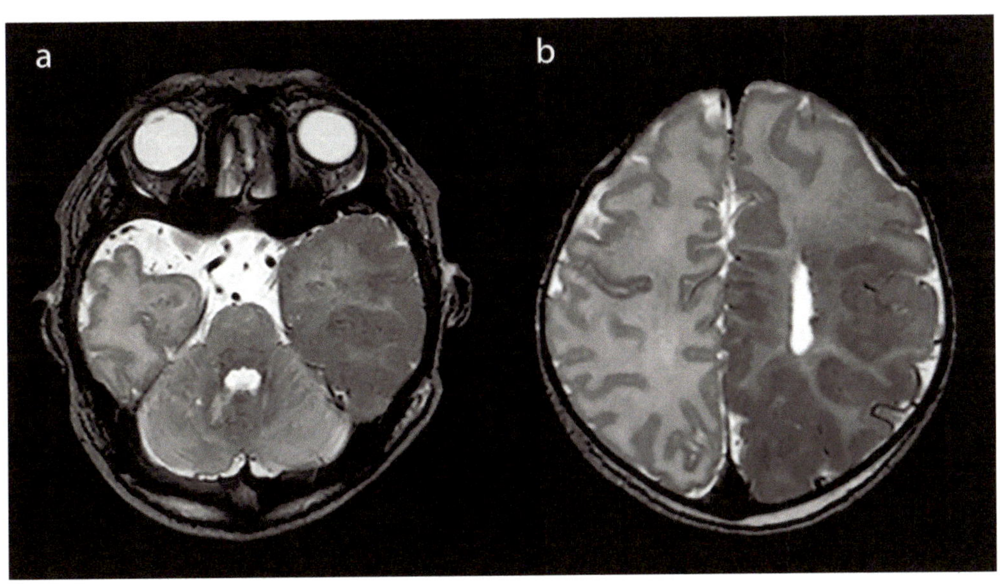

FIGURE 6.13C

Case 6.14 Full-Term Infant with Hemimegalencephaly

This infant was born at 39 weeks' gestation with a birthweight of 3550 g. Apgar scores were 4, 7 and 9 at 1, 5 and 10 minutes, respectively. The infant was macrocephalic (head circumference 36 cm) and developed seizures within 12 hours after birth. Several antiseizure medications were administered in an attempt to control the seizures, but none were able to do so. No mutation was found using whole exome sequencing.

The *aEEG* showed an asymmetry in the background pattern with more discontinuous and high-voltage amplitude, and high-voltage bursts, on the affected right side (Figure 6.14A). After adjusting the y-axis scale, the upper voltage margin of the aEEG trace can be seen (Figure 6.14B). A seizure discharge is seen on the right side (* at time 14:54), and the evolution of the seizure discharge is shown in the four EEG panels later (Figure 6.14C). Ongoing seizure activity is seen during the period highlighted by the red band (Figure 6.14D). A standard EEG was performed, and continuous epileptiform abnormalities were seen in the right hemisphere, with intermittent seizure discharges. Seizures recurred, and midazolam was given after 10 seizures (Figure 6.14E) with immediate response and change of background to a more burst-suppression–like pattern.

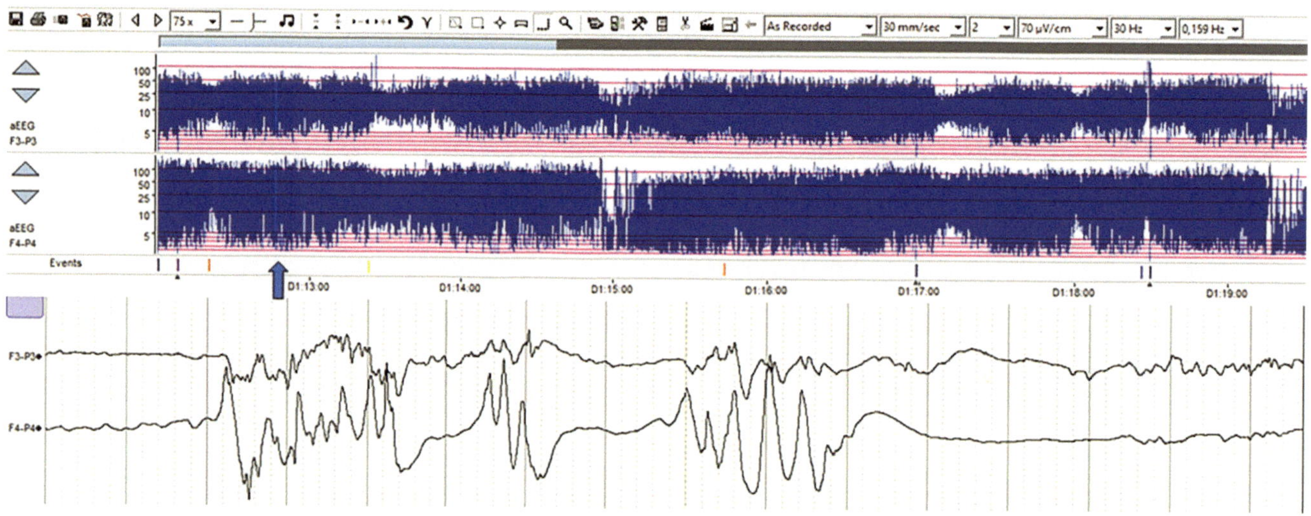

FIGURE 6.14A

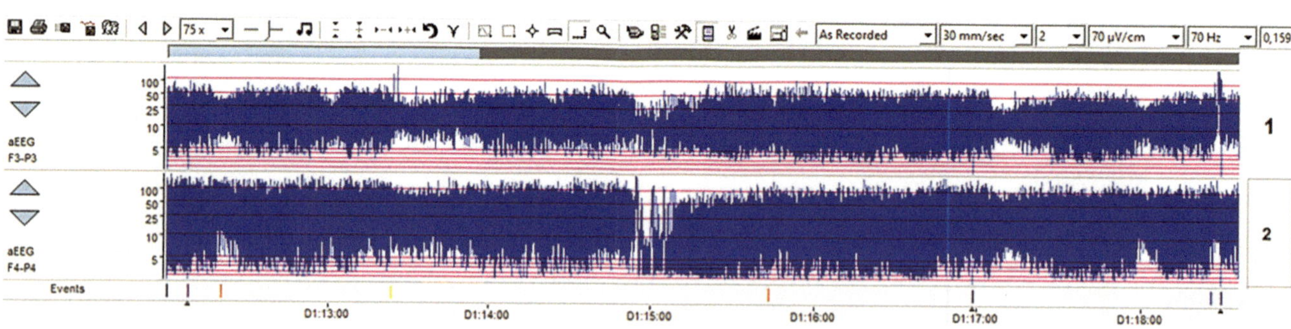

FIGURE 6.14B

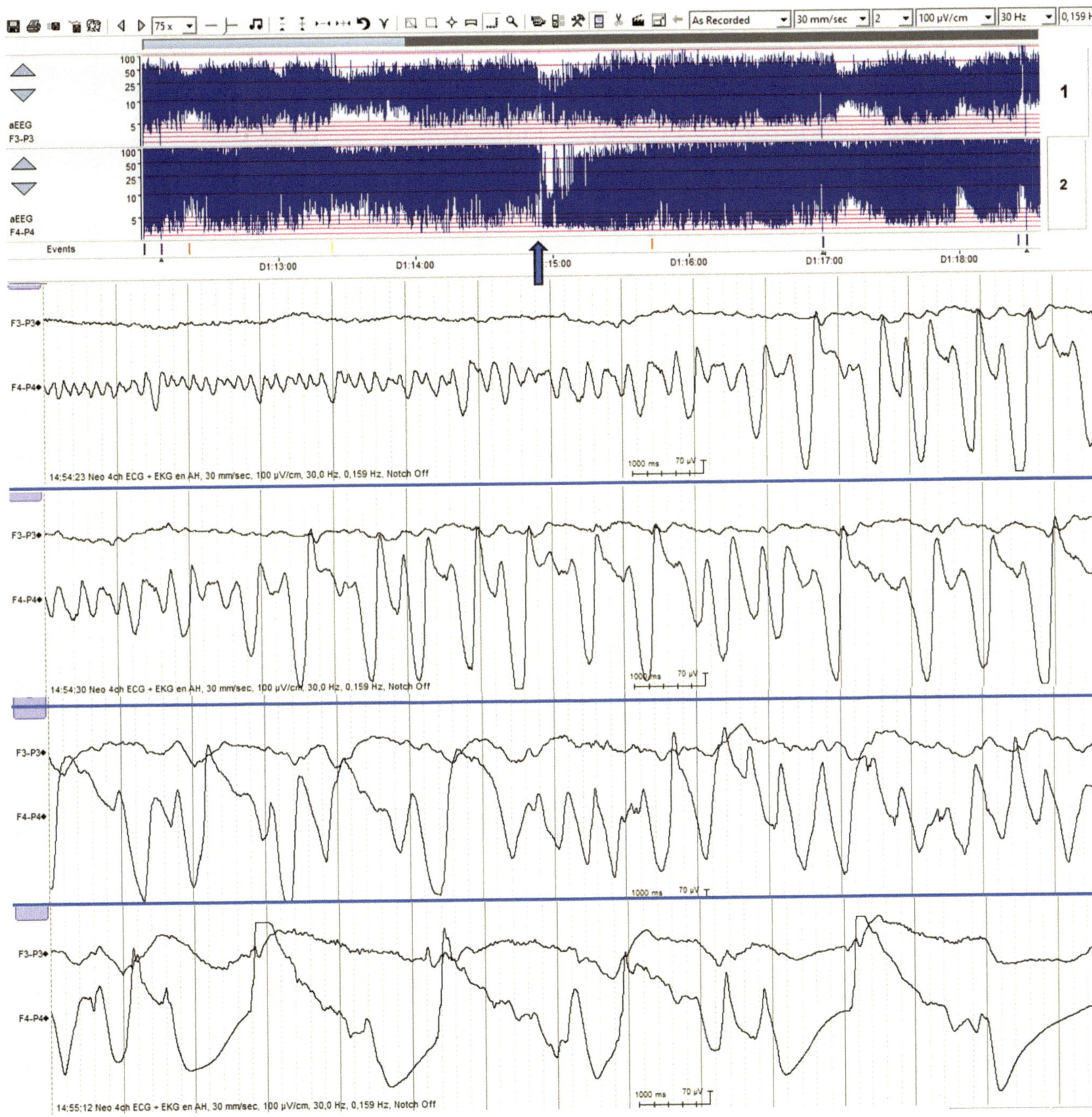

FIGURE 6.14C

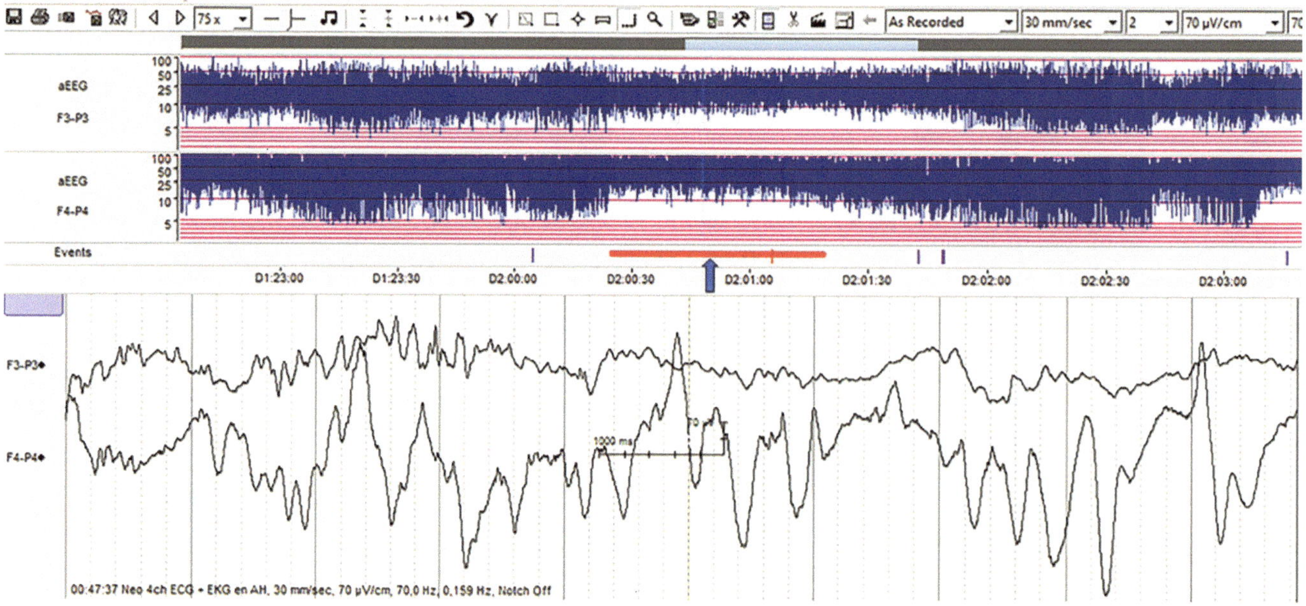

FIGURE 6.14D

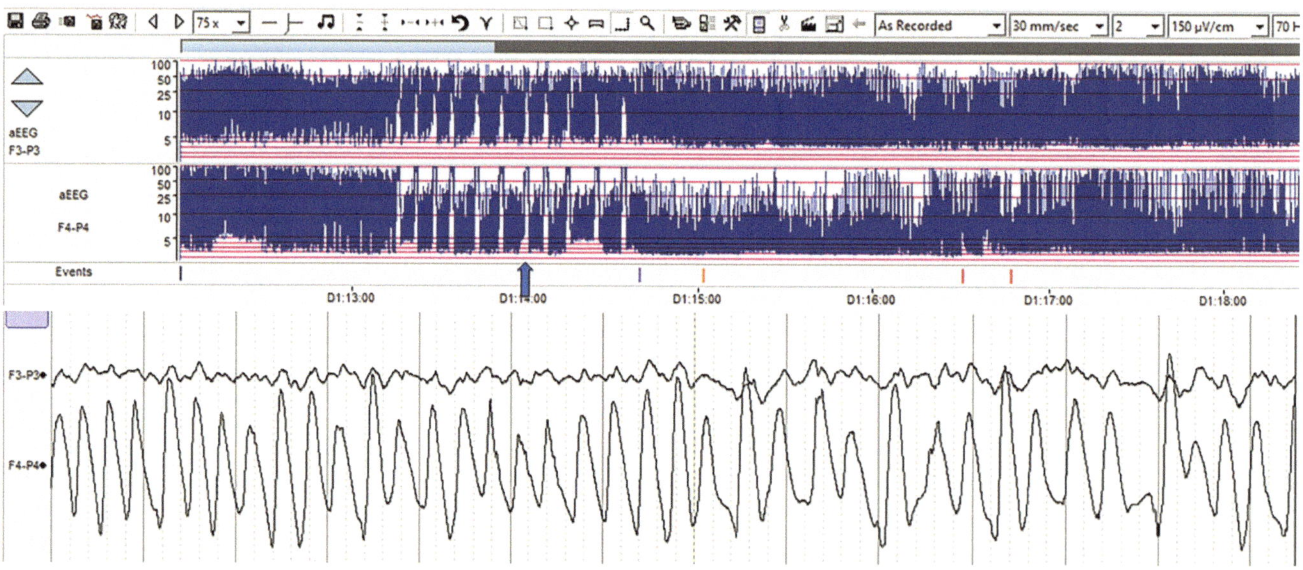

FIGURE 6.14E

Case 6.15 Full-Term Infant with Cortical Malformation

This infant was born by C-section at 38 weeks' gestation. There was a prenatal diagnosis of cortical malformation. At birth, the infant was diffusely hypotonic and received one minute of positive pressure ventilation (PPV). Apgar scores were 4 and 8 at 1 and 5 minutes, respectively. She was admitted to the NICU on room air. Within a few hours, there were multiple respiratory events and concern for abnormal movements. No explanatory mutation was found using whole exome sequencing. In view of the poor prognosis, care was redirected.

aEEG monitoring was started and showed evidence of seizures. Patient received 20 mg/kg iv of phenobarbital. In between the seizures, the background activity shows a DNV pattern. The number of ictal discharges increases in this first figure (Figure 6.15A). The recording is shown with the seizure detection algorithm in Figure 6.15B (short orange markers above the aEEG) and also showing when phenobarbital and fosphenytoin are administered. The right-sided seizure in the EEG later displays the activity in one of the first seizures in the aEEG (orange vertical line through aEEG trace). As the discharges continued, midazolam was given (Figure 6.15C) with a good effect on the seizures and a change of the electrocortical background to a BS pattern.

MRI was performed (Figure 6.15D) and showed severe ventricular dilation and a cortical malformation on the T2-weighted images, axial (a) and coronal (b) view, and a small rotated vermis on the midsagittal view (c).

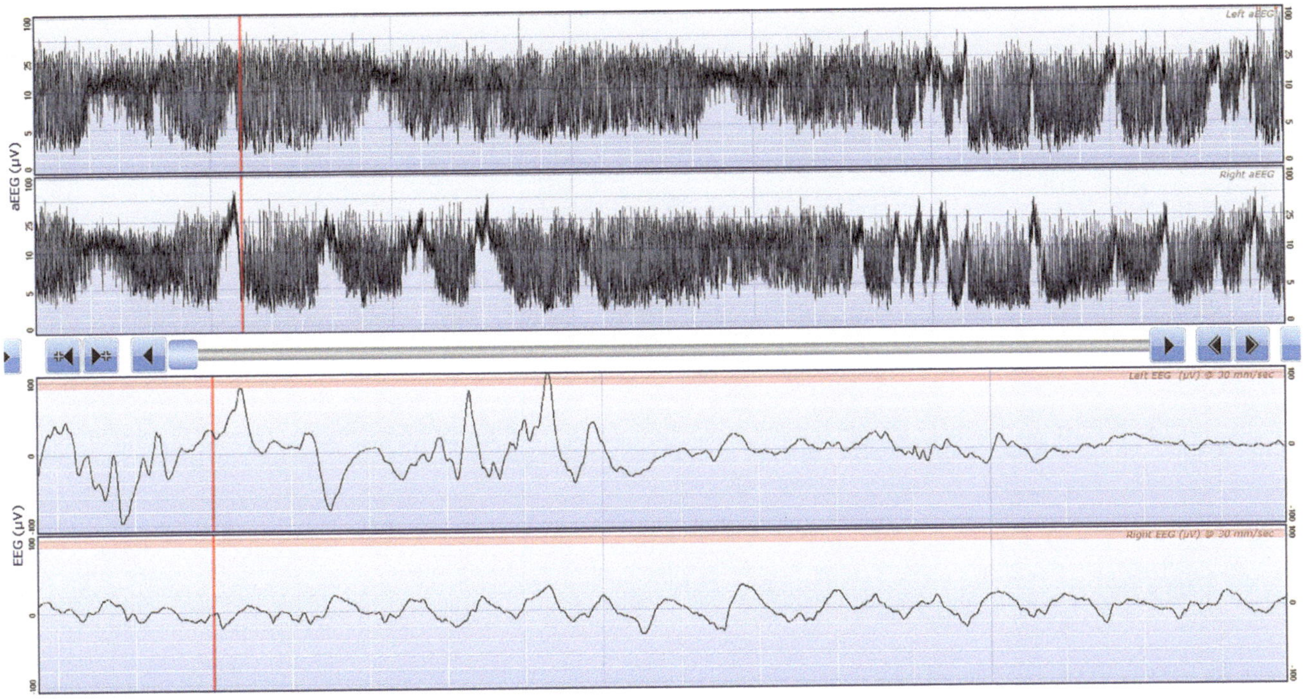

FIGURE 6.15A

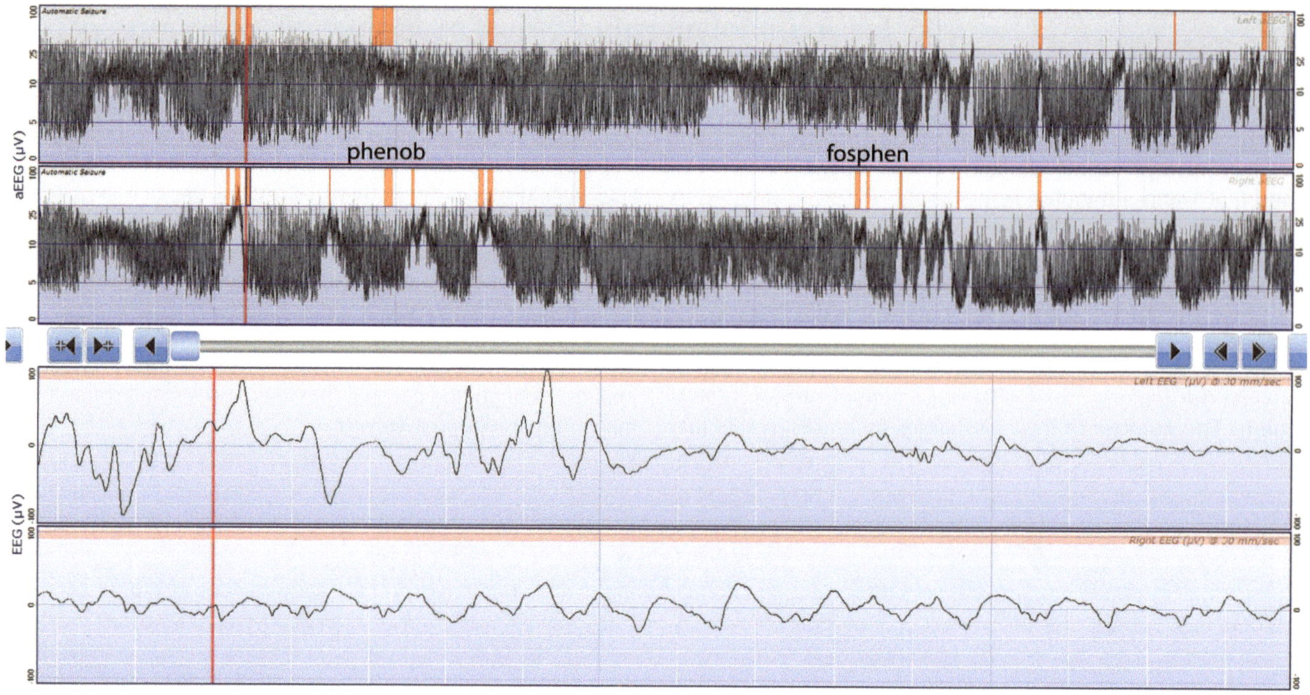

FIGURE 6.15B

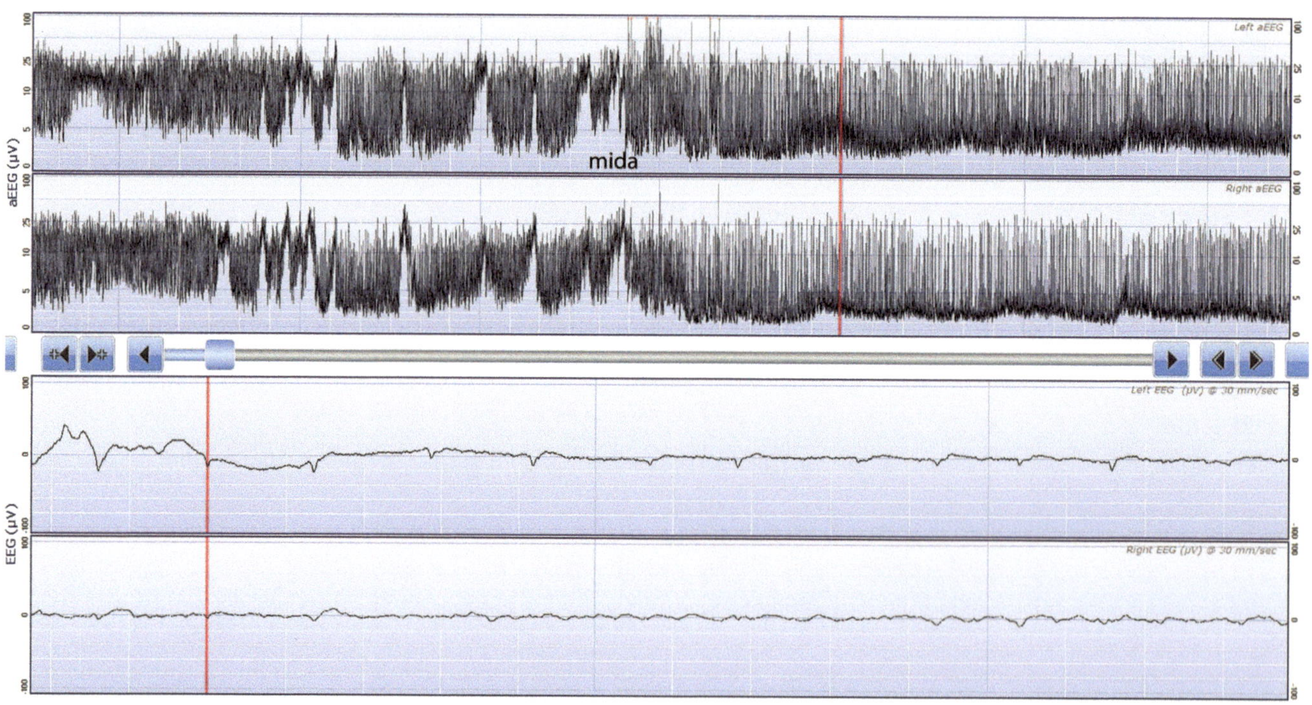

FIGURE 6.15C

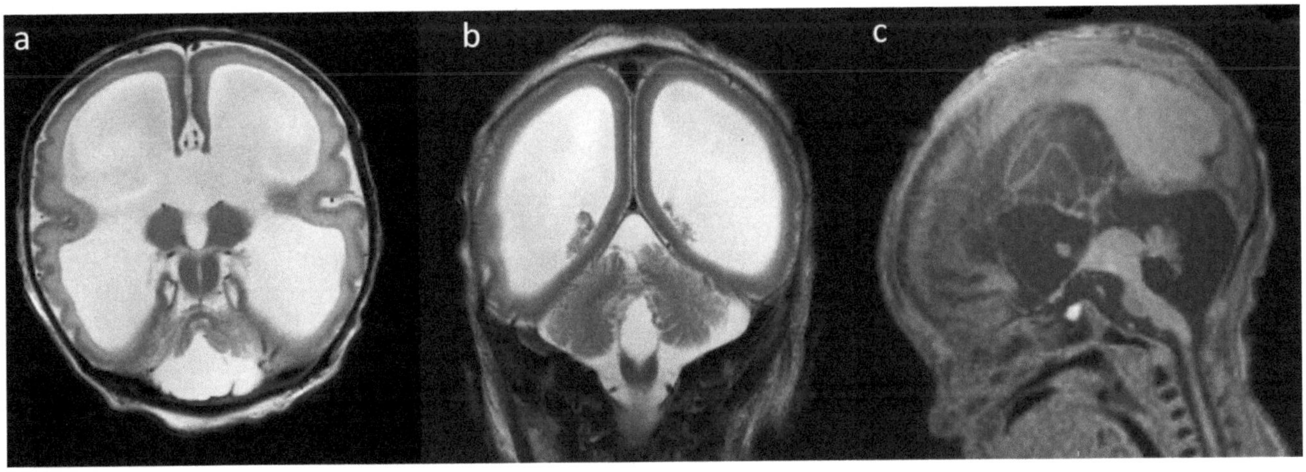

FIGURE 6.15D

Case 6.16 Full-Term Infant with Channelopathy

This infant was born at term with a birthweight of 3600 g. The delivery was uncomplicated. The Apgar scores were 6 and 9 at 1 and 5 minutes, respectively. The umbilical artery pH was 7.35 with a base excess of −6.3 mmol/L. Twelve hours after birth, tonic movements with turning the head to one side were noted, followed by clonic limb movements. A loading dose of phenobarbital (20 mg/kg iv) was administered, and the infant was transferred to the NICU for neuromonitoring.

aEEG showed an increasing number of clinical and electrographic seizures following admission. Phenobarbital (40 mg/kg), levetiracetam (60 mg/kg) and midazolam (0.3 mg/kg/h) were administered but all were ineffective. The suspected seizures in the aEEG had a very characteristic appearance that has been associated with channelopathies. The brief interruptions of the aEEG pattern represent seizures and are followed by a short postictal suppression (Figure 6.16A; see also Video 6.16). In Figure 6.16B, lidocaine was given, and this ASM was able to control the seizures. The initial background activity was slightly discontinuous in Figure 6.16A but showed a CNV pattern in Figure 6.16B, and in Figure 6.16C, this improved further with established SWC. After the lidocaine was stopped, there was recurrence of seizures, and three seizures are shown in Figure 6.16D. Finally, carbamazepine and pyridoxine were given, and the seizures were controlled. Following the results of genetic testing, showing *KCNQ2* mutation (c 997 C>T;pArg 333 Trp), pyridoxine was stopped and carbamazepine was continued.

This infant was born almost 10 years ago, well before a paper was published reporting the typical pattern for infants with a channelopathy. The same aEEG pattern is seen in infants with SCN2A and KCNQ3 mutations.

Bibliography

Pijpers JA, Au PYB, Weeke LC, et al. Early recognition of characteristic conventional and amplitude-integrated EEG patterns of seizures in SCN2A and KCNQ3-related epilepsy in neonates. *Seizure.* 2023;110:212–219.

Vilan A, Mendes Ribeiro J, Striano P, et al. A distinctive ictal amplitude-integrated electroencephalography pattern in newborns with neonatal epilepsy associated with KCNQ2 mutations. *Neonatology.* 2017;112(4):387–393.

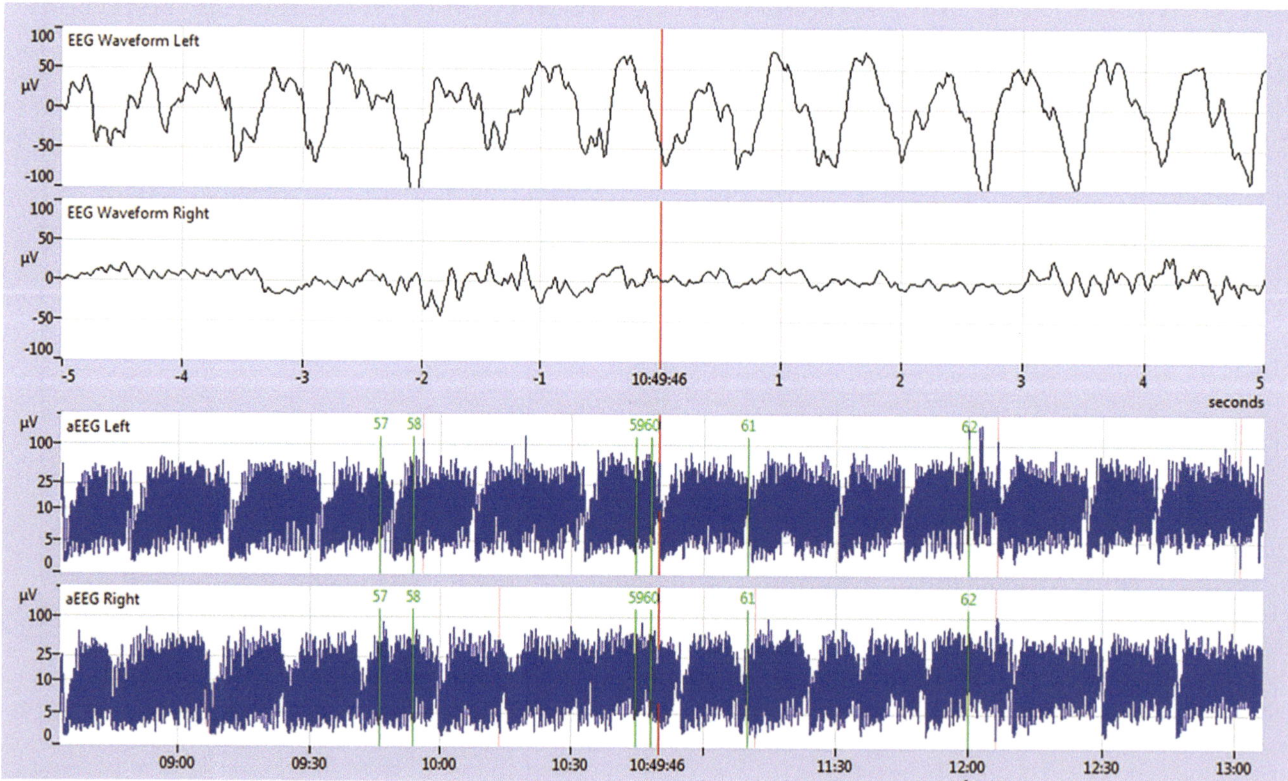

FIGURE 6.16A

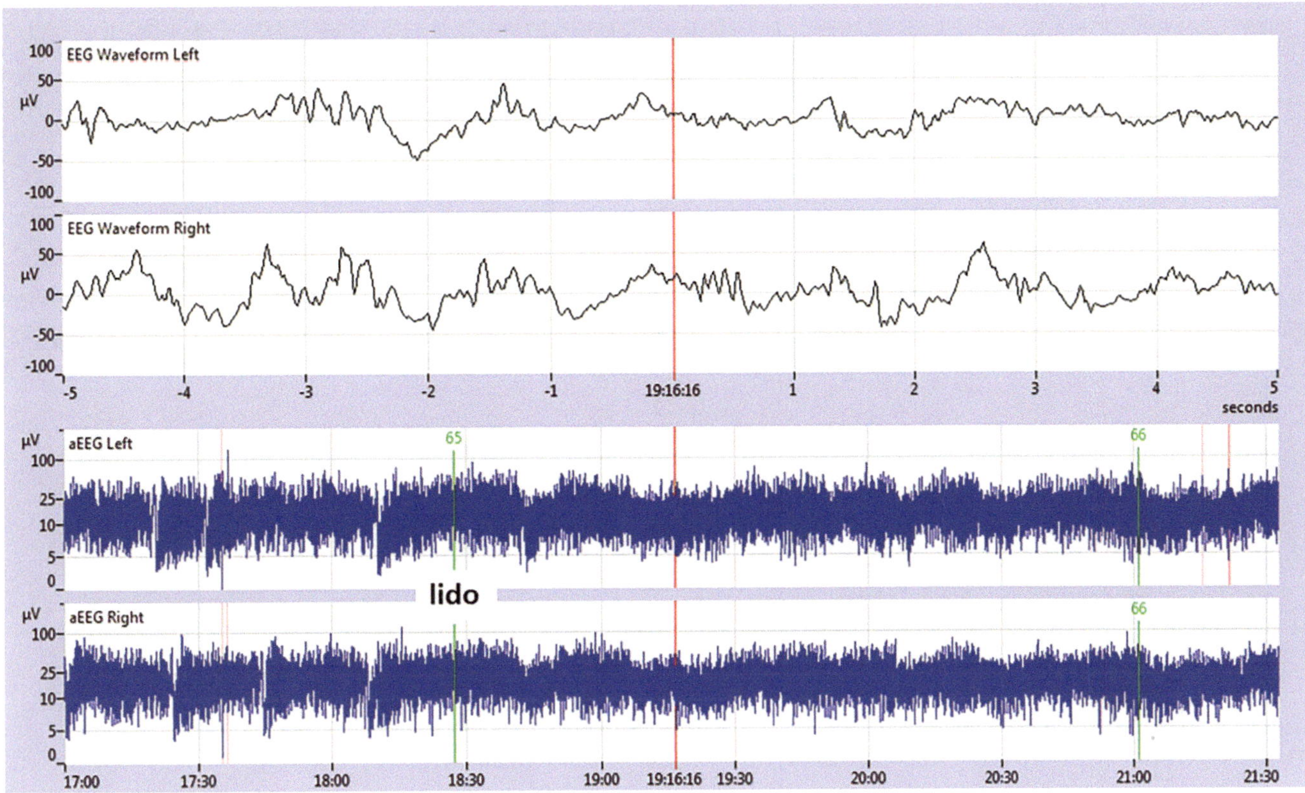

FIGURE 6.16B

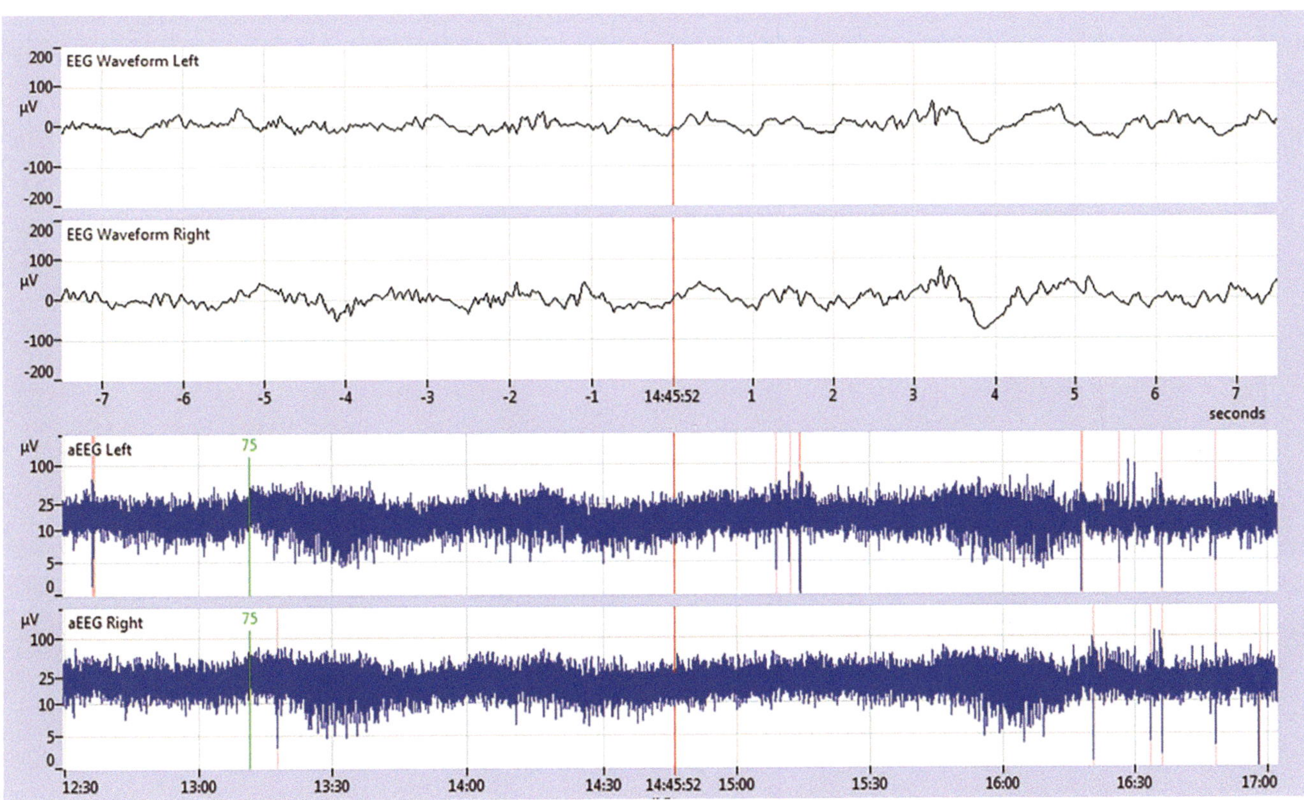

FIGURE 6.16C

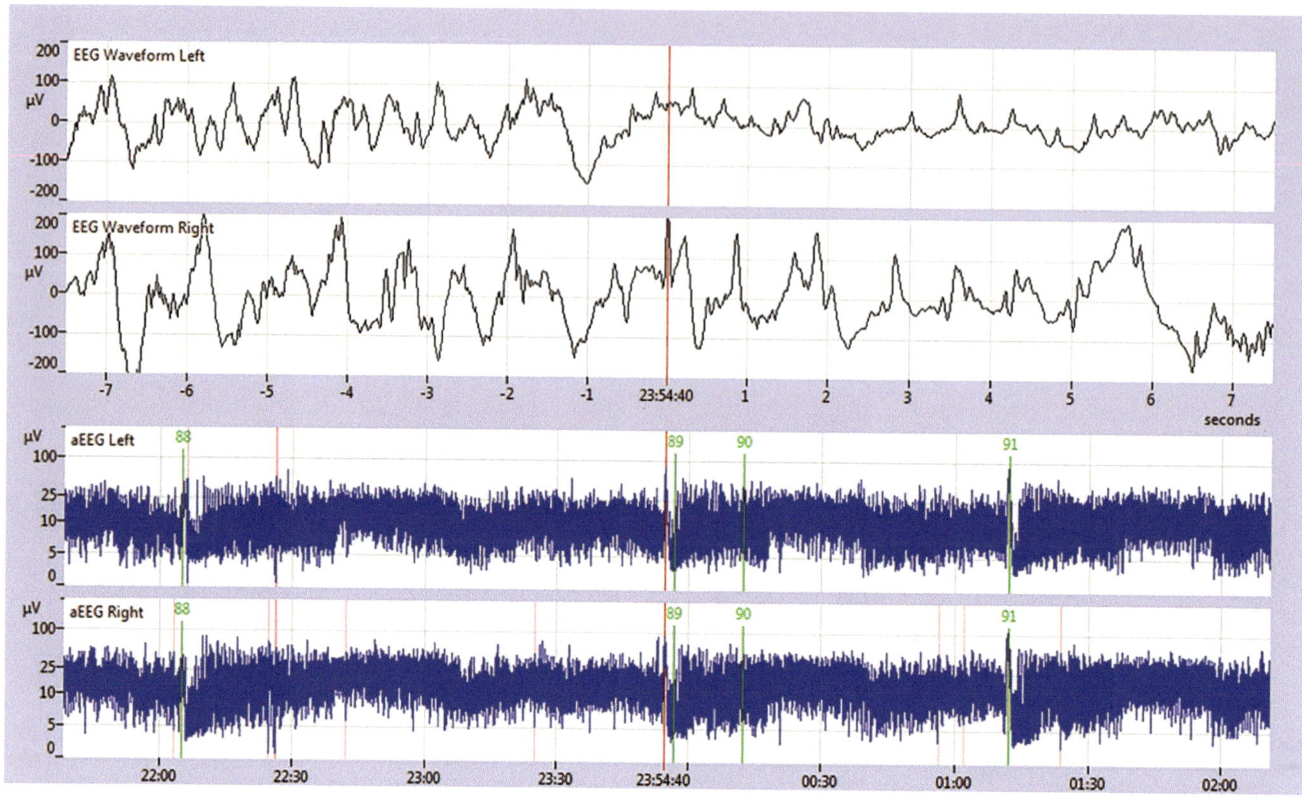
EEG Waveform Left
200
100
µV
0
-100
-200
EEG Waveform Right
200
100
µV
0
-100
-200
-7 -6 -5 -4 -3 -2 -1 23:54:40 1 2 3 4 5 6 7
seconds
µV
aEEG Left
100
25
10
5
0
88 89 90 91
µV
aEEG Right
100
25
10
5
0
88 89 90 91
22:00 22:30 23:00 23:30 23:54:40 00:30 01:00 01:30 02:00

FIGURE 6.16D

Case 6.17 Full-Term Infant with Developmental and Epileptic Encephalopathy (DEE)

This infant was the third child of healthy non-related parents. The pregnancy and delivery at 38 weeks' gestation were normal. Birthweight was 3610 g, and Apgar scores were 9, 10 and 10 at 1, 5 and 10 minutes, respectively. She was initially doing well but was readmitted to the hospital at 6 days due to lethargy and feeding problems, with a weight loss > 10%. Brief suspected clonic seizures were noted 3–4 times per day. Repeated initial EEGs showed BS but no seizures. An extensive neurometabolic investigation was performed but did not give a specific diagnosis. From 1 month of age, an increasing number of myoclonic seizures developed, sometimes accompanied by apneas. The infant received anti-seizure medication, including corticosteroids and pyridoxine, without improvement of the seizures, and died at 3 months of age. The clinical picture together with the continuing BS on EEG led to the diagnosis of Developmental and Epileptic Encephalopathy (DEE), previously referred to as Ohtahara syndrome. The infant was born before the era of whole exome sequencing.

The neonatal *MRI* was considered to be normal. The 4-hour *aEEG* was recorded on postnatal day 10 and showed BS but no seizures (Figure 6.17A) (Courtesy of Katarina Strand-Brodd).

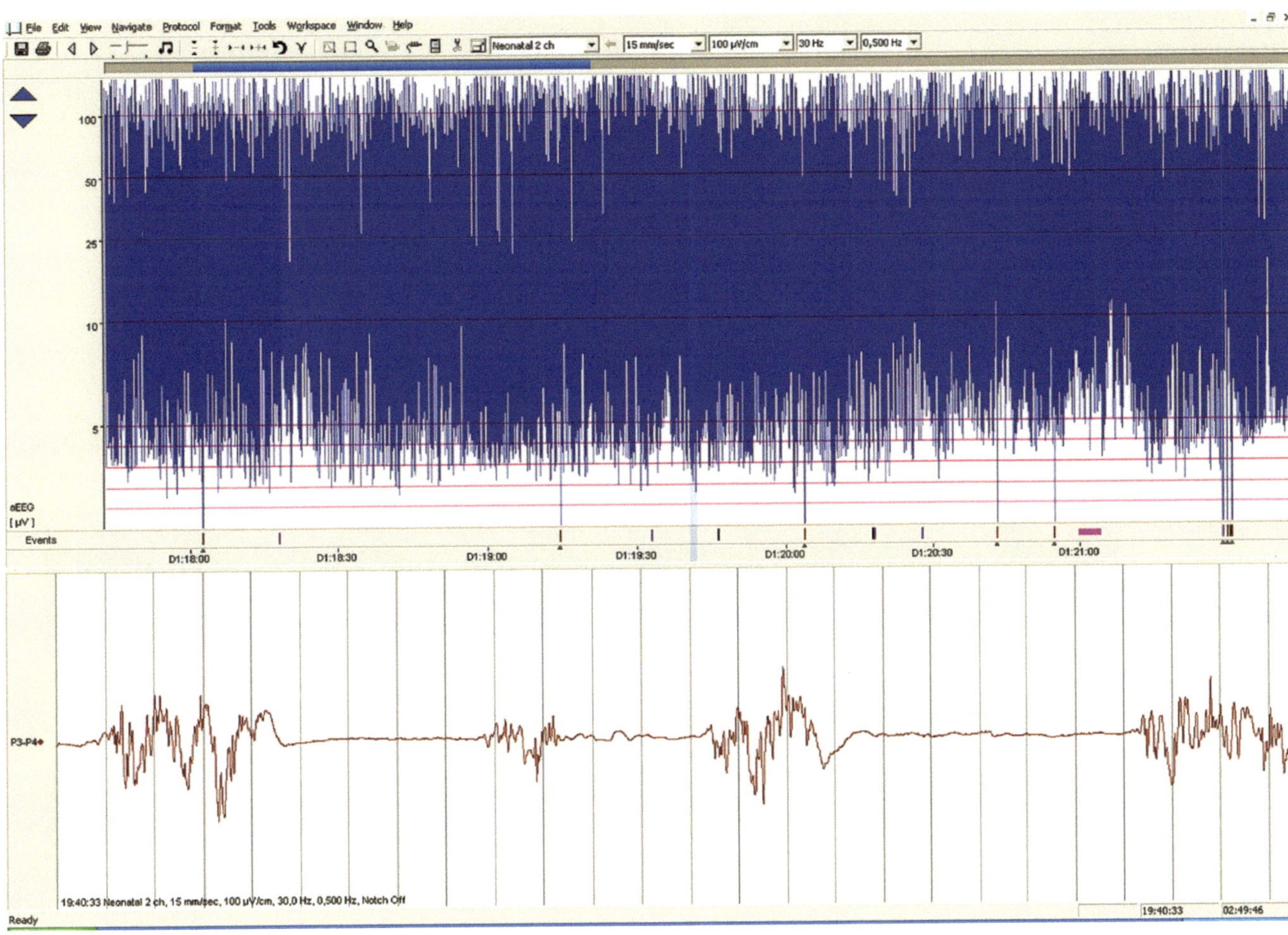

FIGURE 6.17A

Case 6.18 Full-Term Infant with Intracranial Tumor (Teratoma)

This infant was born at 36 weeks' gestation by ventouse extraction, as there was poor progress of labour. The Apgar scores were 6 and 9 at 1 and 5 minutes, respectively. The birthweight was normal, 3000 g, but the head circumference was enlarged, 37 cm (>2.5 SD). The infant developed seizures within some hours after delivery and was referred to the NICU, where the infant died a few weeks later.

aEEG was started soon after admission and showed a unilateral status epilepticus of the affected right hemisphere (Figure 6.18A). The left hemisphere, which is under pressure, starts with a continuous voltage pattern and changes to a more discontinuous voltage pattern following administration of a loading dose of phenobarbitone at marker 3. The discharges do not resolve completely but are less frequent and less prominent and mainly right-sided, although the seizure detection (orange blocks) continues to detect discharges from both hemispheres.

Cranial ultrasound on admission showed a large echogenic mass with an irregular outline, mainly seen in the right hemisphere. An *MRI* (inversion recover sequence; Figure 6.18B) confirmed the finding of a brain tumor, a suspected teratoma. Surgery was not performed; postmortem histology confirmed the diagnosis of a teratoma.

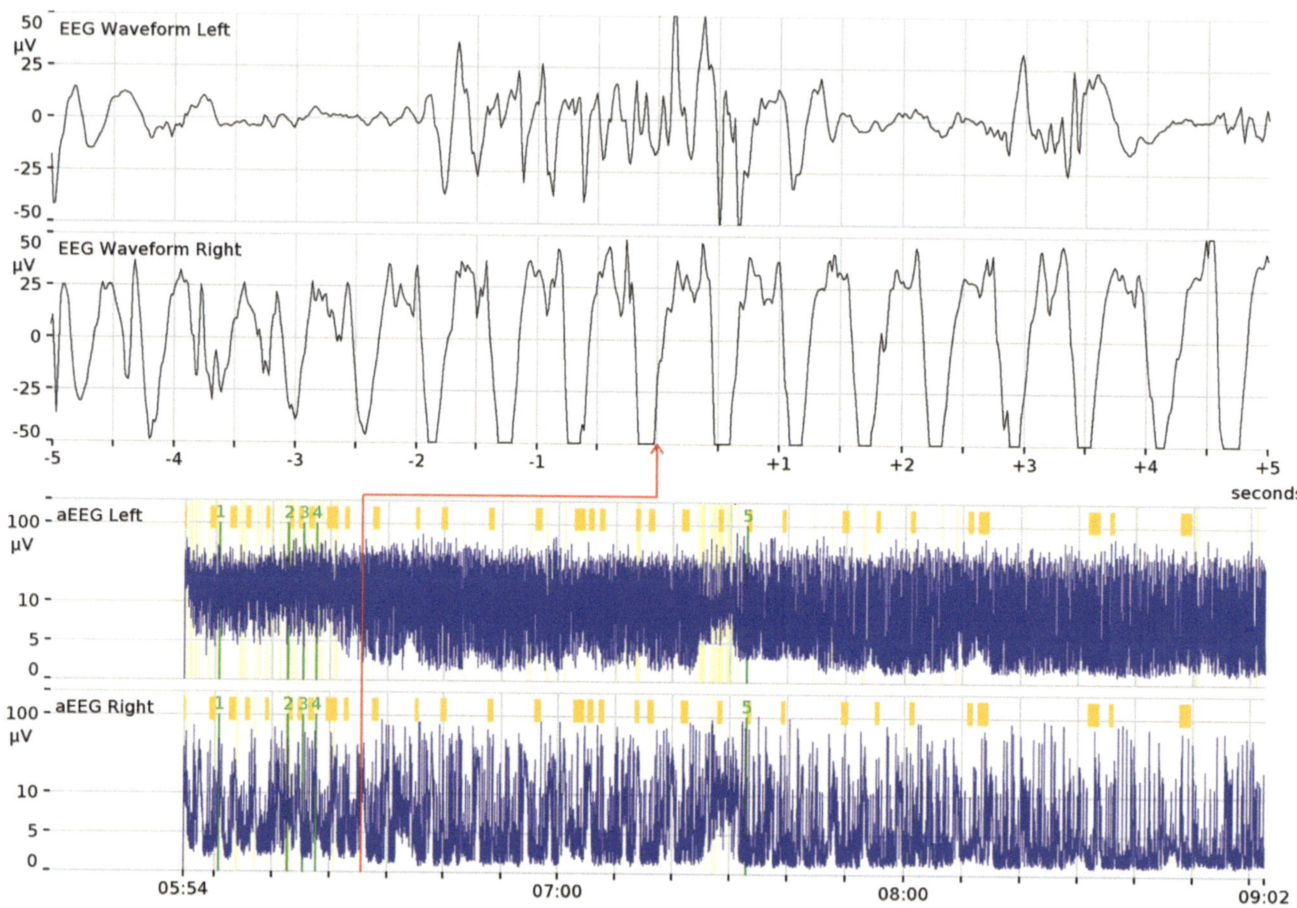

FIGURE 6.18A

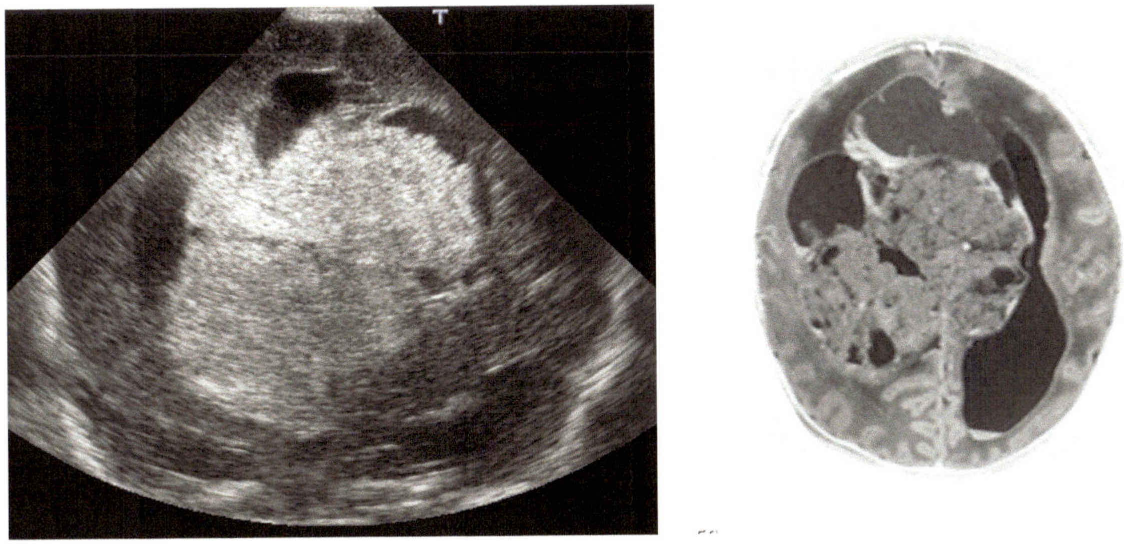

FIGURE 6.18B AND C

7 THE PRETERM aEEG

Lena Hellström-Westas, Linda S de Vries and Sampsa Vanhatalo

SUMMARY

- The aEEG gives valuable information about the current "brain function" of preterm infants.
- From 22 to 36 gestational weeks, the electrocortical activity shows weekly maturation, evolving from a very discontinuous to a continuous pattern.
- The gradual rise of the aEEG lower border is the strongest maturational feature of the aEEG.
- Alternating vigilance states are seen in the aEEG very early, but more stable sleep-wake cycling emerges from 30–32 weeks of gestation.
- Preterm infants are more sensitive to sedative and analgesic medications than term infants, as demonstrated by more severe, although transient, depression of the aEEG.
- During and after a cerebral insult (e.g. asphyxia, IVH), the aEEG trend responds with transient depression and sometimes seizures. The time to aEEG recovery is also predictive of outcome in very preterm infants.

Infants born before 37 gestational weeks are defined as being born preterm. Due to the ongoing structural growth and organization of the brain, the youngest viable preterm infants (born at around 22 weeks of gestation) differ very much from the less preterm infants. While the extremely preterm infants (GA < 28 weeks) may be at increased risk for several months, a majority of the moderately and late preterm infants (GA 32–36 weeks) do well and develop well. Consequently, most of the current knowledge of aEEG in preterm infants is focused on the extremely preterm infants. These infants usually require prolonged intensive care treatment, and they are at risk of developing germinal matrix and intraventricular hemorrhages (IVH) during the first week, as well as white matter injury (WMI). Contributing to these complications is the immature lung function and circulation and risk for sepsis and other infections that may affect brain development and function.

7.1 aEEG Monitoring of Preterm Infants

Several studies have assessed early and repeated aEEGs of very preterm infants in relation to both short-term (acute) and long-term (maturation) outcomes. Dominating pathologies in these populations are IVH and WMI, but also, hypoxic-ischemic injury may occur during difficult deliveries or acute collapse, e.g. due to sepsis. In such cases, the early aEEG and EEG background activity is closely associated to the severity of brain injury and also predictive of long-term outcomes. Late preterm infants (GA 34–36 weeks) may also become compromised by perinatal asphyxia, severe infections and congenital malformations. It was accordingly shown that the electrocortical background activity in the early aEEG of asphyxiated late preterm infants is predictive of long-term outcomes in non-cooled infants with GA 34–36 weeks.

In preterm infants, we recommend the F3, F4, P3 and P4 electrode positions for aEEG monitoring since other electrode positions may lead to technical challenges in the aEEG interpretation due to the following:

- Short interelectrode distance reducing signal amplitudes. This effect is particularly important in the very preterm infants with small heads, as the relative difference between electrode pairs (e.g. between hemispheres) may become substantial and lead to misinterpretations (Figure 7.1).
- Electrodes over prefrontal or temporal or occipital sites capture muscle activity or arterial pulsations, while occipital locations often contain movement interference coming from head movements, respiration or care.

7.2 Normal Maturational Changes

The aEEG trend undergoes characteristic maturational changes until some weeks after term equivalent age. The developmental changes in preterm cortical activity reflects growth and organization of neuronal networks, and fluctuation of vigilance states, and is highly reactive to several physiological and pathological challenges. Therefore, it is possible to assess the infants' overall cortical maturation from the EEG and, to a lesser extent, also from the aEEG reading.

The earliest scalp-recorded activity seen in the extremely preterm EEG is characterized by a highly discontinuous signal ('tracé discontinu')—i.e. intermittent high-voltage activity (i.e. bursts; also known as spontaneous activity transients, or SAT) alternating with periods of very low-voltage (interburst intervals, IBI). Higher burst rates (SAT counts) in extremely preterm infants are related to better brain growth. In the aEEG trend, the physiologically discontinuous activity (tracé discontinu pattern) of the early premature infants may resemble a burst-suppression pattern (see Chapter 2). However, it is distinguished from burst-suppression by a variable lower border.

During extreme prematurity, the bursts typically co-occur accross both hemispheres, and their frequency changes with vigilance states. After growth of the thalamo-cortical connections by gestational weeks 28–35, the bursts become reactive to sensory activity or stimulation (e.g. touch, flash, auditory), which can be readily elicited bedside. The discontinuous activity becomes more continuous over weeks, thus the strongest maturational features in the EEG and aEEG relate to continuity as follows:

- Increasingly longer and more frequent bursts
- Shorter IBIs
- Increasing amplitude during the IBI periods

DOI: 10.1201/b22858-7

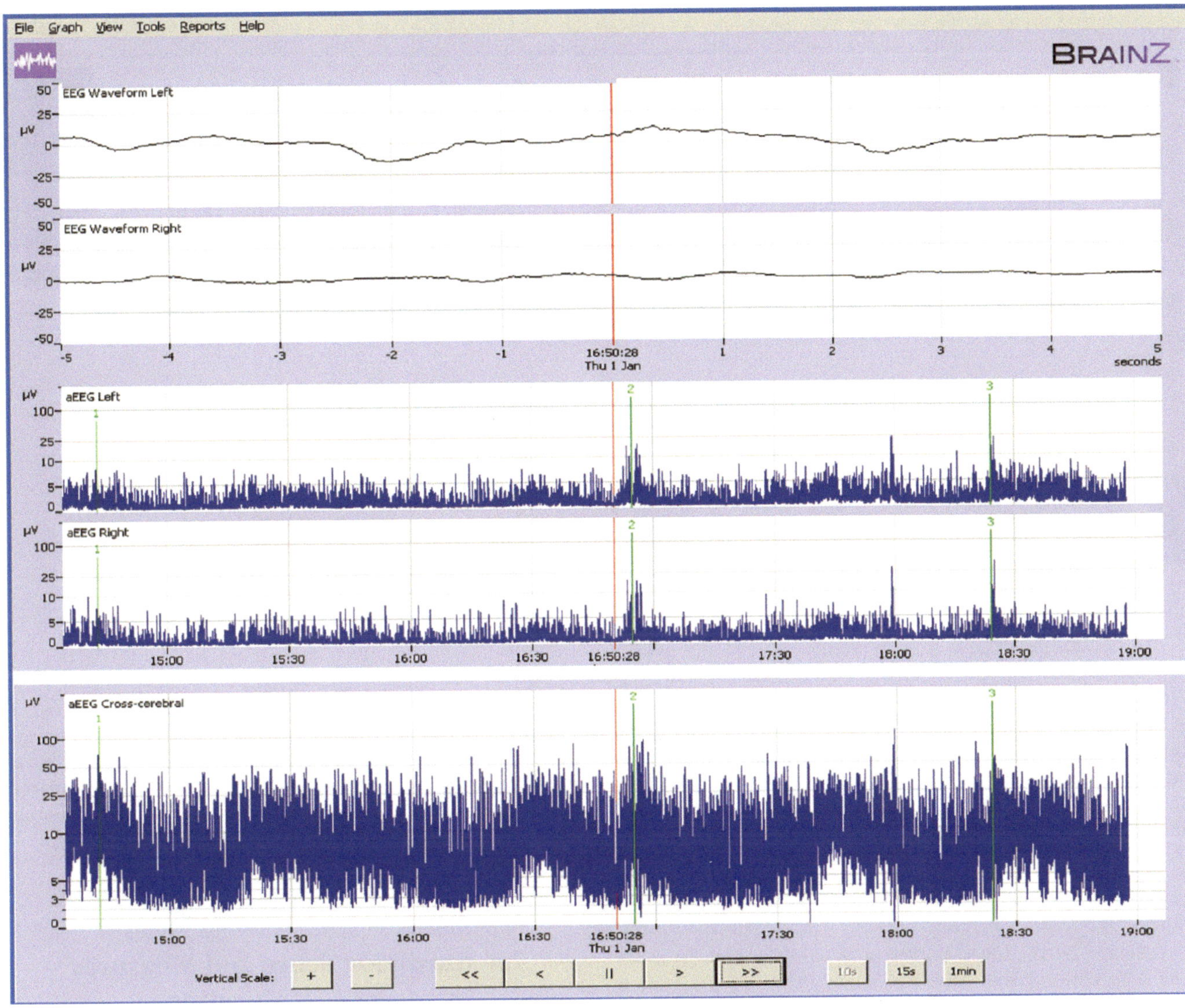

FIGURE 7.1 This figure shows an example of a falsely flat bilateral EEG (10 seconds) and aEEG (4 hours). This was caused by an inadvertent positioning of frontal and parietal electrodes over each hemisphere being placed too close to each other. However, the simultaneous cross-cerebral aEEG from biparietal electrodes with sufficient interelectrode distance, shows normal discontinuous activity and well-developed cyclicity in this very preterm infant.

Several studies have demonstrated that the EEG and aEEG activity in very preterm infants increases during the first postnatal days. This effect is mainly observed in stable infants, and the changes are relatively small. The underlying mechanism is not known, and it has been hypothesized that it may represent recovery after the delivery or postnatal adaptation associated with the birth.

7.3 Assessing Continuity in the Preterm aEEG

One of the most important maturational features in the EEG and aEEG is the increasing continuity of cortical activity, which corresponds to a gradual increase of the amplitude of the lower aEEG border. In extremely preterm infants with a normal, mainly discontinuous pattern, the increase of the lower border is caused by a combination of higher burst rates, progressively shorter IBIs and increasing amplitudes during the IBIs.

In stable extremely preterm infants, EEG bursts give rise to the high-amplitude peaks in the aEEG, resulting in a discontinuous burst-suppression–like pattern. However, the lower border amplitude should normally show some age-dependent variability (called tracé discontinu or tracé alternant pattern, respectively, in the EEG). Pathological burst-suppression is characterized by a flat aEEG lower border that reflects the inactivity during IBIs.

There are no unambiguous and universally applicable criteria for either normal bursts or IBI in the preterm aEEG or EEG. Thus, for scientific evaluations, the thresholds need to be calibrated separately for each study cohort (Figure 7.2).

The level of continuity of the recorded aEEG can also be crudely assessed by the proportion of low-amplitude activity,

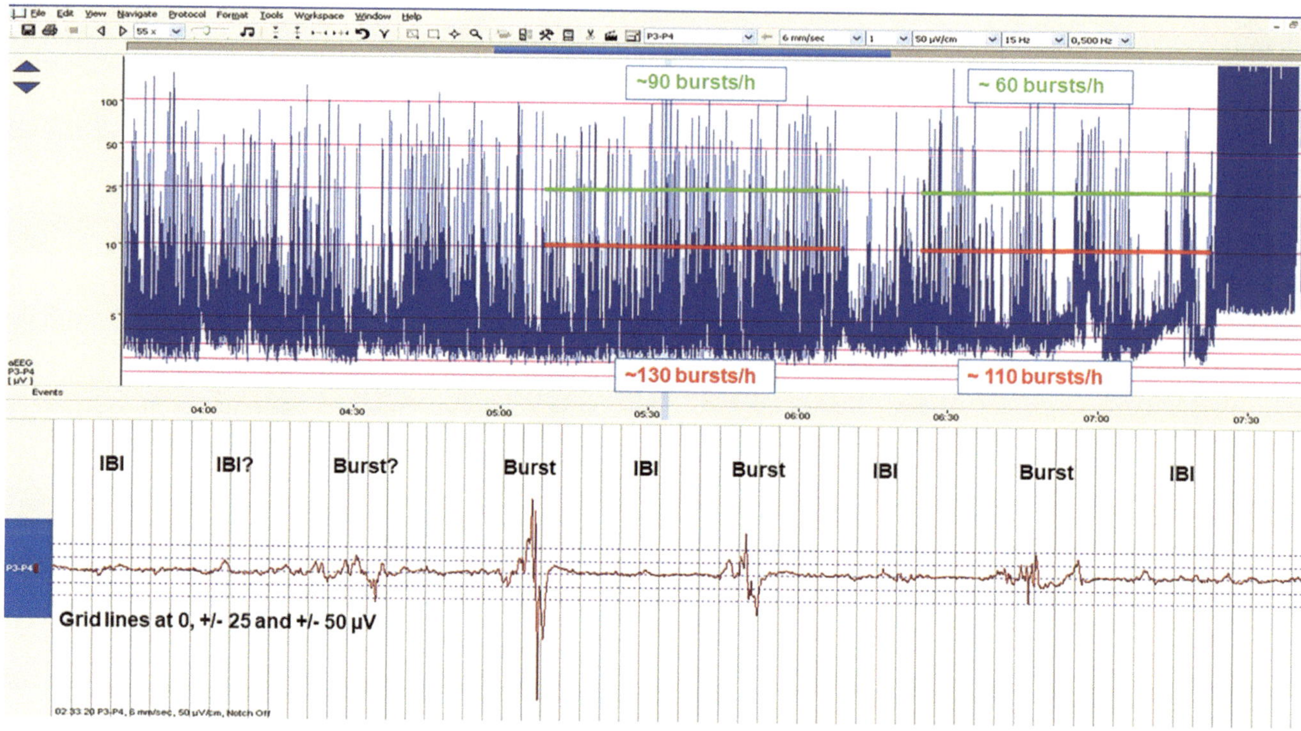

FIGURE 7.2 This figure shows 4 hours of aEEG and 64 seconds of the raw EEG at the time of the light blue vertical line in the aEEG trend. Both the aEEG and EEG show a discontinuous pattern. Depending on the criteria chosen for classification of bursts and IBIs, the burst counts will differ (see burst rates related to the green and red cut-off lines in the aEEG trend). Also, the burst rates and IBIs in the raw EEG will differ according to chosen criteria. Therefore, the exact burst rates should not be compared between different monitors, although the relative changes over time in an individual, or between infants recorded with the same device, are strongly correlated.

as reflected by the lower border of the aEEG trend. In practice, a persistent lower aEEG border amplitude < 5 µV is often interpreted as a discontinuous EEG pattern, and a lower border amplitude < 2 µV would be taken as depressed electrocortical activity. However, these approximate cut-off levels only apply to aEEG that is computed from an artefact-free EEG signal.

7.4 aEEG Recordings in Extremely Preterm Infants

During the first days of life, skin conductance is high (i.e. electrode impedance is low), and it is usually very easy to record aEEG with hydrogel electrodes in extremely preterm infants. Stable extremely preterm infants should not be disturbed more than necessary, but some compromised infants can probably benefit from the information gained from aEEG monitoring.

7.5 Burdjalov Score and Measures of aEEG Maturation

The so-called Burdjalov score offers a structured method for analyzing maturational aEEG features in the preterm infants. The Burdjalov score can be used for repeated evaluation of maturational changes that may be reflected in the overall neurodevelopment. The Burdjalov score distinguishes normal recordings from infants of different gestational ages and also delayed maturation in infants with, for example, significant white matter injury. While this score is relatively easy to learn and it may be powerful in assessing maturation (see Figure 7.3), it does not offer direct information about acute events, such as background depression and seizures. Figure 7.4 further defines the main developmental changes. The three cases in Figure 7.5 A,B,C were chosen in order to represent stable babies and what can be expected as being "normal" in these immature infants.

aEEG trace (4 hours)	Co	Cy	LB	B	Total BS	True PMA
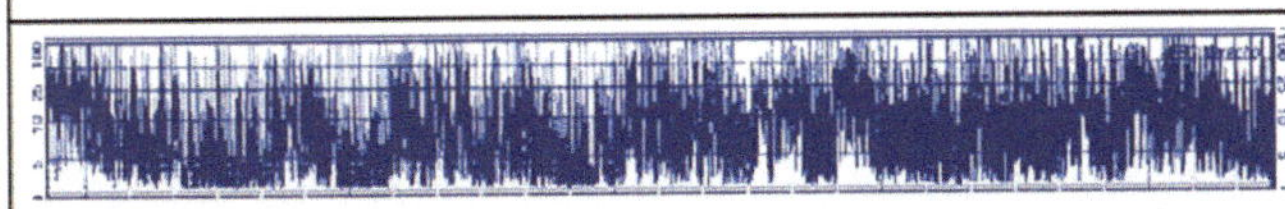	0	0	1	1	**2** *(24-25wks)*	25.3 weeks
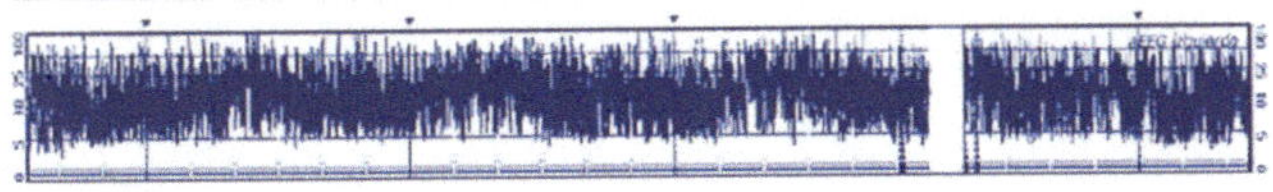	1	1	2	2	**6** *(27-28wks)*	26.6 weeks
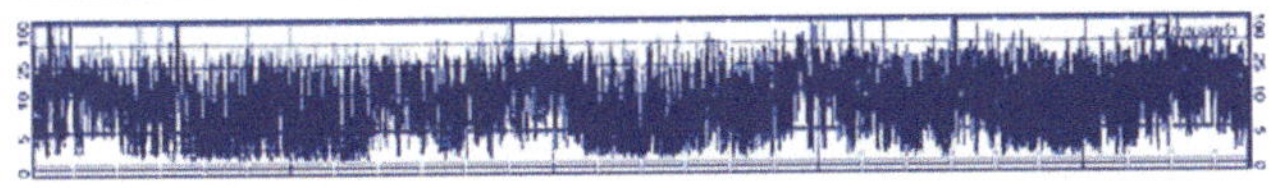	2	2	2	2	**8** *(29-30wks)*	30.0 weeks
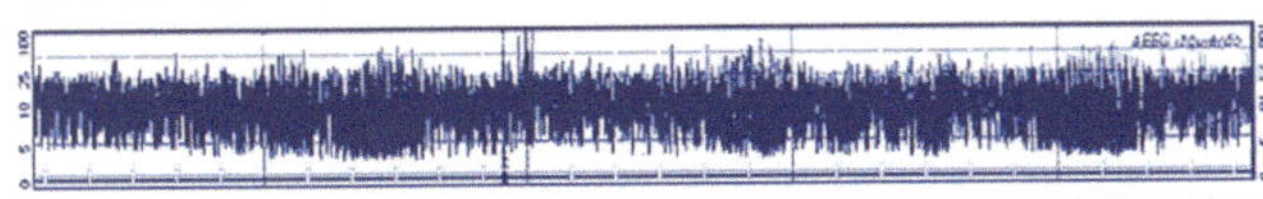	2	3	2	3	**10** *(31-32wks)*	32.0 weeks
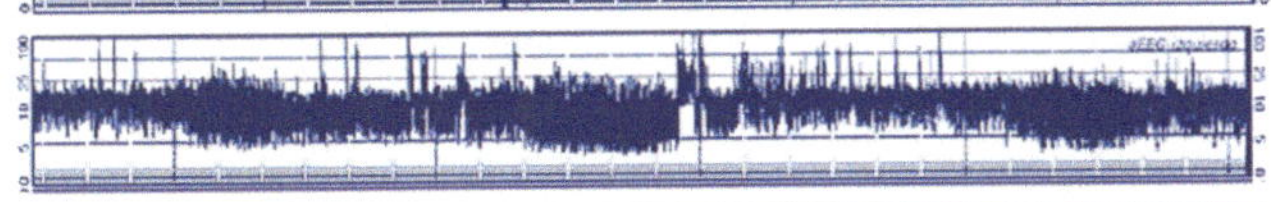	2	4	2	3	**11***(33-34wks)*	34.0 weeks
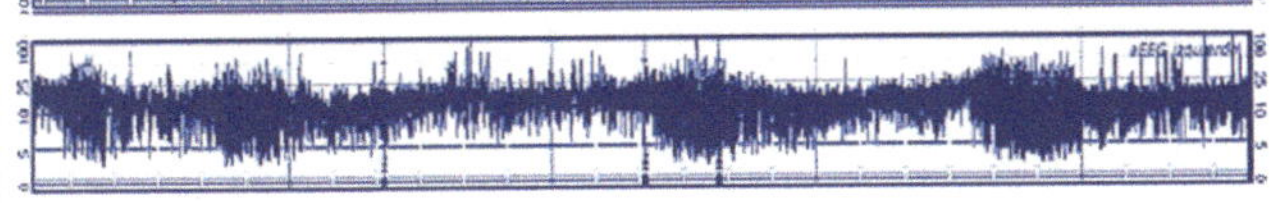	2	5	2	4	**13** *(36-37wks)*	37.0 weeks

FIGURE 7.3 Rationale of the Burdjalov score (BS) in assessing developmental changes in the preterm aEEG. It is based on four items identified in the aEEG: continuity (Co), cyclicity (Cy), level of lower border (LB) and bandwidth (B). The typical summary score (total BS) for specified postmenstrual ages (PMA) is also shown. Please see later typical aEEG traces from infants who were recorded at 25.3 to 37.0 weeks (true PMA). (Courtesy of Ana Alarcon and Mar Velilla.)

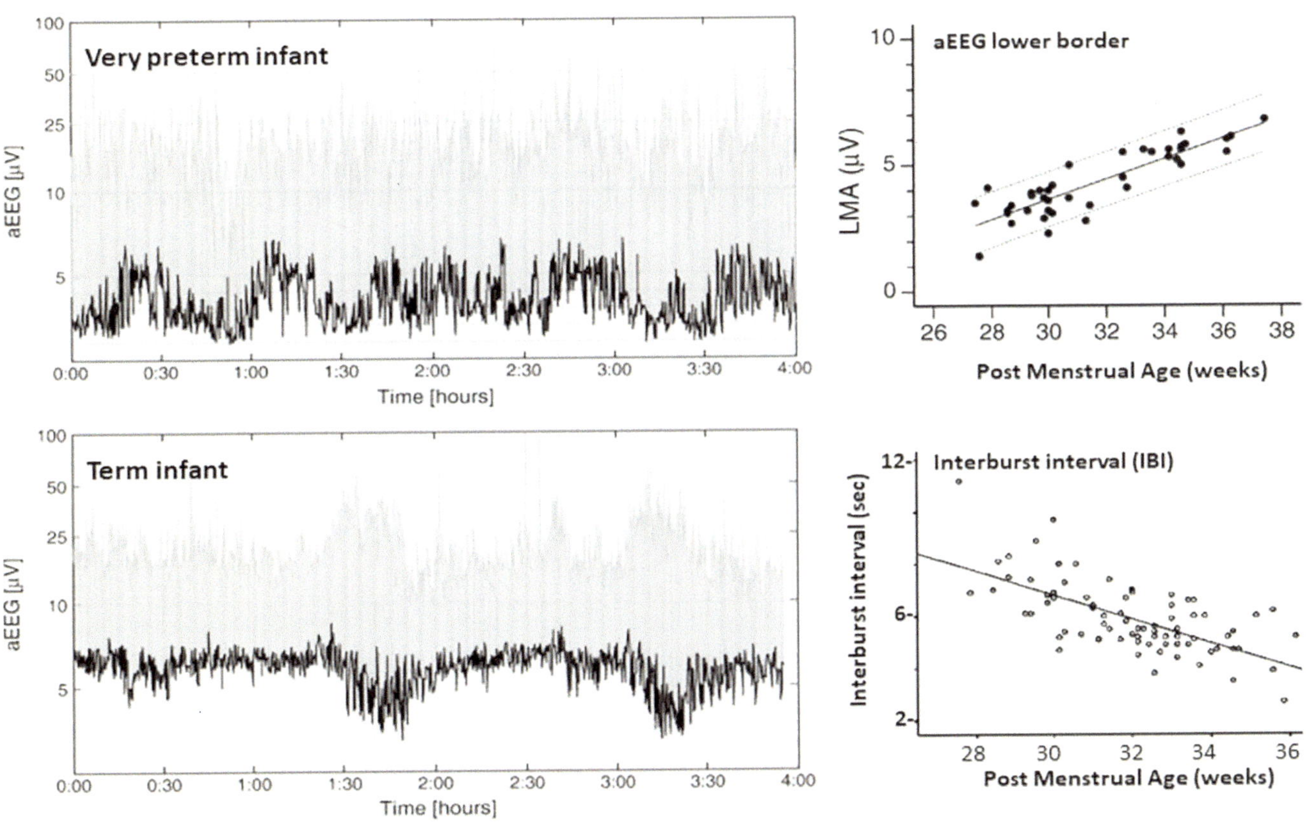

FIGURE 7.4 On the left side of this figure are two examples of normal variability of the lower border: the upper trace from a very preterm infant and below from a term infant with sleep-wake cycling. On the right side are two graphs describing normal developmental changes in continuity: the upper example shows the gradually increasing amplitude of the lower border (LMA: lower margin amplitude, µV), and the lower graph shows the decreasing IBI (in seconds) with increasing maturation. Please note that the decreasing IBI is a general finding, but the IBI numbers are mainly indicative since studies using other IBI criteria may come to slightly different numbers. (Re-arranged figure from *Niemarkt et al. 2012, with permission.*)

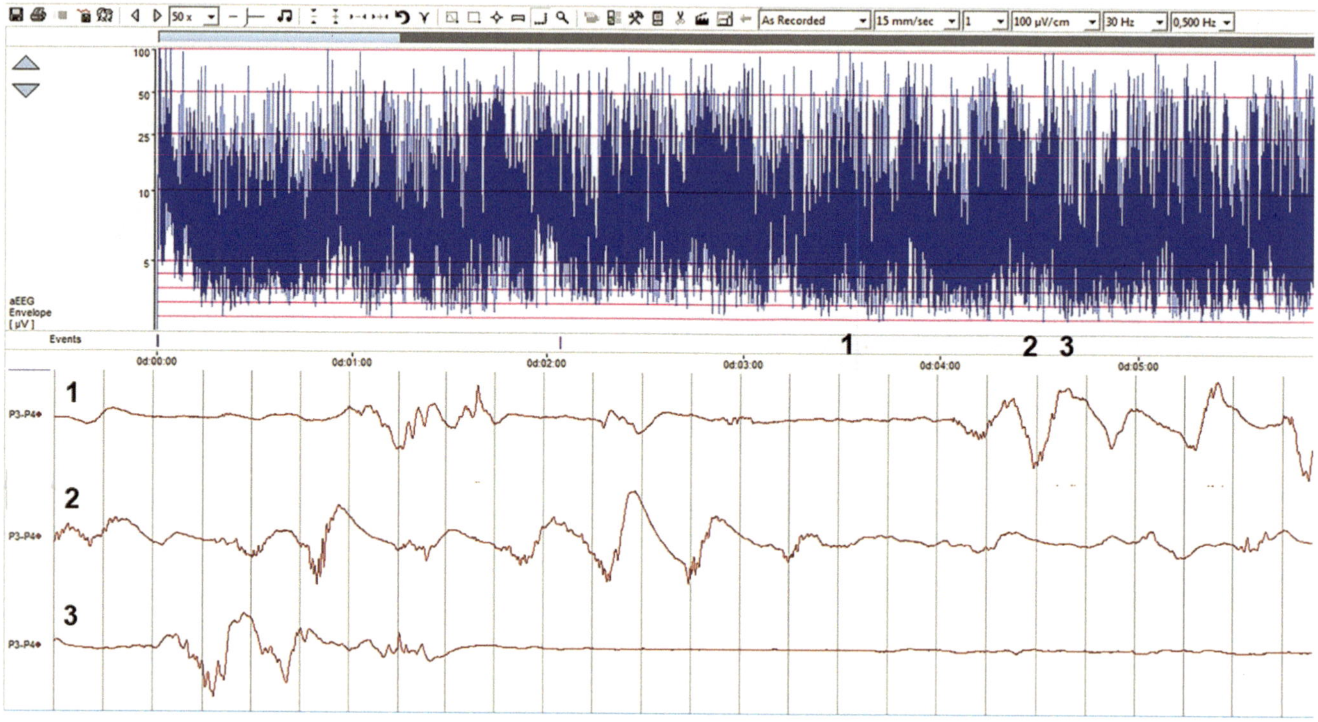

FIGURE 7.5A This infant, born at a GA of 23 + 6 weeks (+ day) was stable on CPAP and did not develop any IVH. The aEEG on days 1 to 2 was characterized by discontinuous activity, relatively frequent bursts, short IBIs and variability of the lower border but no cyclicity (the duration of aEEG was 6 hours, and the corresponding EEG traces were 25 seconds).

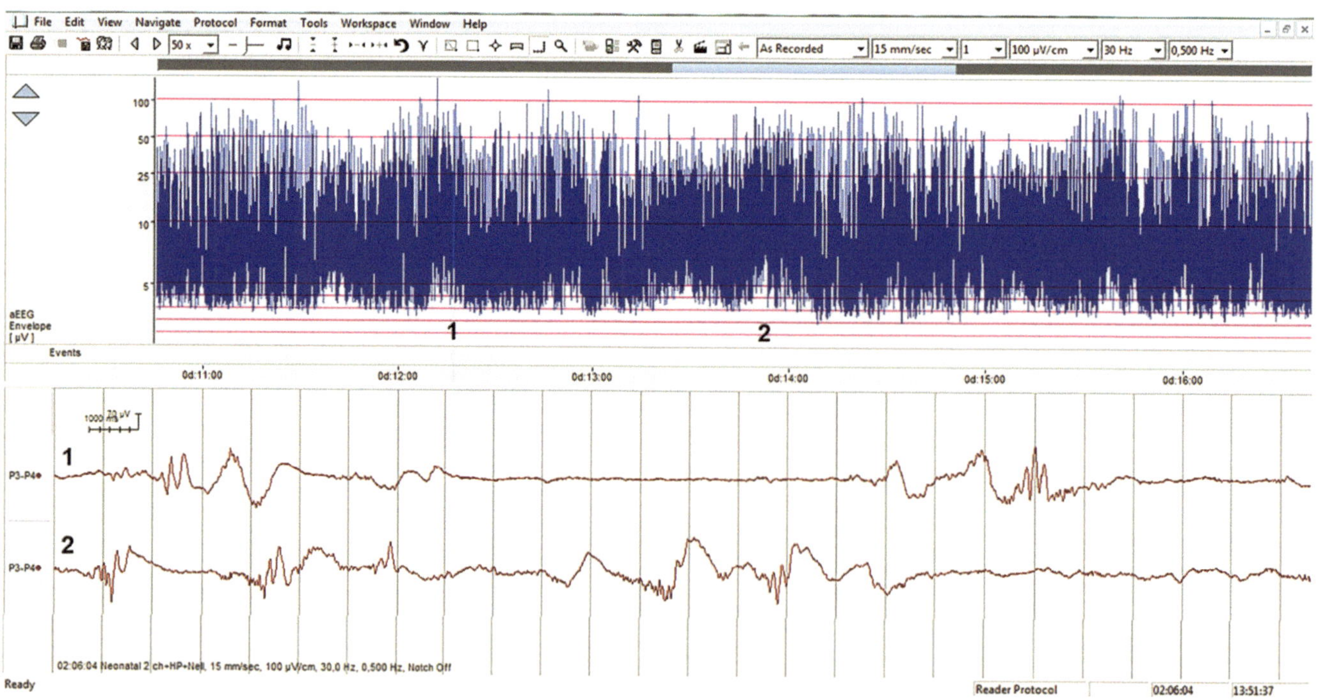

FIGURE 7.5B This infant was born at a GA of 25 + 5 weeks and was stable on day 1. The aEEG shows a discontinuous pattern with some variability of the lower border. Please note that the EEG shows longer bursts and shorter IBIs than in the previous infant born at 23 + 6 weeks (the duration of aEEG was 6 hours, and the EEG traces were 25 seconds).

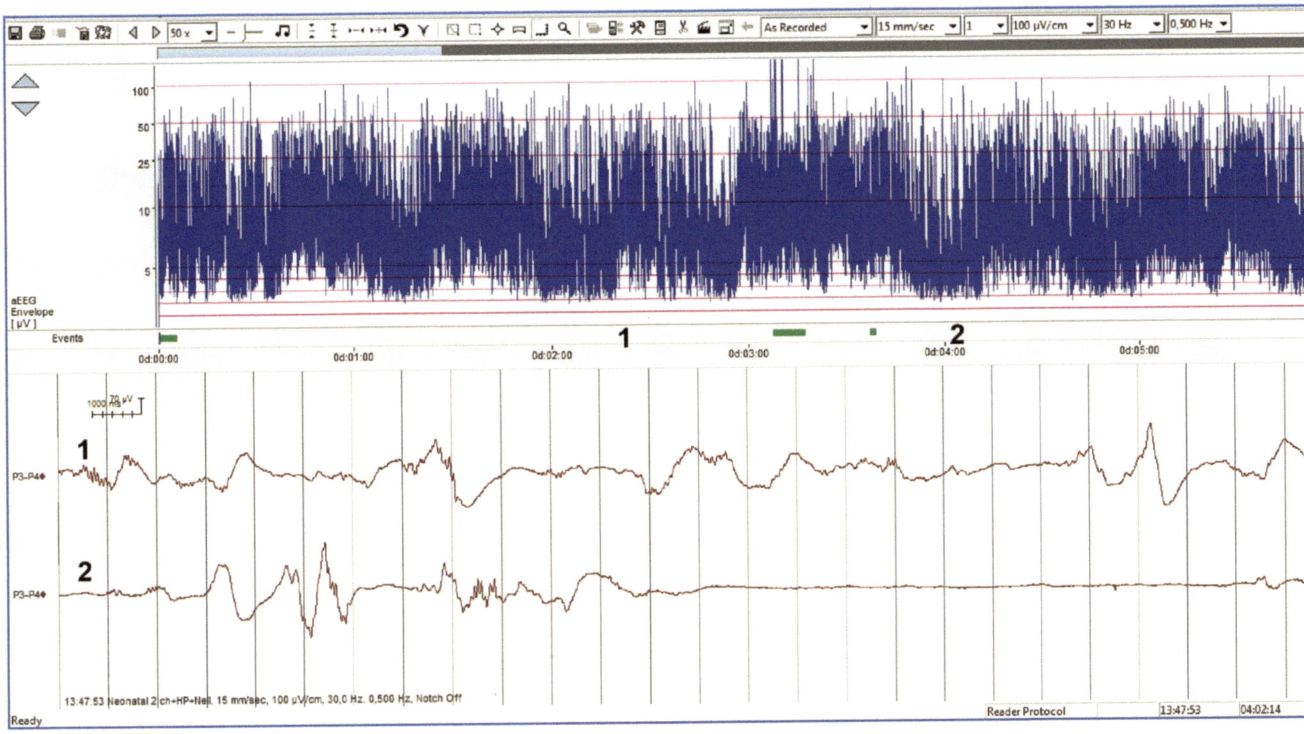

FIGURE 7.5C This infant, born at GA of 27 + 0 weeks, was stable when recorded on day 2. The aEEG shows a cyclical pattern that could represent immature sleep-wake cycling, with periods of continuous activity (1) mixed with discontinuous activity (2) (the duration of aEEG was 6 hours, and the EEG traces were 25 seconds).

7.6 Sleep-Wake Cycling (SWC)

Spontaneously alternating vigilance states (wakefulness, active and quiet sleep) are considered to reflect neurological stability in newborn infants. Well-defined sleep states emerge in the EEG at around 30 gestational weeks, soon after the growth of thalamo-cortical connections. Sleep-wake cycling can also be seen in the aEEG from around 30–32 gestational weeks and appears as periods with more discontinuous activity (broad band) representing quiet sleep, alternating with more narrow continuous parts representing wakefulness or active sleep. Brief transitional periods can be seen between the changing background patterns. Direct observation of the infant is required in order to distinguish wakefulness and active sleep since the aEEG patterns are similar. In less mature infants, "cyclicity"—i.e. smooth cyclical variations of the lower border—can be observed and probably represents developing sleep-wake cycling.

With increasing maturation, sleep-wake states become increasingly separated and the cycle length becomes longer and more stable, from around 15–30 min in very preterm infants to 60–90 min in term infants. Cyclicity in the aEEG trace of relatively mature infants is usually easily recognized/easy to recognize and appears gradually in previously compromised infants. There are no established criteria for cycle length, its variability over successive sleep cycles or how many sleep cycles are needed for declaring the presence of SWC. See further Table 7.1 and Figure 7.6.

TABLE 7.1 **Clinical and aEEG Characteristics of Sleep-Wake States in Newborn Infants**

Sleep-wake states in stable newborn infants from 30–32 weeks PMA to full-term		aEEG Characteristics
Awake	Open eyes, alert or drowsy, calm or agitated, active movements	Continuous pattern
Transitional sleep	Brief period when sleep-wake state changes	Gradual, relatively brief, change in continuity/discontinuity during state change to/from quiet sleep
Quiet sleep	Closed eyes, regular breathing, regular heart rate, few movements	Broader bandwidth, more discontinuous pattern
Active sleep	Closed eyes, eye movements, irregular breathing, regular heart rate, low muscular tone with intermittent movements	Continuous (the aEEG cannot distinguish wakefulness and active sleep)

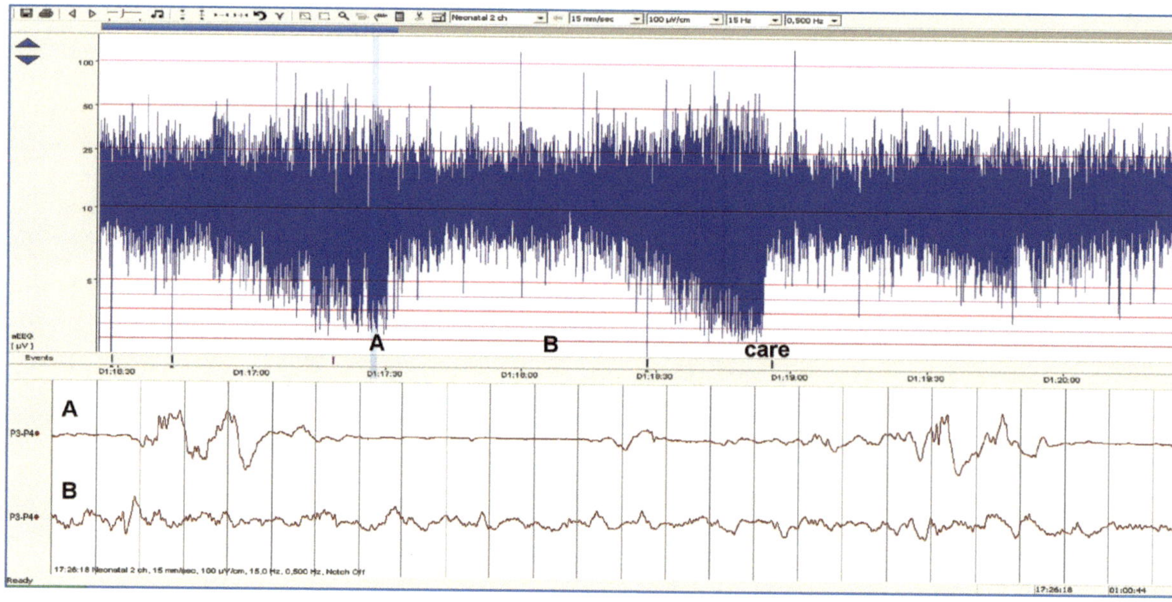

FIGURE 7.6 This is an example of developed sleep-wake cycling in a preterm infant (GA 35 weeks) who was stable. The infant was known to have a Dandy-Walker malformation. The background activity in this 4-hour recording is continuous, and there are two well-developed quiet sleep periods [(A) shows the first]. It is not possible to distinguish whether period (B) represents wakefulness or active sleep from the aEEG; that requires clinical observation. The second quiet sleep period is abruptly interrupted by a care procedure.

7.7 aEEG Monitoring in Sick and Unstable Preterm Infants

aEEG monitoring in sick and unstable preterm infants can give valuable information about the infant's current "brain state". Depressed electrocortical activity and seizures may be related, e.g. delivery complications, intracranial hemorrhages, hemodynamic instability, sepsis, hypoglycemia, pulmonary problems and hypercapnia or medication. The aEEG findings are usually non-specific, and the etiology must be investigated with other means. In contrast, well-preserved aEEG activity during or after a severe acute event can indicate that the infant's brain function was less affected. See further Figure 7.7.

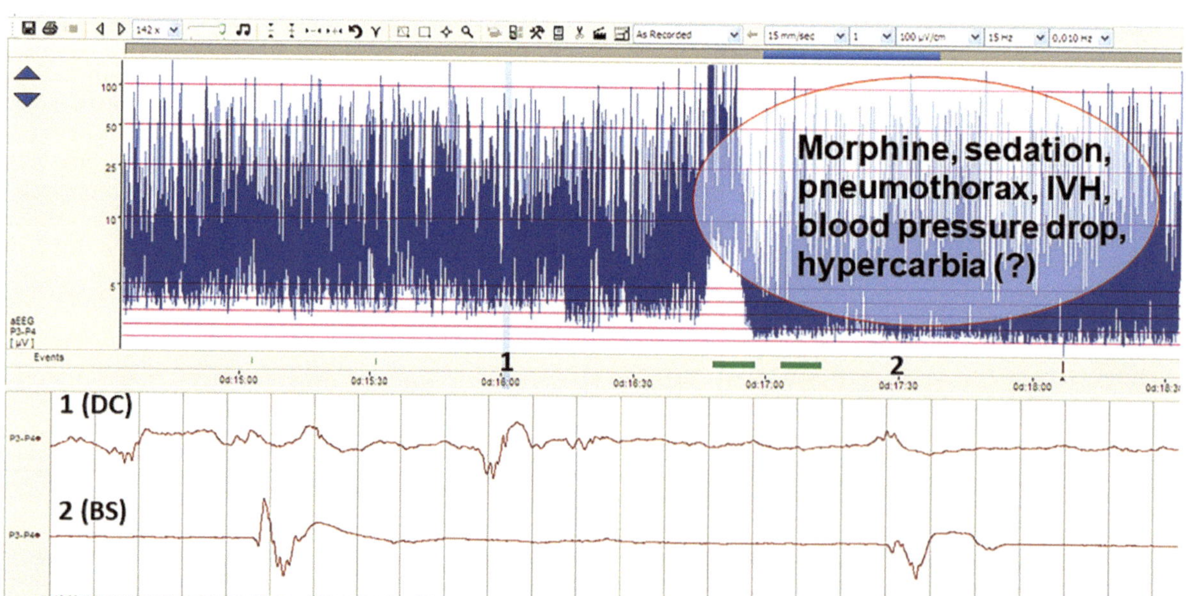

FIGURE 7.7 This 4-hour aEEG recording and 25 seconds of EEG signals from an extremely preterm infant shows a sudden change of the aEEG background pattern from discontinuous to burst-suppression. It is not possible to tell from the aEEG response what the implication of this abrupt change of cerebral activity represents since it has to be considered together with the clinical situation. A list of potential causes is shown in the figure. The raw EEG traces below the aEEG were extracted from the correspondingly numbered parts of the aEEG above (1: showing a discontinuous pattern and 2: showing a more depressed burst-suppression–like pattern).

In extremely preterm infants, it can sometimes be difficult to appreciate if the aEEG pattern is normal or abnormal. An easy rule of thumb is that the lower border should normally have some variability and the burst pattern should be so dense that individual bursts are difficult to count in the aEEG trend. Other trends such as burst frequency and IBI, present in some monitors, may also assist in sorting out the relevance of relatively subtle aEEG findings (Figure 7.8 A,B).

In twin A, the aEEG trace is discontinuous with a relatively dense burst pattern and variability of the lower border amplitude. After 3 hours, there is a 30-minute artefact. The burst count is around 5 bursts per minute, and most IBIs are shorter than 25 seconds (marked by red lines).

In twin B, with the large IVH, the aEEG is more depressed with no variability of the lower border. The burst frequency is mainly below 5 bursts per minute, and the IBIs are longer, frequently 60 seconds or more.

The aEEG in twin A can probably be considered as "normal" at this early gestational age, while the aEEG from twin B is depressed. The difference between normal and depressed electrocortical activity can be difficult to evaluate in an extremely preterm infant. However, the mainly flat lower border with long interburst intervals indicates depressed activity.

Although aEEG/EEG changes related to brain injury in very preterm infants can be relatively subtle, they can be recognized, usually in the flat lower border and sparse burst activity (Figure 7.9). Additional trends such as IBI and burst counts can sometimes be helpful in estimating the overall activity. However, please note that different monitors may have different algorithms for quantifying burst activity, and the numbers may not be directly comparable.

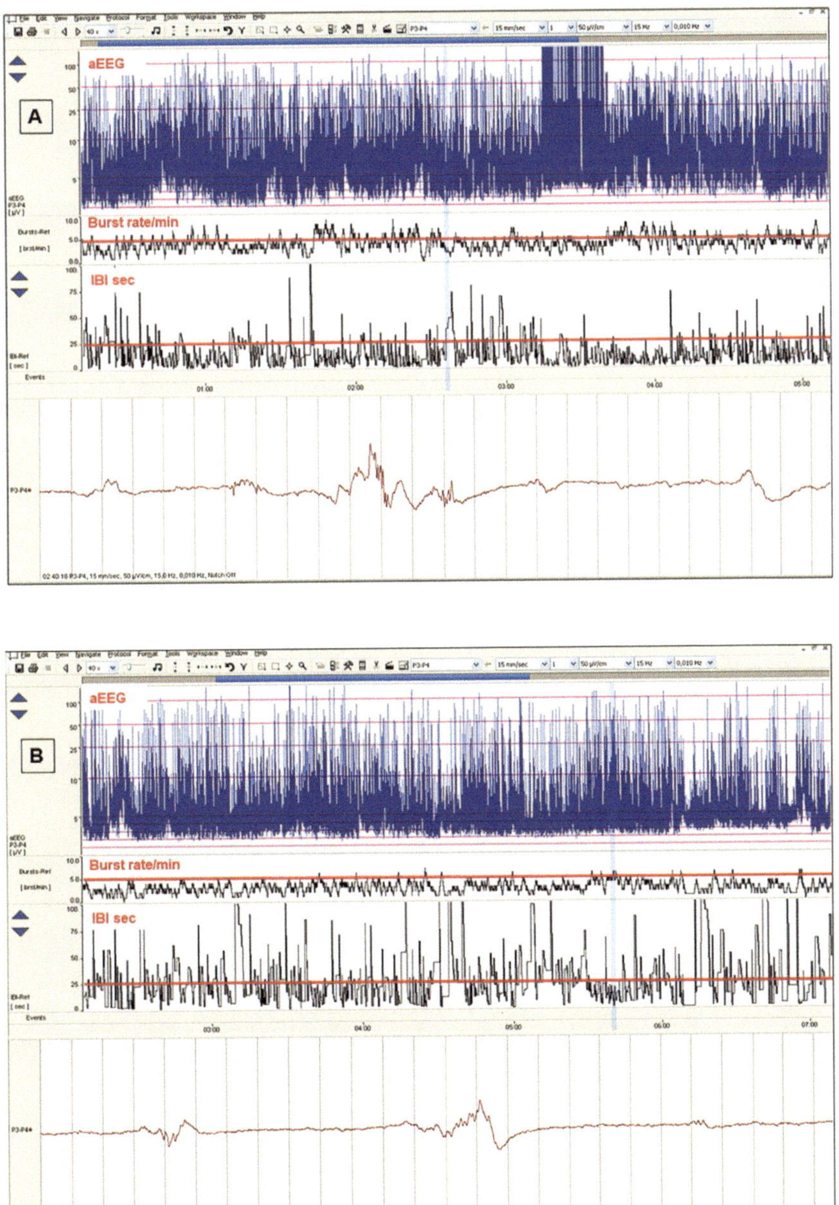

FIGURES 7.8A and B This example is from a pair of twins, born at 24 gestational weeks and recorded during the first days of life. Twin A (top) did not develop brain injury, while twin B (bottom) developed a large IVH grade III. The figures show 5 hours of aEEG and two other trends created from the raw EEG: "bursts per minute" and "interburst interval (IBI)". Below is 25 seconds of the raw EEG.

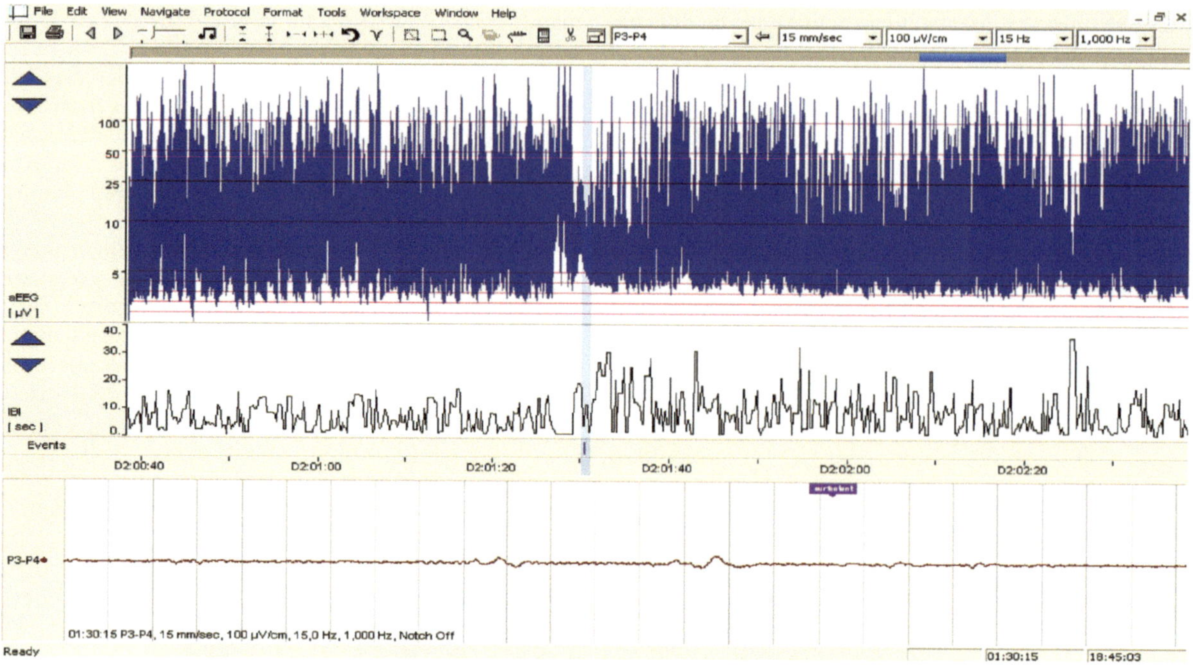

FIGURE 7.9 This figure shows the aEEG (2 hours) and EEG (25 sec) response to surfactant administration. The initial aEEG pattern looks good (dense bursts, some variability of the lower border) and stable in this very immature infant with a gestational age of 24 weeks. In the middle of the recording, just before the vertical light blue line, the infant received an intratracheal bolus of surfactant. This was followed by around 10 minutes of depressed aEEG/EEG activity, with increasing interburst intervals (IBI trend below the aEEG). Similar responses to surfactant have been described in several studies, but the etiology is not clear.

7.8 Acute Changes

The preterm cortical activity reacts to all challenges by suppression, which is best seen relative to the state before the challenge. In the aEEG trend, this is seen as an acute depression of the background amplitude and/or a decrease in the number of bursts ("aEEG spikes"). Such challenges include, for instance, development of large IVH, hemodynamic or respiratory collapse, sepsis, pneumothorax, administration of sedative and analgesic medications, hypercapnia or other severe medical conditions (e.g. sepsis). See Figures 7.10–7.12.

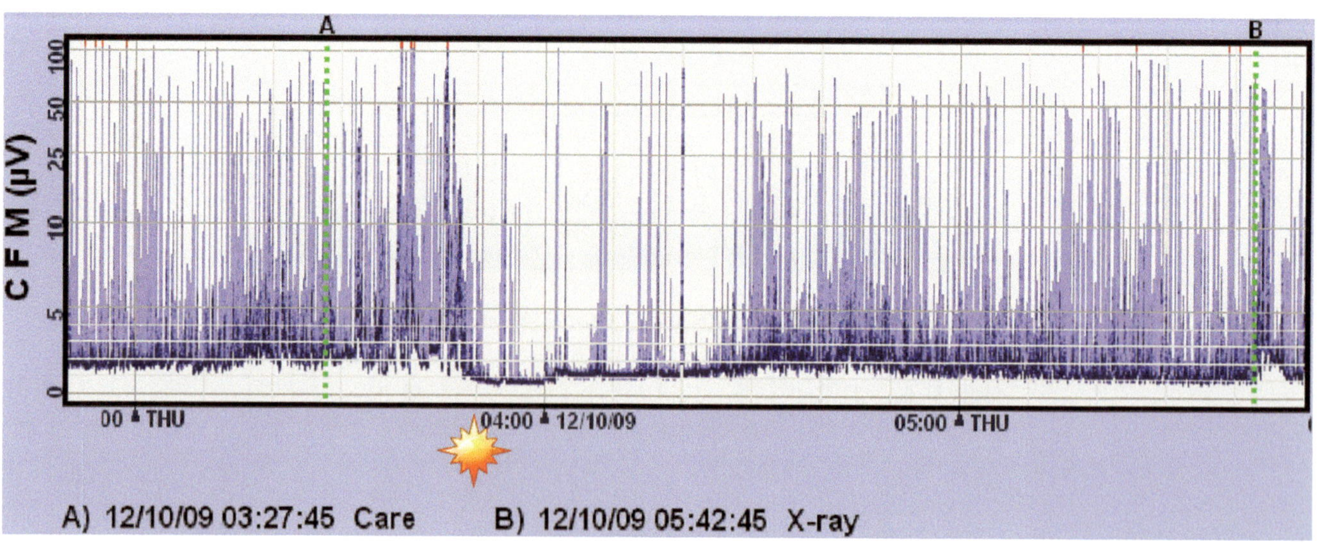

FIGURE 7.10 This figure shows a very preterm infant (29 weeks of gestational age) with necrotizing enterocolitis (NEC) who also required surgery for persistent ductus arteriosus (PDA) and was sedated on high-frequency oscillation ventilation (HFOV). The overall aEEG pattern is severely depressed from the beginning but becomes even more depressed (in the middle of the trace) due to acute severe hypercarbia ($PaCO_2$ 99 mmHg), followed by recovery after 30–40 minutes as the $PaCO_2$ decreased with improved ventilation. The reversible depressive effect of hypercarbia on the newborn infant's electrocortical activity has been shown in several publications.

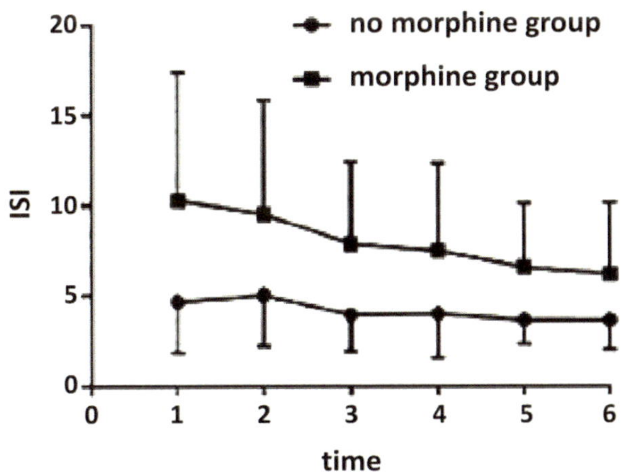

FIGURE 7.11 This figure shows the depressive effect of morphine sedation during mechanical ventilation in a population of *174* extremely preterm infants, of whom 89 received morphine. The y-axis shows ISI, i.e. interSAT intervals in seconds (EEG measure comparable to IBI), here presented over the first 72 hours (six time points: 4–6 h, 10–12 h, 20–24 h, 32–36 h, 44–48 h and 68–72 h). (From *Tataranno et al. 2020, with permission.*)

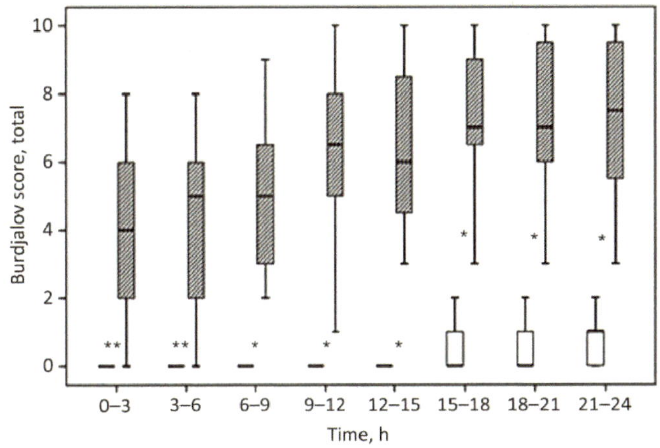

FIGURE 7.12 A small randomized study compared effects of morphine with thiopental/remifentanil as premedication for intubation of very preterm infants. Morphine caused EEG depression that was measurable for 24 hours, while the effect of thiopental/remifentanil lasted up to 6 hours. The graph shows the effects on the Burdjalov score during the first 24 hours. Morphine is shown as white bars and thiopental/remifentanil as grey bars. (Courtesy of Elisabeth Norman.)

7.9 Chronic Changes

Diffuse white matter injury is common in very preterm infants, while cystic white matter injury is now rarely seen. The onset of diffuse white matter injury is seldom acute or related to a specific event, and the timing is rarely known. Consequently, there is usually no acute detection of these injuries. However, several studies, including aEEG and EEG, have demonstrated that significant white matter injury is associated with delayed electrocortical maturation in the aEEG and EEG, including delayed sleep-wake cycling.

Evaluation of chronic changes is better with EEG. Multiple studies have extensively described delayed or abnormal EEG maturation ("dysmaturation") and presence of abnormal waveforms (e.g. positive rolandic sharp waves in cystic PVL) in the EEG in infants with neurological adversities, such as white matter injury.

7.10 Seizures

Seizures may appear after acute severe events such as perinatal asphyxia, hemodynamic collapse, sepsis and in conjunction with developing brain injury such as IVH. In moderately preterm infants, seizures appear in the aEEG in a similar fashion as in term infants. Seizures in extremely preterm infants are dominated by slow waveforms, which makes them difficult or impossible to recognize in the aEEG trend that attenuates waveforms < 2 Hz.

Seizures in preterm infants should preferably be detected from the raw EEG. It is important that frequent clinical notes are made when monitoring preterm infants with suspected seizures because many kinds of artefacts (e.g. parental patting) can easily be misinterpreted as seizures. See Figures 7.13–7.14 (see also Chapter 4).

Please note, for confirmation of seizure activity, three criteria are required (see also Chapter 4). The seizure should be the following: 1) "sudden", i.e. show a clear beginning and end; 2) "repetitive" or "stereotyped", i.e. waveforms that keeps repeating; and 3) "evolving", over time.

7.11 Prediction of Outcome

Several studies have shown that features of the early aEEG background contains predictive information in both general populations of very preterm infants and in selected high-risk populations (e.g. with large IVH) already during the first 24–72 hours. These findings are in line with studies showing that IVH links to EEG depression. A higher aEEG burst count (maximum over 130 per hour) during the first 3 days of life has also been associated with better outcome (survival with no or mild handicap) in preterm infants with large IVH.

aEEG features that are typically evaluated in both stable and compromised very preterm infants for evaluation of brain function:

- Type of background pattern (e.g. continuous, discontinuous, burst-suppression or worse)
- Number of bursts/hour
- Continuity, measured as % of lower border activity above a certain amplitude, e.g. 3 μV or 5 μV
- Seizures

Less is known about the predictive value of aEEG in asphyxiated moderately and late preterm infants; however, the present evidence suggests that aEEG may provide clinical useful prediction of outcome during the first day after birth.

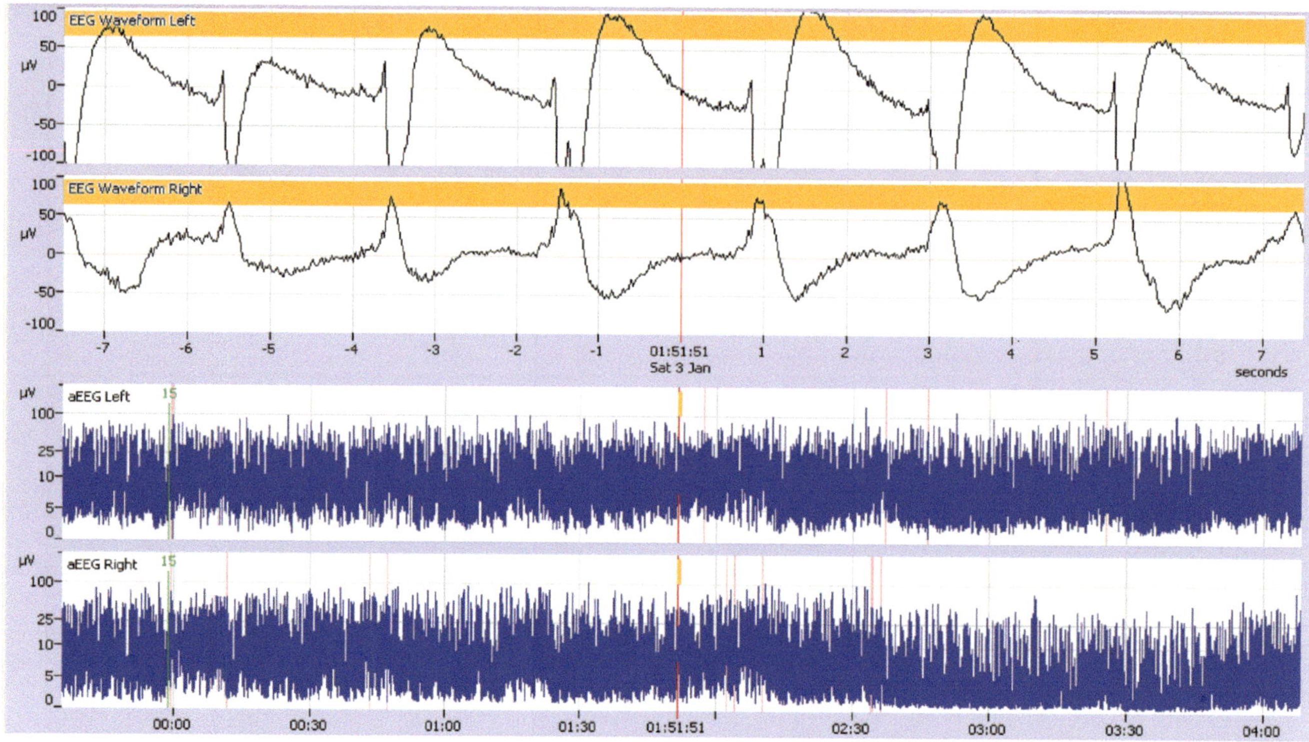

FIGURE 7.13 Example from extremely preterm infant with a suspected seizure, detected by a waveform alarm (yellow marker), indicating possible seizures. The duration of the aEEG is 3.5 hours and the EEG 15 seconds. This event is not visible in the aEEG trend for two main reasons: it is slow (0.5–1 Hz) and, therefore, attenuated or entirely filtered out by the aEEG algorithm and also too brief to make any change in the compressed aEEG trend.

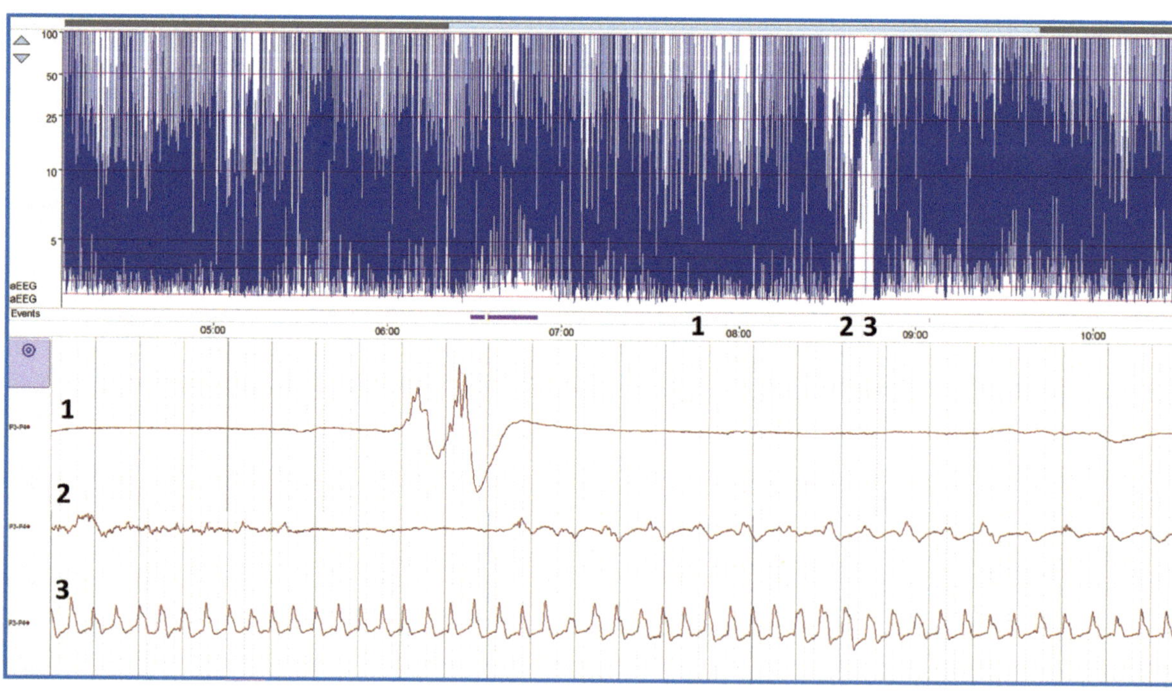

FIGURE 7.14 This figure shows 6 hours of single-channel aEEG (from P3-P4), and below are three 25-second EEG traces from a preterm infant (GA 25 weeks) with periventricular hemorrhagic infarction (PVHI). The overall background pattern (1) is depressed and shows burst-suppression without variability. The initial progression of an electrographic seizure, with no clinical manifestations, and lasting a couple of minutes, is also shown (2, 3).

References

Benders MJ, Palmu K, Menache C, et al. Early brain activity relates to subsequent brain growth in premature infants. *Cereb Cortex.* 2015;25(9):3014–3024.

Burdjalov VF, Baumgart S, Spitzer AR. Cerebral function monitoring: A new scoring system for the evaluation of brain maturation in neonates. *Pediatrics.* 2003;112(4):855–861.

Burger C, Hammerl M, Neubauer V, et al. Early preterm infants with abnormal psychomotor neurodevelopmental outcome at age two show alterations in amplitude-integrated encephalopgraphy signals. *Early Hum Dev.* 2020;141:104935.

Clancy RR, Tharp BR, Enzman D. EEG in premature infants with intraventricular hemorrhage. *Neurology.* 1984;34:583–590.

Connell J, Oozeer R, Regev R, et al. Continuous four-channel EEG monitoring in the evaluation of echodense ultrasound lesions and cystic leucomalacia. *Arch Dis Childh.* 1987;62:1019–1024.

Greisen G, Hellström-Vestas L, Lou H, et al. Sleep-waking shifts and cerebral blood flow in stable preterm infants. *Pediatr Res.* 1985;19(11):1156–1159.

Greisen G, Hellström-Westas L, Lou H, et al. EEG depression and germinal layer haemorrhage in the newborn. *Acta Paediatr Scand.* 1987;76(3):519–525.

Hellström-Westas L, Klette J, Thorngren-Jerneck K, Rosén I. Early prediction of outcome with aEEG in preterm infants with large intraventricular hemorrhages. *Neuropediatrics.* 2001;33:319–324.

Inder TE, Buckland L, Williams CE, et al. Lowered electroencephalographic spectral edge frequency predicts the presence of cerebral white matter injury in premature infants. *Pediatrics.* 2003;111(1):27–33.

Iyer KK, Roberts JA, Hellström-Westas L, et al. Cortical burst dynamics predict outcome early in extremely preterm infants. *Brain.* 2015a;138(Pt8):2206–2218.

Iyer KK, Roberts JA, Hellström-Westas L, et al. Early detection of preterm intraventricular hemorrhage from clinical electroencephalography. *Crit Care Med.* 2015b;43(10):2219–2227.

Jiang CM, Yang YH, Chen LQ, et al. Early amplitude-integrated EEG monitoring 6 h after birth predicts long-term neurodevelopment of asphyxiated late preterm infants. *Eur J Pediatr.* 2015;174(8):1043–1052.

Klebermass K, Olischar M, Waldhoer T, et al. Amplitude-integrated EEG pattern predicts further outcome in preterm infants. *Pediatr Res.* 2011;70(1):102–108.

Niemarkt HJ, Andriessen P, Peters CHL, et al. Quantitative analysis of maturational changes in EEG background activity in very preterm infants with a normal neurodevelopment at 1 year of age. *Early Hum Dev.* 2010;86:219–224.

Niemarkt HJ, Jennekens W, Maartens IA, et al. Multi-channel amplitude-integrated EEG characteristics in preterm infants with a normal neurodevelopment at two years of corrected age. *Early Hum Dev.* 2012;88(4):209–216.

Norman E, Wikström S, Rosén I, et al. Premedication for intubation with morphine causes prolonged depression of electrocortical background activity in preterm infants. *Pediatr Res.* 2013 Jan;73(1):87–94.

Olischar M, Klebermass K, Kuhle S, et al. Reference values for amplitude-integrated electroencephalographic activity in preterm infants younger than 30 weeks' gestational age. *Pediatrics.* 2004;113:61–66.

Parmelee Jr AH, Schulte FJ, Akiyama Y, et al. Maturation of EEG activity during sleep in premature infants. *Electroencephalogr Clin Neurophysiol.* 1968;24(4):319–329.

Richardson J, Goshen S, Meledin I, et al. Predictive value of early amplitude integrated EEG in extremely premature infants. *J Child Neurol.* 2020;35(11):737–743.

Song J, Xu F, Wang L, et al. Early amplitude-integrated electroencephalography predicts brain injury and neurological outcome in very preterm infants. *Sci Rep.* 2015;5:13810.

Tataranno ML, Gui L, Hellström-Westas L, et al. Morphine affects brain activity and volumes in preterms: An observational multi-center study. *Early Hum Dev.* 2020;144:104970.

Watanabe K, Hayakawa F, Okumura A. Neonatal EEG: A powerful tool in the assessment of brain damage in preterm infants. *Brain Dev.* 1999;21:361–372.

Weeke LC, van Ooijen IM, Groenendaal F, et al. Rhythmic EEG patterns in extremely preterm infants: Classification and association with brain injury and outcome. *Clin Neurophysiol.* 2017;128(12):2428–2435.

Wikström S, Pupp IH, Rosén I, et al. Early single-channel aEEG/EEG predicts outcome in very preterm infants. *Acta Paediatr.* 2012;101(7):719–726.

Zhang D, Liu Y, Hou X, et al. Reference values for amplitude-integrated EEGs in infants from preterm to 3.5 months of age. *Pediatrics.* 2011;127:e1280.

Case 7.1 Preterm Infant with Grade III Intraventricular Hemorrhage and Posthemorrhagic Ventricular Dilatation

This preterm infant was born at 29 weeks' gestation by an emergency caesarean section for placental abruption. Apgar scores were 6, 7 and 8 at 1, 5 and 10 minutes, respectively. The infant developed severe respiratory problems, required three doses of surfactant and developed a pulmonary hemorrhage. Following a pulmonary hemorrhage, a repeat cUS showed an IVH grade III. A ventricular reservoir was inserted following the development of posthemorrhagic ventricular dilatation, later followed by a ventriculo-peritoneal shunt.

The *aEEG* recording was started following the IVH diagnosis. The background activity was more discontinuous than expected for the gestational age, and six single seizures were noted during the first 3.5 hours of aEEG recording (Figure 7.1A). Figure 7.1B shows how seizure frequency increased to a more status epilepticus–like pattern, in spite of the administration of phenobarbital iv at markers (c) and (d). Clonazepam was also given (Figure 7.1C) and resulted in a severely depressed, flat background with continuing superimposed seizures. A third antiseizure medication, lidocaine, was given at marker (c) in Figure 7.1D, and no more seizures were seen after the 10-hour period of repetitive seizures. Figure 7.1E was recorded 4 days later and showed good recovery of the background activity with some cyclicity.

An *MRI* was performed at term equivalent age and showed moderate ventricular dilatation in spite of reservoir taps (Figure 7.1F). The MRI at 2 years of age showed no ventricular enlargement and good progression of myelination. The infant did not develop cerebral palsy and was in a mainstream school at 5 years of age. (See also the images on the cover of this edition.)

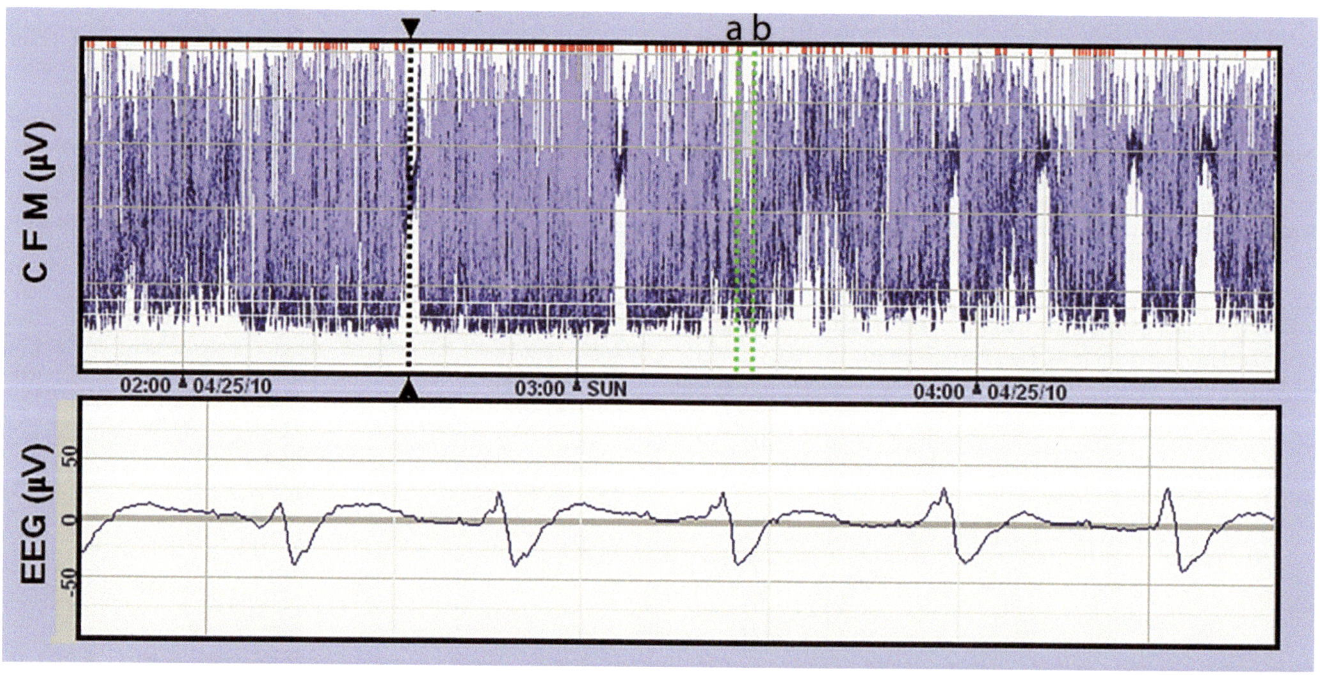

FIGURE 7.1A

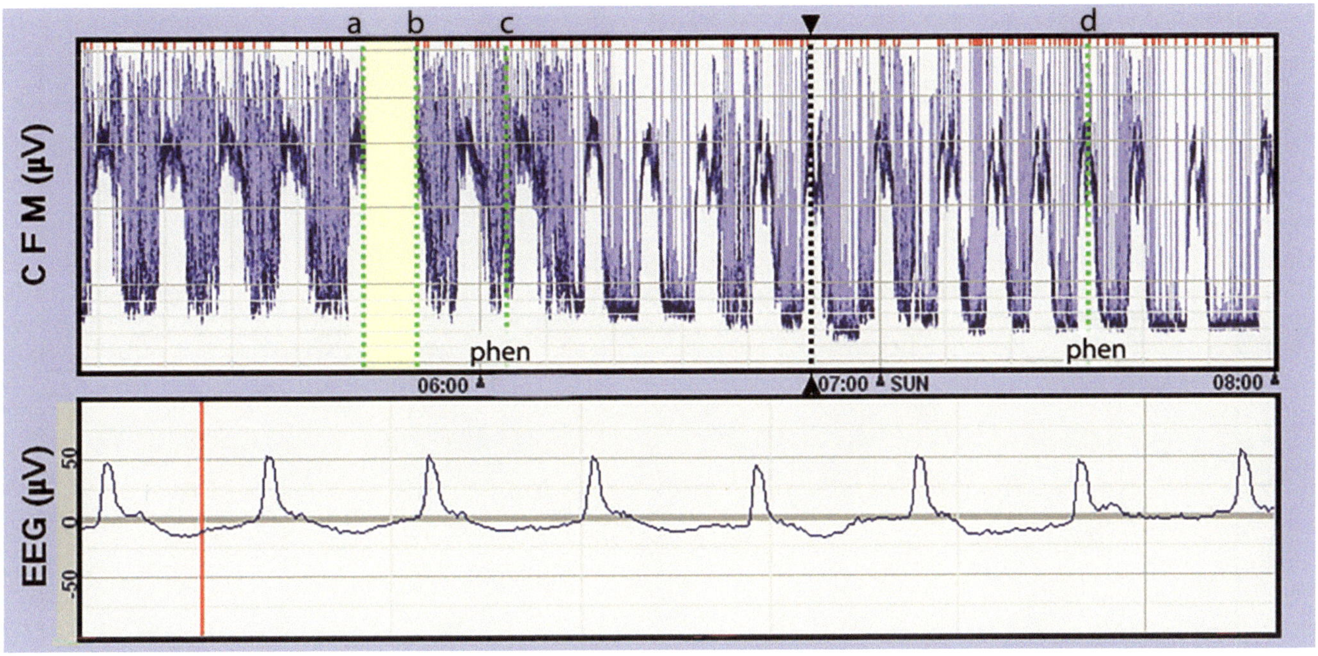

FIGURE 7.1B

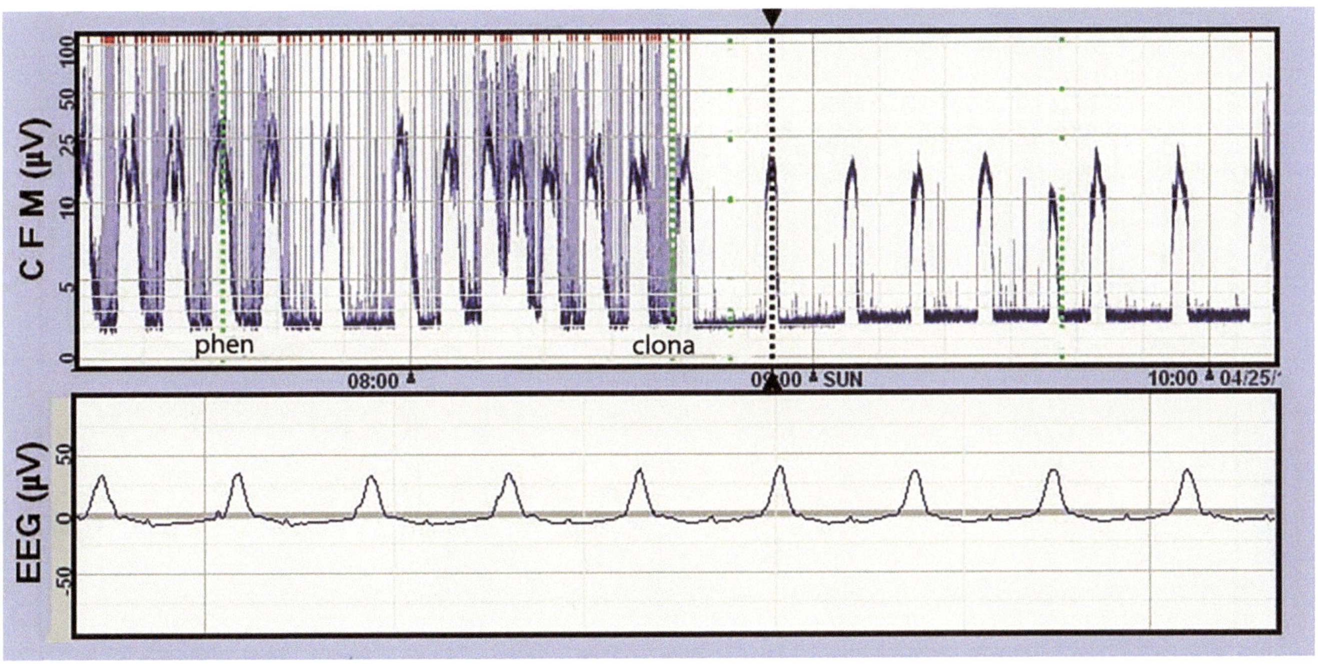

FIGURE 7.1C

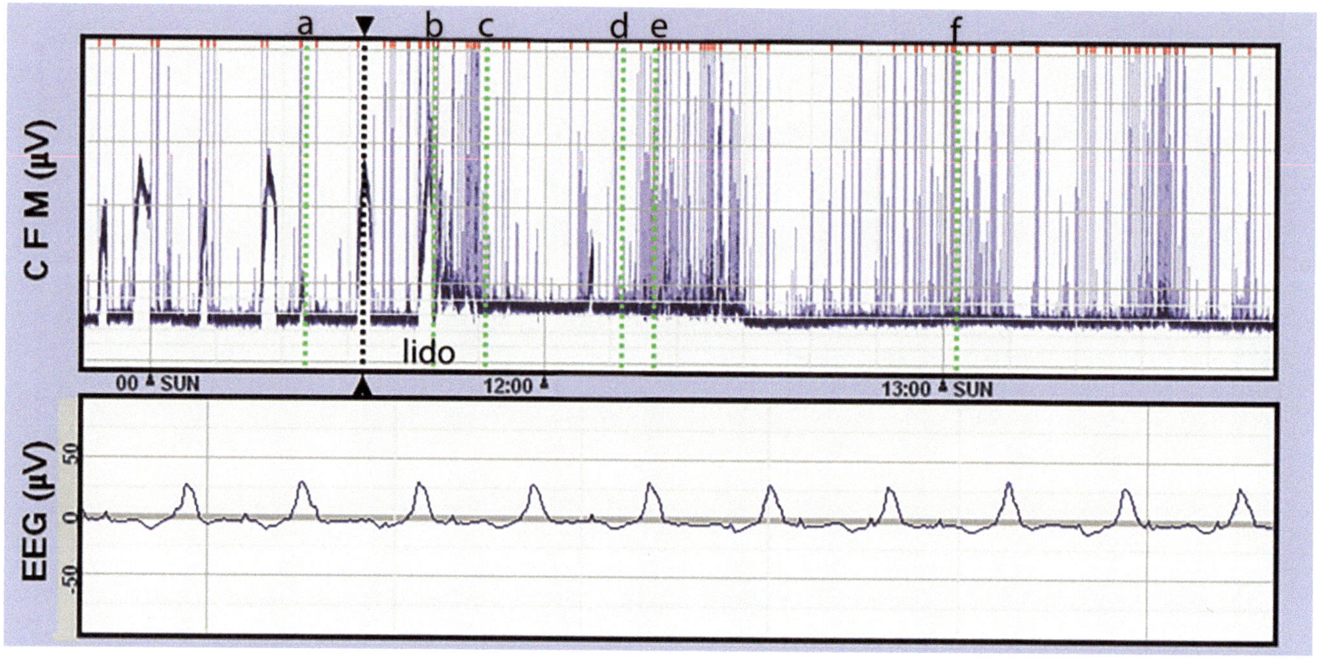

FIGURE 7.1D

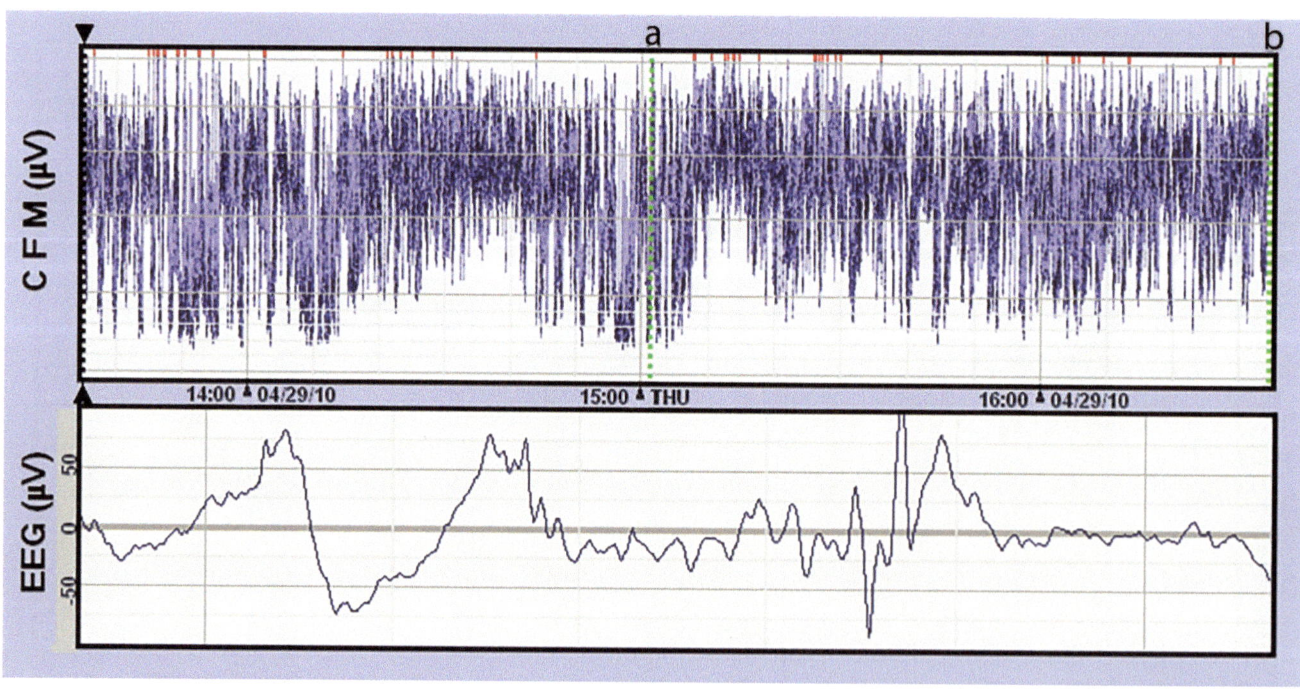

FIGURE 7.1E

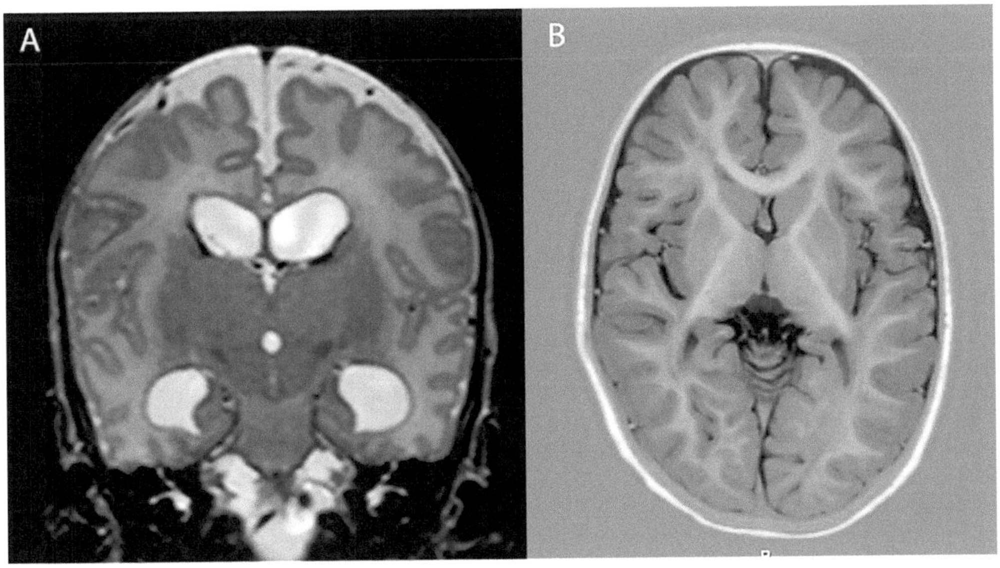

FIGURE 7.1F

Case 7.2 Severe IVH/PVHI and Refractory Seizures

This infant, born at 32 weeks' gestation, was transferred from a level-two unit on day 2 with an intracranial hemorrhage and abnormal neurological exam.

The perinatal history was significant for preterm labor at 31 weeks, and the mother was given betamethasone and magnesium sulfate. On the day of delivery, there was rapid progression of labor, membranes were ruptured at delivery, and there was meconium-stained, foul-smelling fluid and maternal chorioamnionitis. A precipitous delivery followed, and the infant was born with a nuchal cord. There was no respiratory effort, and the HR was below 100. Resuscitation was initiated, and the infant was intubated 3.5 min after birth. The cord blood pH was 6.9 and the BE was −13 mmol/L. Apgar scores were 3, 6 and 8 at 1, 5 and 10 minutes. Umbilical lines were placed. The placenta was foul-smelling and grew Gram-negative rods.

The initial neurologic exam after birth was documented as normal (i.e. normal tone, normal response to tactile stimuli, normal spontaneous movements, symmetry of exam, normal truncal tone, negative for myoclonus). On the following day, the neurologic exam changed and cUS showed a significant left-sided parenchymal hemorrhage involving the deep white tissue of the left cerebral cortex in addition to blood within the left lateral ventricle. The infant was transferred to the level-three unit for further evaluation and brain monitoring. During transfer, there was abnormal posturing and development of a bulging fontanelle.

The *EEG/aEEG* monitoring was started just after admission, continued over the following days (Figures 7.2A to 7.2D) and displayed a three-channel aEEG (left, right, cross-cerebral) and below the raw EEG from the aEEG time point in green numbers.

At the start of the recording (Figure 7.2A, aEEG duration was 3 hours and EEG was 8 seconds), the electrocortical background is suppressed and discontinuous with numerous elevations of the lower margin highlighted by * which on EEG were verified to be seizures. The seizures were best identified on the upper aEEG panel. Phenobarbital 20 mg/kg iv was given twice, at 00:35 and at 02:08 hrs, and resulted in a more depressed background pattern.

Despite a total of 40 mg/kg iv of phenobarbital, there were ongoing seizures (Figure 7.2B, aEEG duration was 8 hours and EEG was 17 seconds), and levetiracetam was administered at 05:00 hrs but did not resolve the seizures.

Due to ongoing seizures, fosphenytoin was administered at 10:30 hrs (Figure 7.2C, aEEG duration was 4 hours and EEG was 9 seconds). After that, seizures became less frequent, and a dense burst-suppression pattern emerged. The seizures had a sawtooth appearance, suggestive of a status epilepticus that lasted 10 hours.

A repeat cUS was done, and a midline shift was noted, and thus, an MRI was requested by the neurosurgical team (Figure 7.2D). The *MRI* was performed the next day. The T2-weighted images confirmed the left-sided periventricular hemorrhagic infarction (PVHI) extending over several lobes (Figure 7.2E). Ultimately, the infant required placement of a VP shunt. At 5 years of age, there was an abnormal development with cerebral palsy. This example also shows how the scales can be adjusted according to individual needs. The displayed aEEG in Fig 7.2A is 3 h and the EEG below 8 sec. In Fig 7.2B the aEEG is 7 h and the EEG below 18 sec. In Fig 7.2C the aEEG is a bit longer than 4 h and the EEG 9.5 sec.

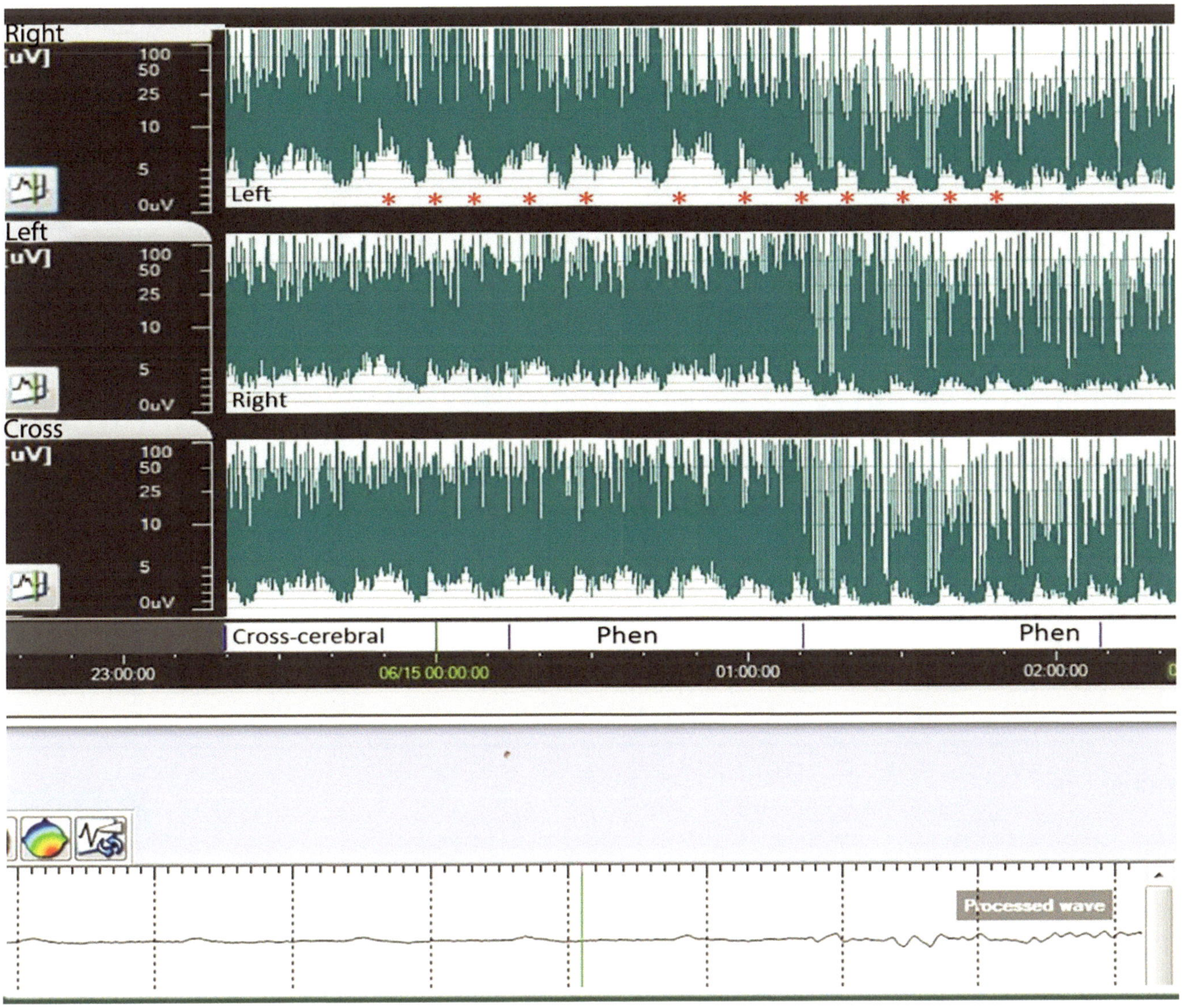
Right
[uV]
100
50
25
10
5
0uV
Left
Left
[uV]
100
50
25
10
5
0uV
Right
Cross
[uV]
100
50
25
10
5
0uV
Cross-cerebral
Phen
Phen
23:00:00
06/15 00:00:00
01:00:00
02:00:00
Processed wave

FIGURE 7.2A

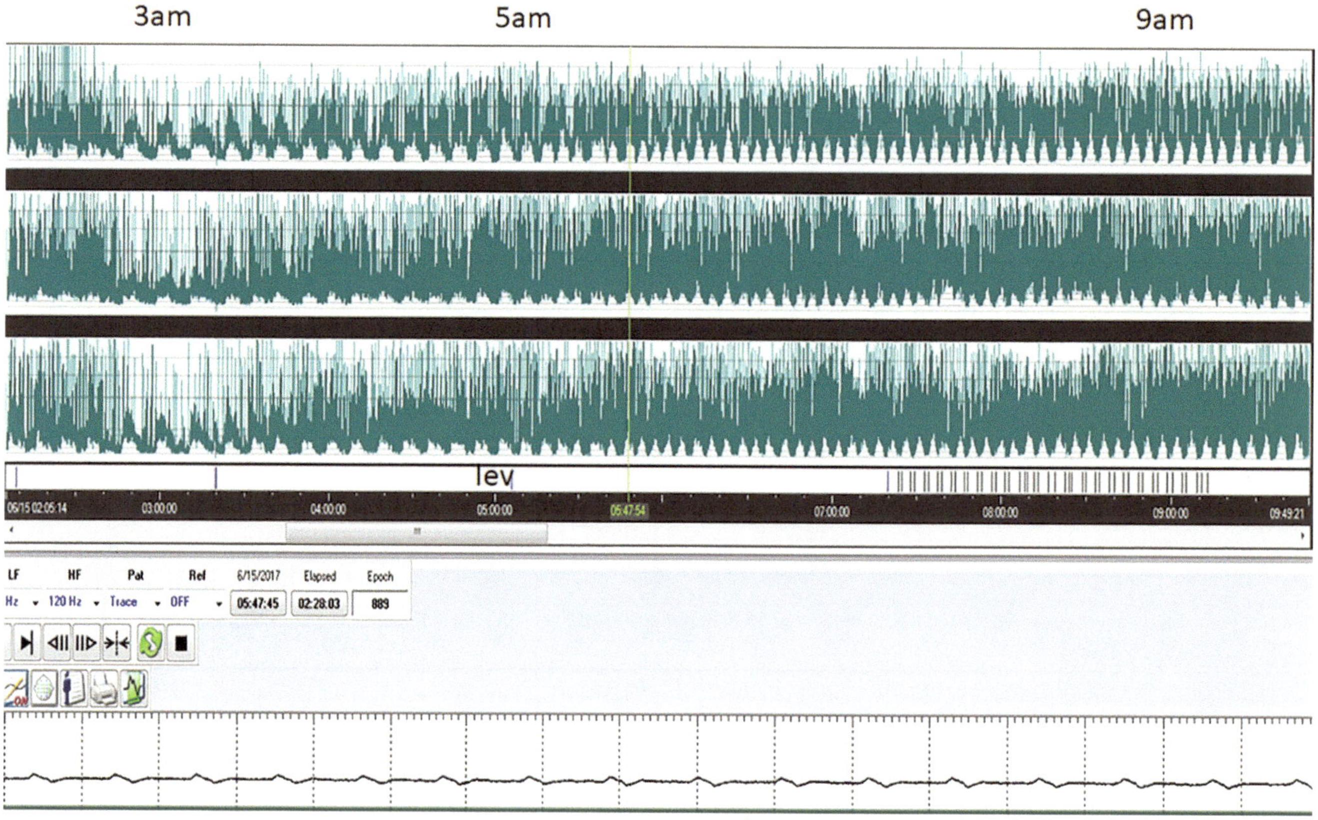
3am
5am
9am
lev
06/15 02:05:14
03:00:00
04:00:00
05:00:00
05:47:54
07:00:00
08:00:00
09:00:00
09:49:21
LF
HF
Pat
Ref
6/15/2017
Elapsed
Epoch
Hz
120 Hz
Trace
OFF
05:47:45
02:28:03
889

FIGURE 7.2B

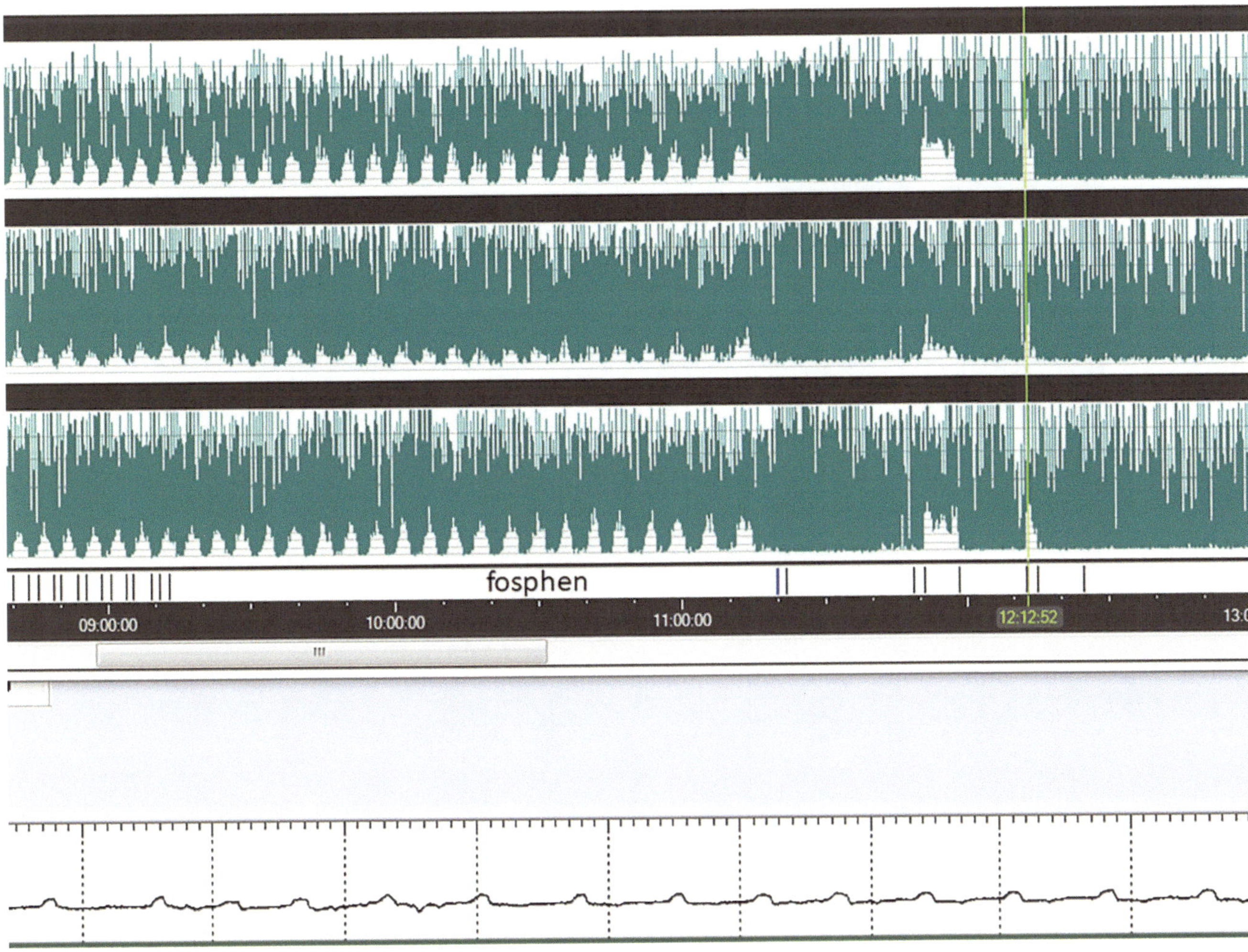

FIGURE 7.2C

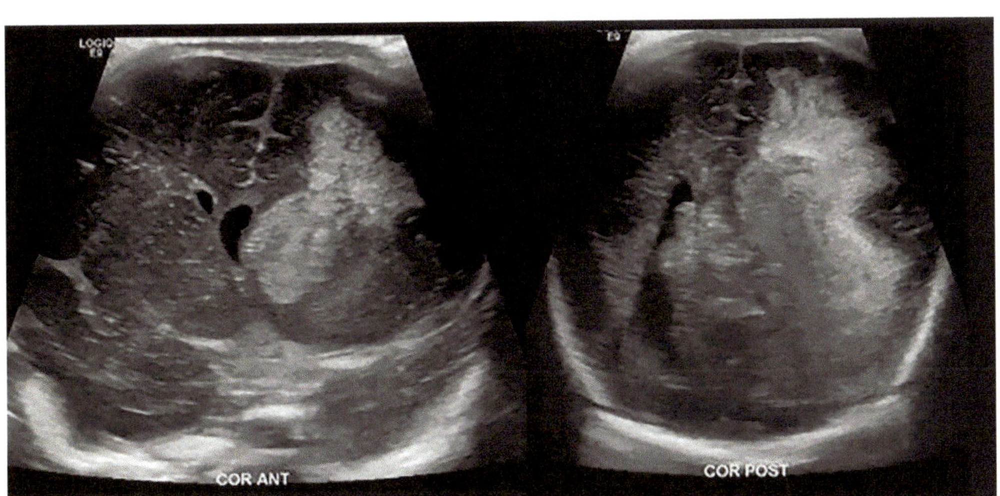

FIGURE 7.2D

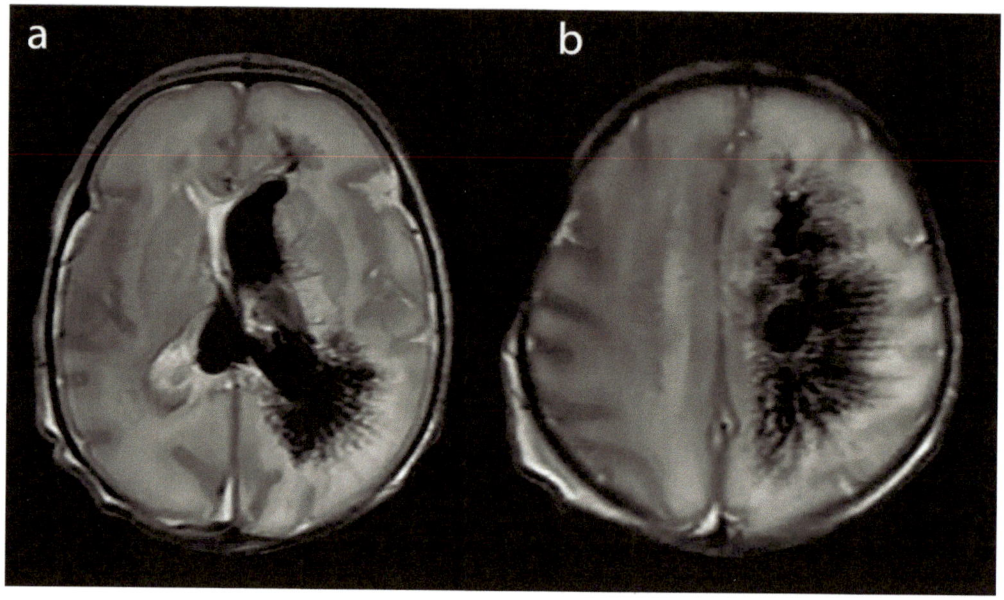

FIGURE 7.2E

Case 7.3 Very Preterm Infant with Severe Asphyxia

This very preterm infant was born at 30 weeks' gestational age by emergency caesarean section because of placental abruption and a severely abnormal CTG. Apgar scores were 0, 1 and 6 at 1, 5 and 10 minutes, respectively. The first arterial lactate was 14.7 mmol/L. Extensive resuscitation was required, including intubation and administration of adrenaline iv. A bilateral IVH grade III developed on the first day of life.

The recording started at 9 hours after birth and showed a severely depressed, flat trace with superimposed seizures. The seizures were seen on the aEEG trace and recognized by the waveform (seizure) detection algorithm (yellow band). Lidocaine was administered at marker 3 (Figure 7.3A). As the repetitive seizures continued, clonazepam was given (Figure 7.3B; see also Video 7.3) followed by phenobarbital (Figure 7.3C), which resulted in an entirely flat trace. Seventeen hours later, there was recurrence of the seizures, and levetiracetam was given (Figure 7.3D). Intermittent seizures continued on a mainly flat background, and as the electrocortical background activity did not show recovery, care was redirected on day 2.

Cranial *ultrasound* was normal on admission but showed a bilateral IVH grade III the next day (Figure 7.3E).

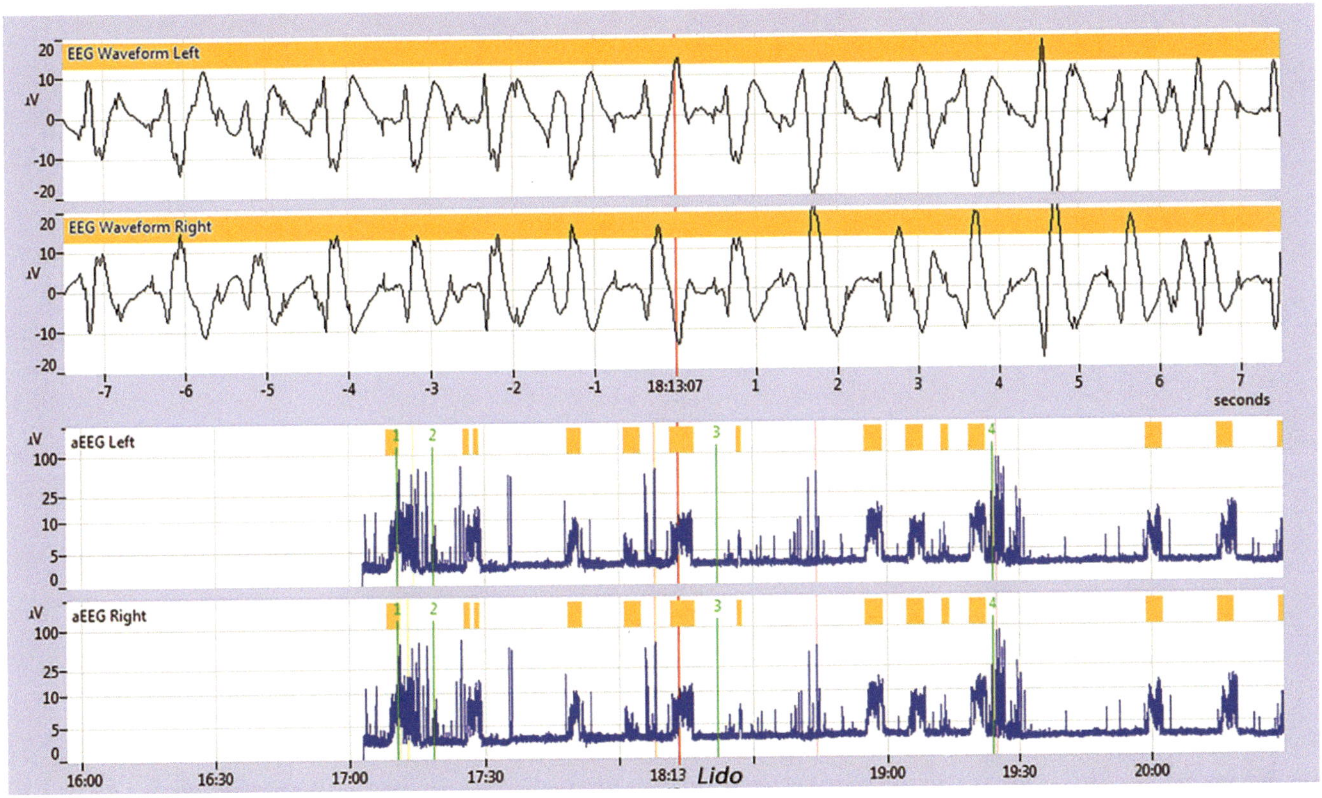

FIGURE 7.3A

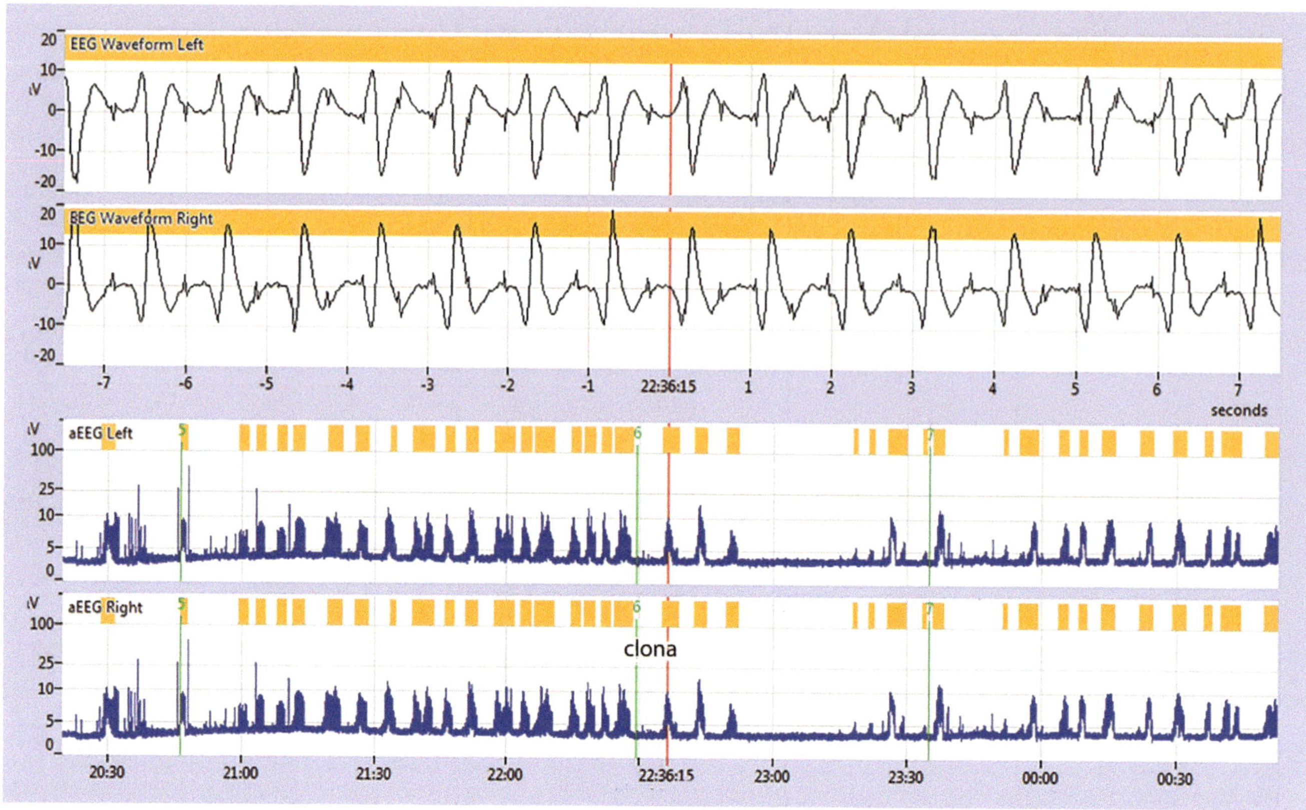

FIGURE 7.3B

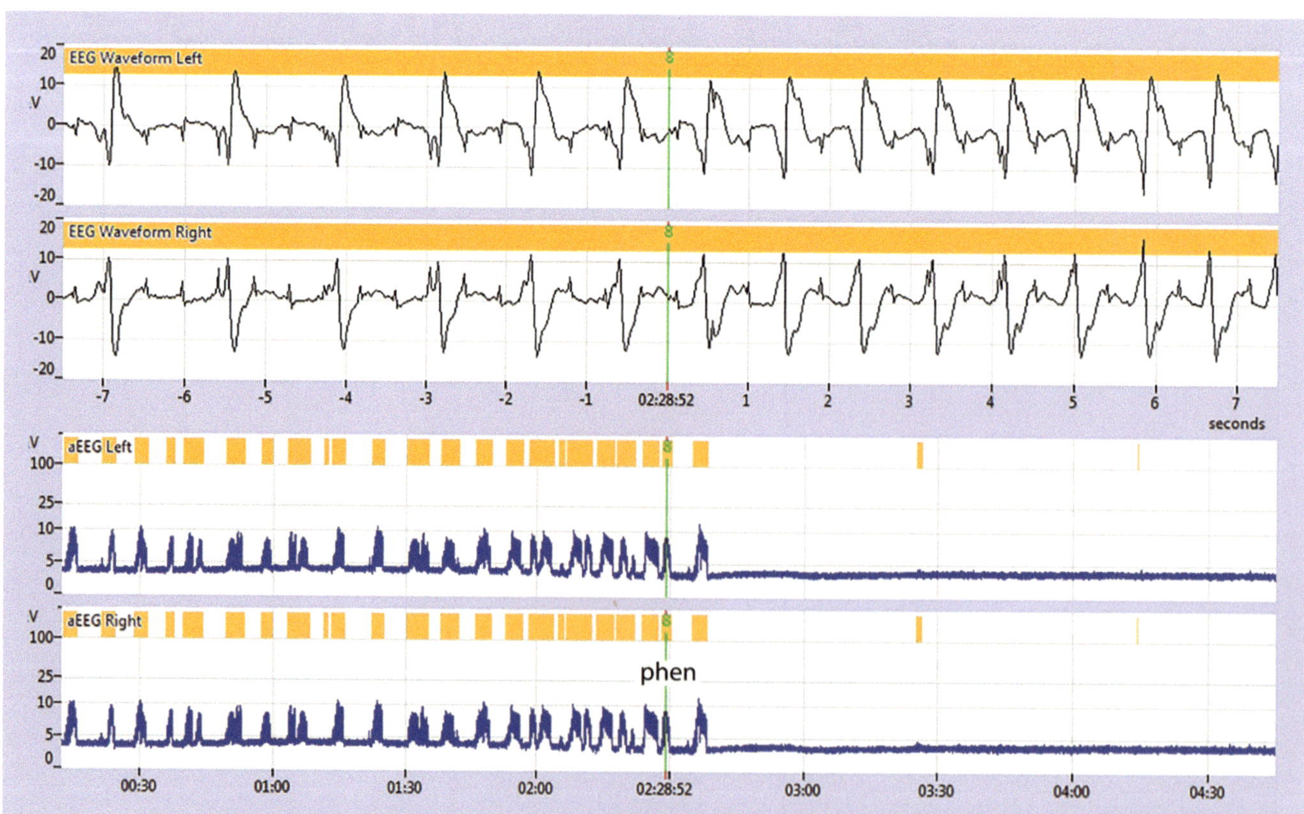

FIGURE 7.3C

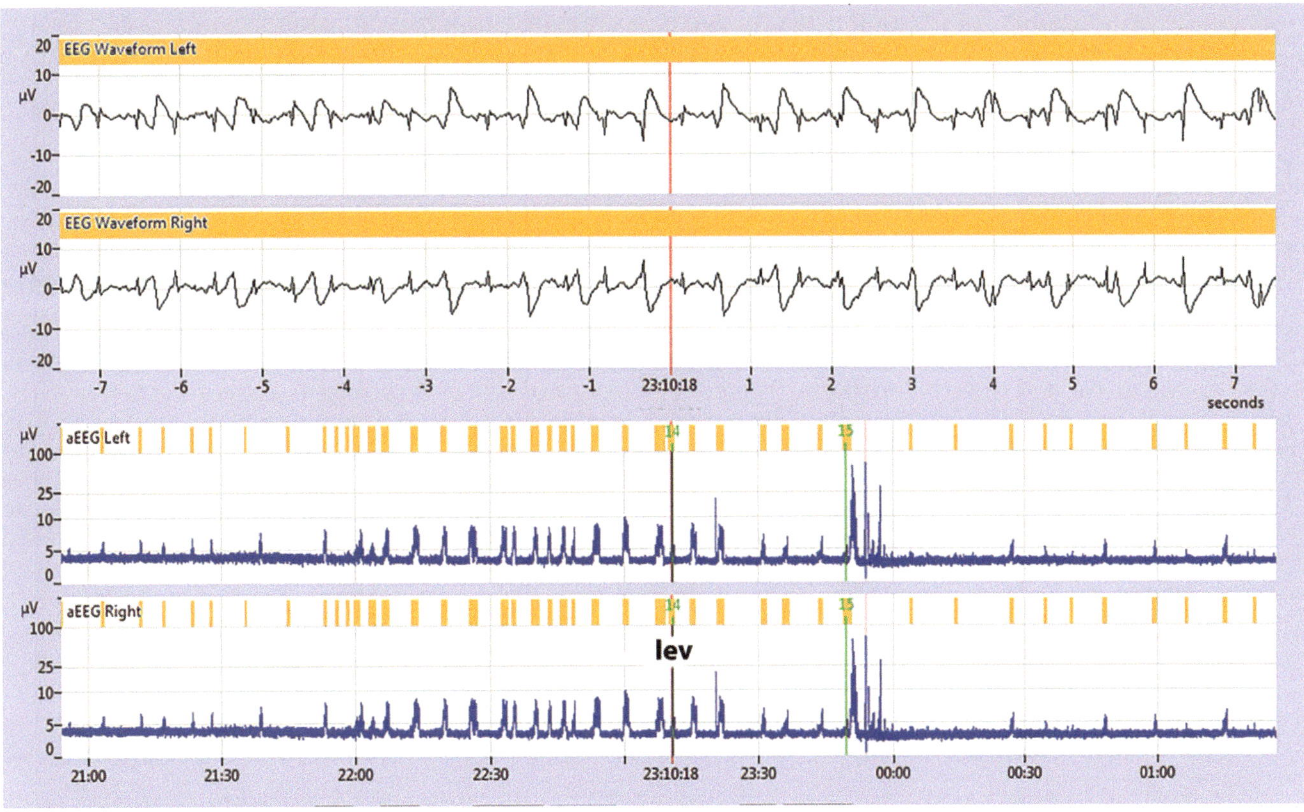

FIGURE 7.3D

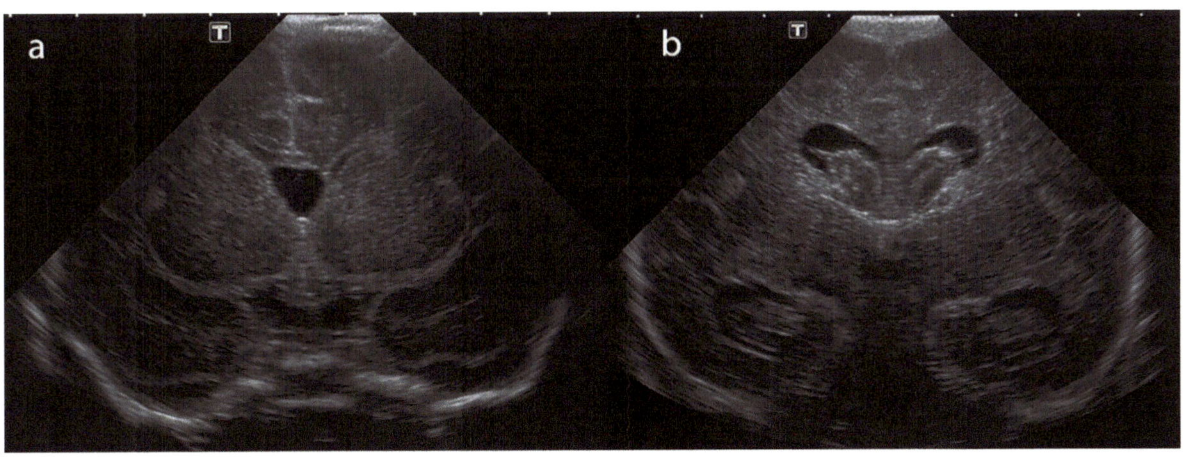

FIGURE 7.3E

Case 7.4 Preterm Infant with Severe Intrapartum Asphyxia

This preterm infant, was born at 32 weeks' gestation by a complicated vaginal breech delivery. Apgar scores were 0, 1 and 2 at 1, 5 and 10 minutes, respectively. Extensive resuscitation was required. The umbilical artery pH was 6.92. The first arterial lactate was 8.2 mmol/L. The infant developed therapy-resistant hypotension, renal failure and severe respiratory problems for which high-frequency ventilation (HFV) and nitric oxide (NO) for pulmonary hypertension were required. Care was redirected after 4 days due to a combination of multi-organ failure and severe brain injury.

The *aEEG* recording was started 7 hours after birth and showed an almost flat trace (Figure 7.4A) with intermittent (several minutes between) low-amplitude, burst-like activity of uncertain origin. Also note the HFV artefact on F3-P3 between 03.10 till 04.30.

Following recovery to a BS pattern (Figure 7.4B; see also Video 7.4), repetitive seizures were noted. Midazolam was given (bolus and continuous infusion), followed by lidocaine that stopped the seizures. The raw EEG shows three consecutive 26-second traces demonstrating the evolution of a right-sided seizure at the time of the midazolam administration (blue arrow).

The sparse burst-suppression pattern (with interburst intervals lasting several minutes) persisted till the end of the recording on day 6 (Figure 7.4C), when midazolam was no longer administered, but the infant was still on a low dose of continuous morphine. The EEG below the aEEG shows 13 seconds of a flat interburst interval.

Both *cranial ultrasound* and *MRI* (Figure 7.4D) showed extensive ischemic injury, especially in the right hemisphere, but there was no clear laterality on the aEEG/EEG.

cUS (a) also showed agenesis of the septum pellucidum, ventriculomegaly and increased echogenicity in the territory of the right middle cerebral artery. *MRI* (b, c) was performed on day 4, and areas of restricted diffusion were seen, especially in the right hemisphere and more marked in the right posterior limb of the internal capsule than the left.

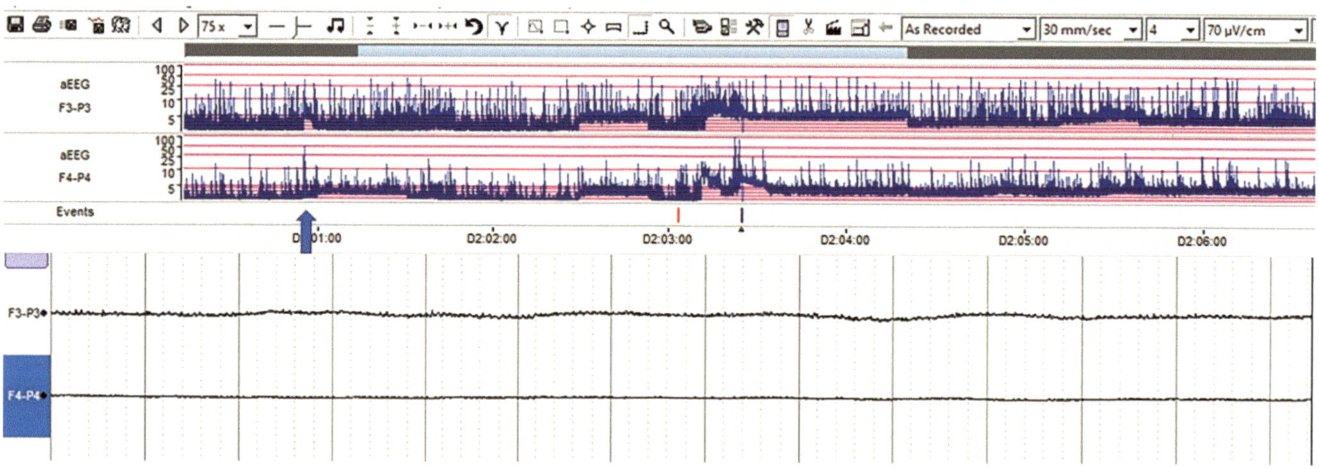

FIGURE 7.4A

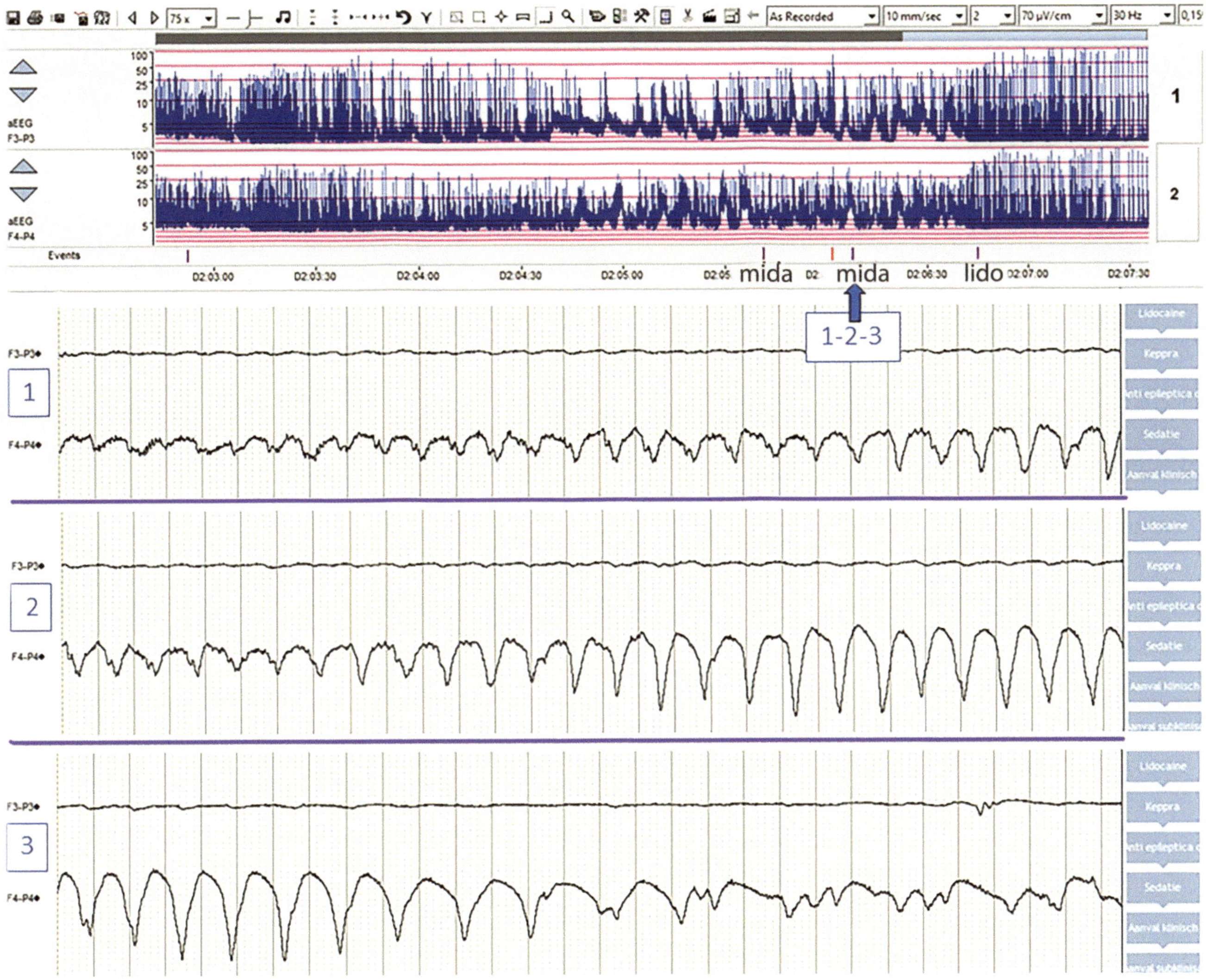

FIGURE 7.4B

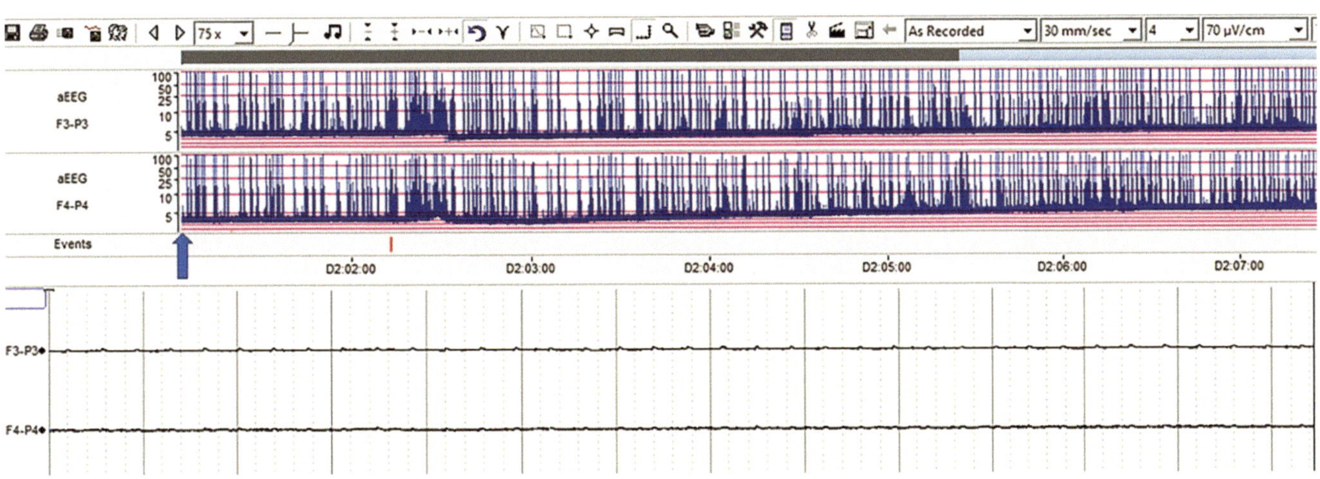

FIGURE 7.4C

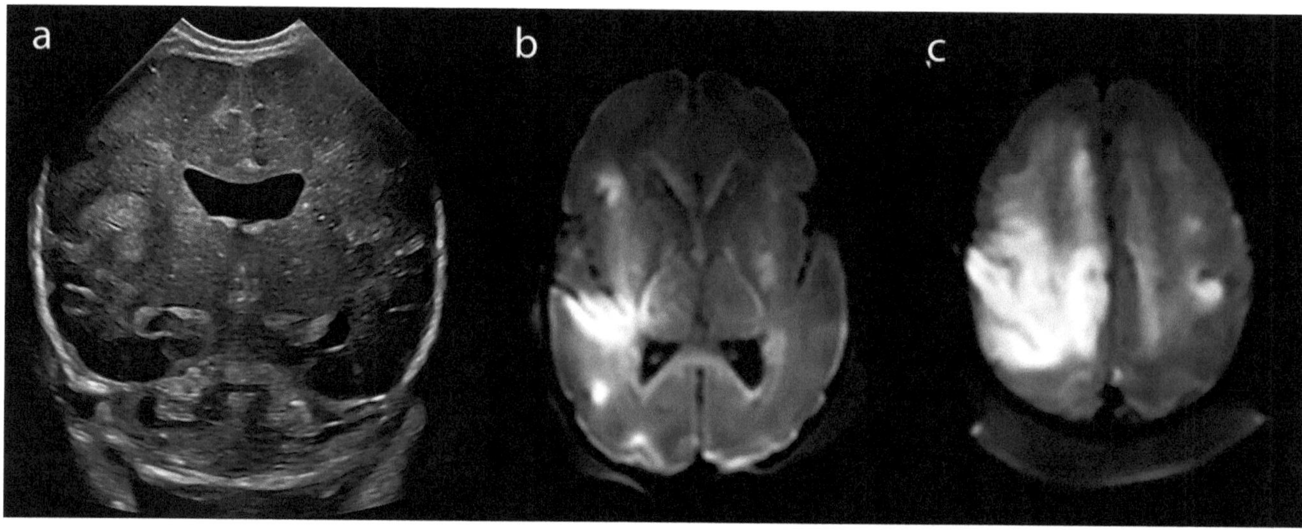

FIGURE 7.4D

Case 7.5 Vein of Galen Malformation in Late Preterm Infant

This infant was born at 35 weeks' gestation. An antenatal ultrasound and fetal MRI confirmed vein of Galen malformation (VOGM) with ensuing in utero heart failure. Attempted in utero intervention with coiling proceeded to emergency caesarean section and the need for extensive resuscitation. At the NICU, the infant required respiratory support with high-frequency ventilation. In view of the extensive resuscitation, it was decided to start therapeutic hypothermia.

The *aEEG* recording started at 5 hours after birth and showed a BS pattern. The recording from the left hemisphere shows some drift of the baseline that could be due to the high-frequency ventilation, maybe with the infant lying with the head to the left. It could, however, also be due to the malformation positioned in the left hemisphere with a turbulent blood flow (Figure 7.5A).

No seizures developed, and the background pattern gradually recovered to a DNV, more convincing on the left side (Figure 7.5B), but there was no clear sleep-wake cycling.

The fetal *MRI* (Figure 7.5C) (T2 sequence) shows the malformation but no apparent injury to the white matter. The postnatal cranial *ultrasound* (Figure 7.5D) shows the large cystic lesion (A, B). Using color Doppler ultrasound clearly shows the turbulent flow within (C). The postnatal MRI, done on the second day of life (Figure 7.5E), was reassuring regarding the absence of significant acute brain injury: the T2 sequence (A) shows the maximum caliber of the VOGM in the axial midline. The susceptibility weighted imaging (SWI) sequence on the MRI (B) shows small hypodensities in the ventricles and subdural regions indicating hemorrhage (hemosiderin). The flowing blood in the VOGM appears bright (hyperdense) on the SWI. The DWI sequence (C) does not demonstrate any significant restriction indicating ischemic injury, only small foci in the left occipital cortex (arrow) and the right frontal periventricular white matter.

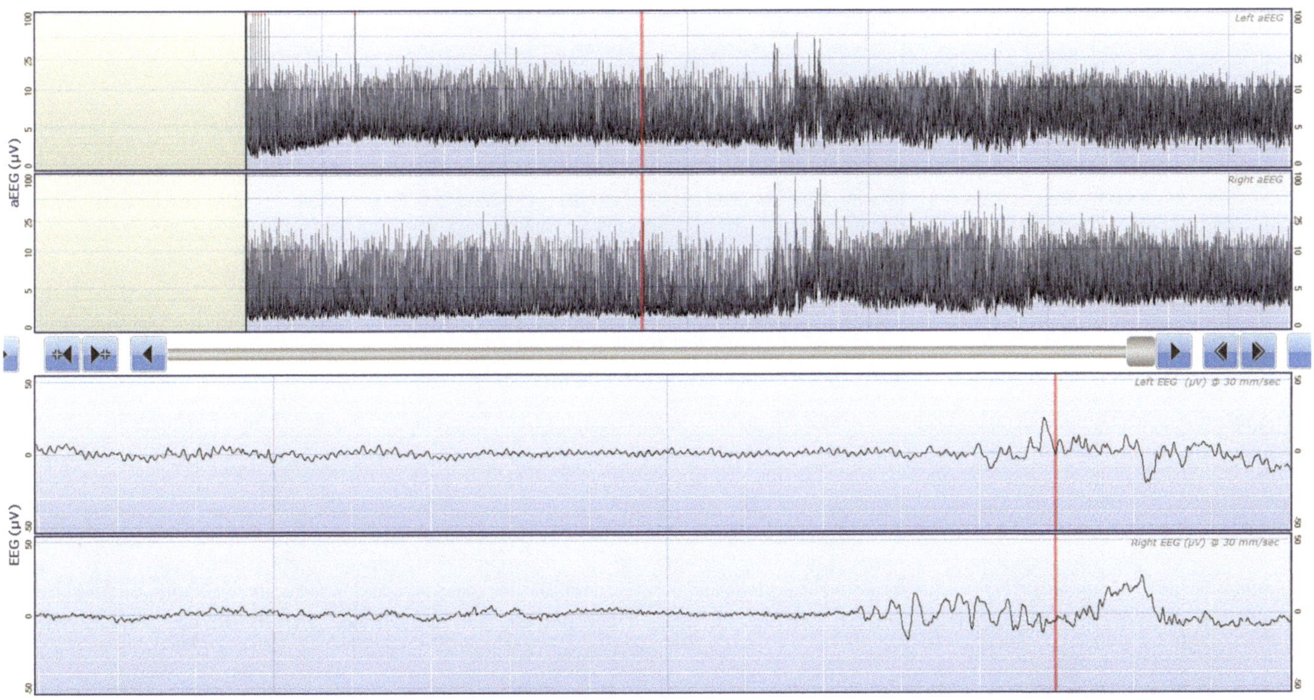

FIGURE 7.5A

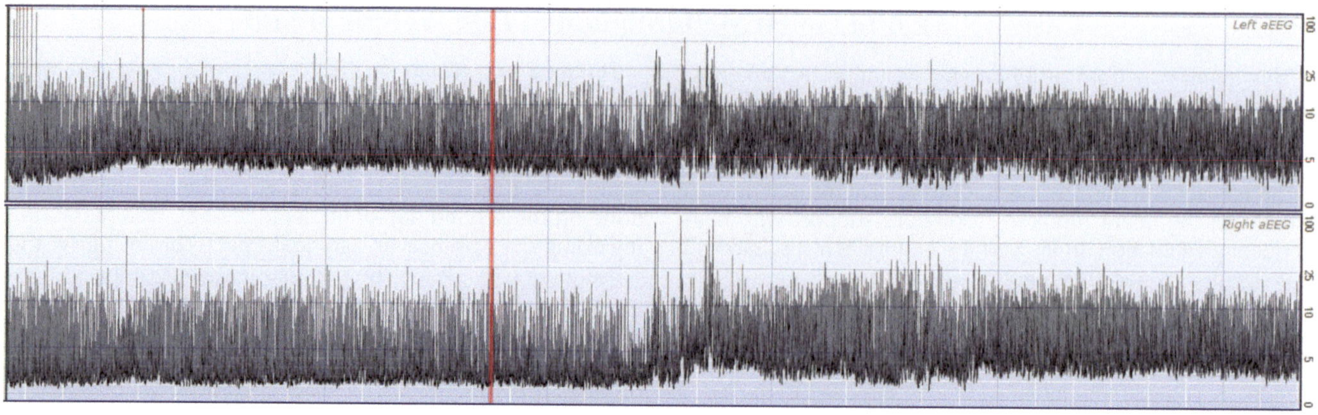

FIGURE 7.5B

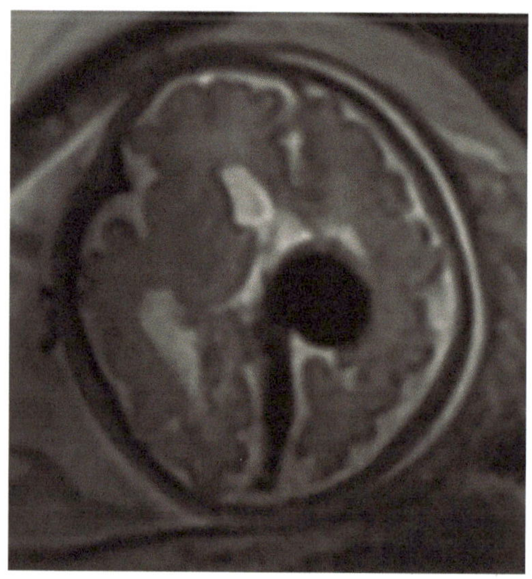

FIGURE 7.5C

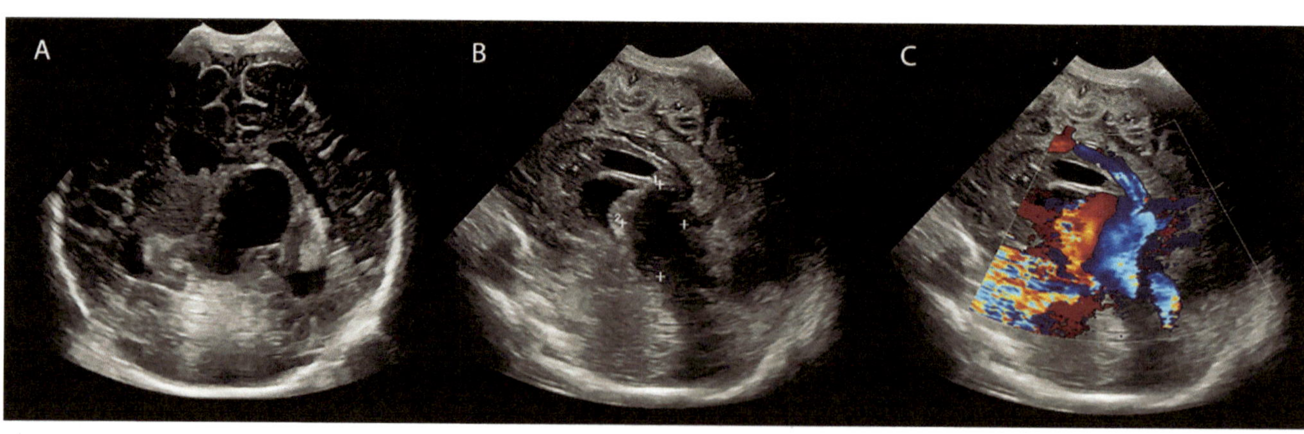

FIGURE 7.5D

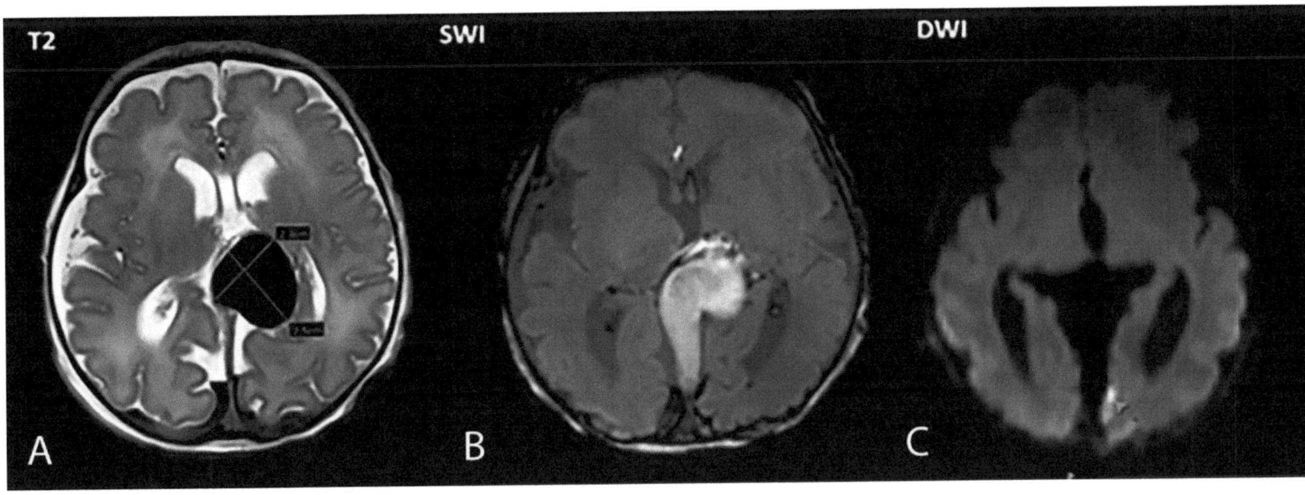

FIGURE 7.5E

Case 7.6 Encephalitis with *Bacillus cereus* in a Preterm Infant

This male infant was born at 31 weeks' gestation, with a birthweight of 1600 g. He was initially doing well but developed a rapidly progressing sepsis and meningoencephalitis with *Bacillus cereus* on day 3. He died 36 h after the onset of the infection in spite of full intensive care support.

A single-channel *aEEG* was started following the onset of the septicemia and encephalitis, showing a sawtooth pattern with repetitive seizures (Figure 7.6A). Following the administration of phenobarbitone (A), the background pattern changed to a very depressed BS pattern, with sparse bursts appearing with intervals of several minutes. There was a recurrence of the seizures, and a loading dose of lidocaine was administered without effect (A) in Figure 7.6B. In spite of the lidocaine, a status epilepticus developed. A loading dose of clonazepam was given (B) which stopped the seizures and resulted in a flat background activity. In Figure 7.6C, the status epilepticus recurred on a flat background, and the clonazepam was increased several times without any effect. Figure 7.6D shows an almost isoelectric recording with some very low-voltage possible ictal discharges.

Cranial ultrasound was normal on admission, but the white matter became severely echogenic (coronal views, Figure 7.6E; a and b), and cystic evolution was seen within the following 12 h (arrow) (c).

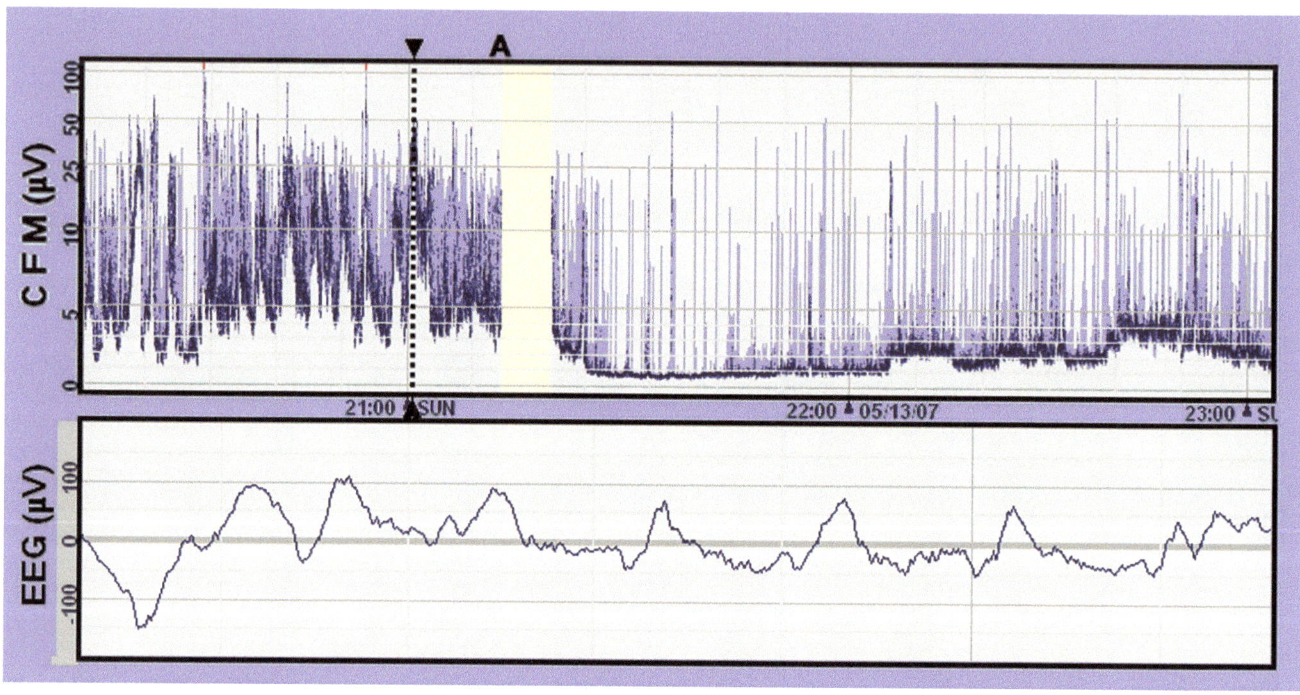

FIGURE 7.6A A, phenobarbitone.

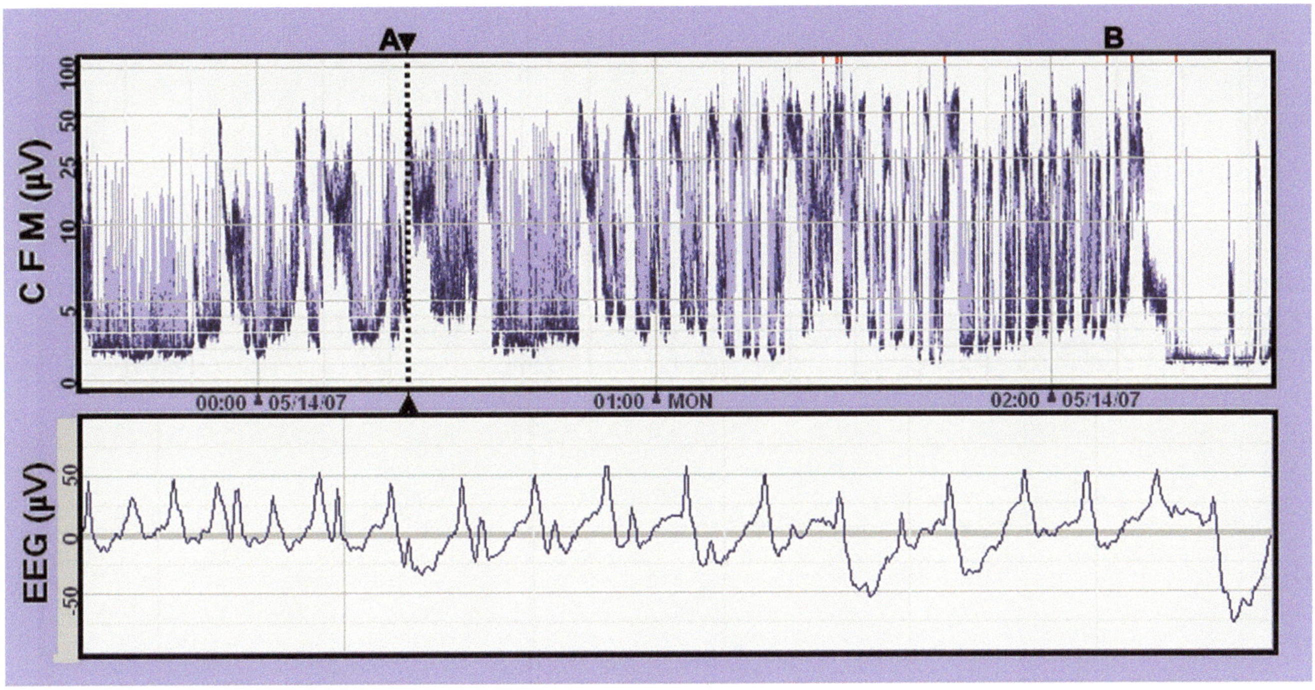

FIGURE 7.6B A, lidocaine loading dose; B, clonazepam loading dose.

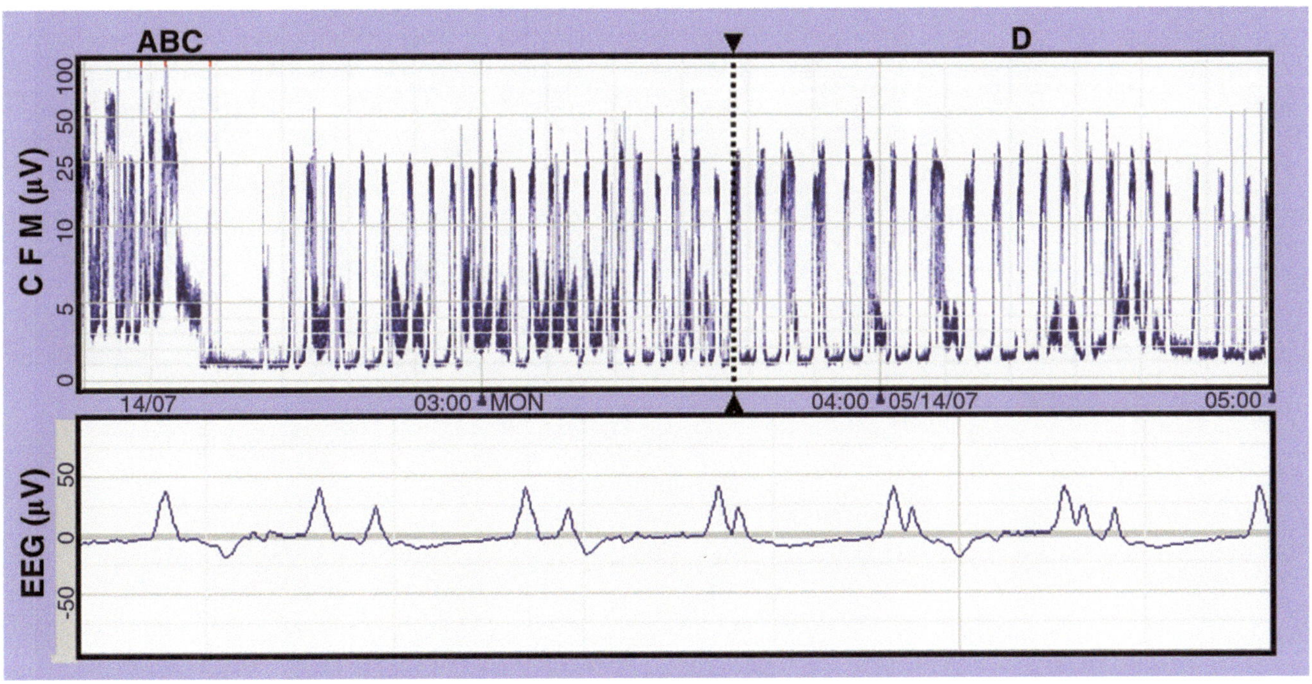

FIGURE 7.6C Clonazepam was increased at A, B, C and D.

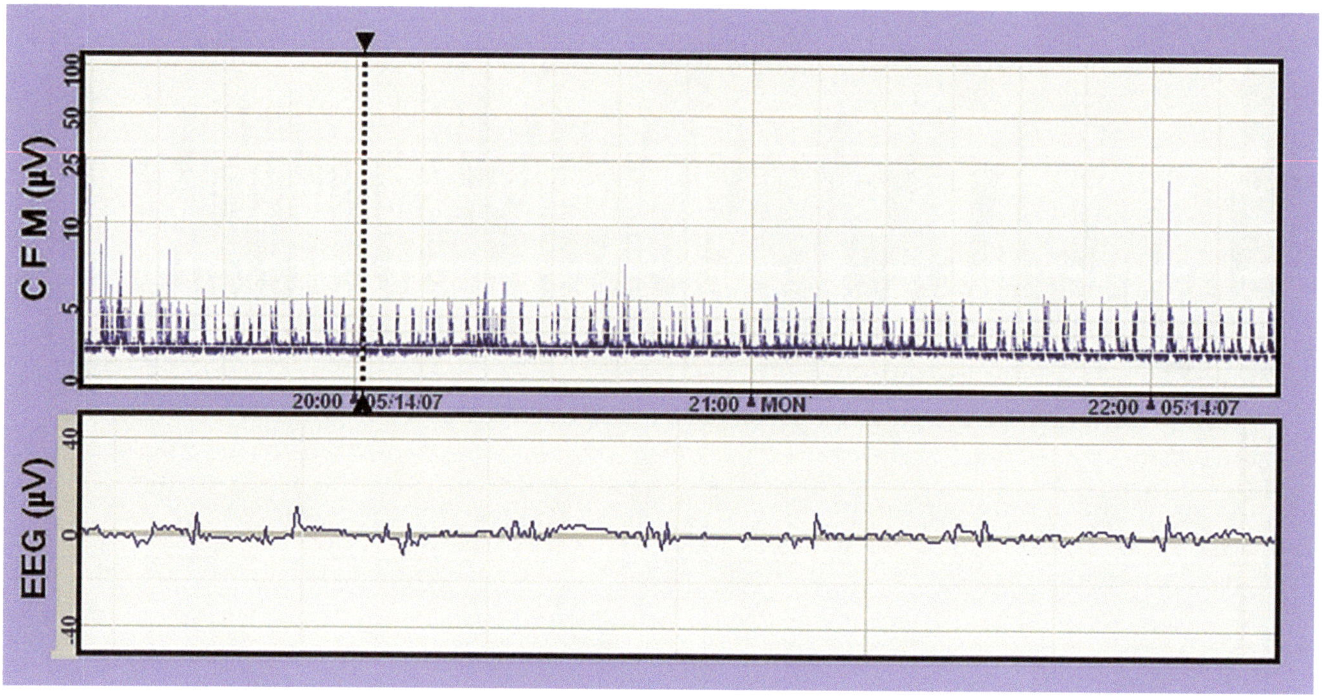

FIGURE 7.6D

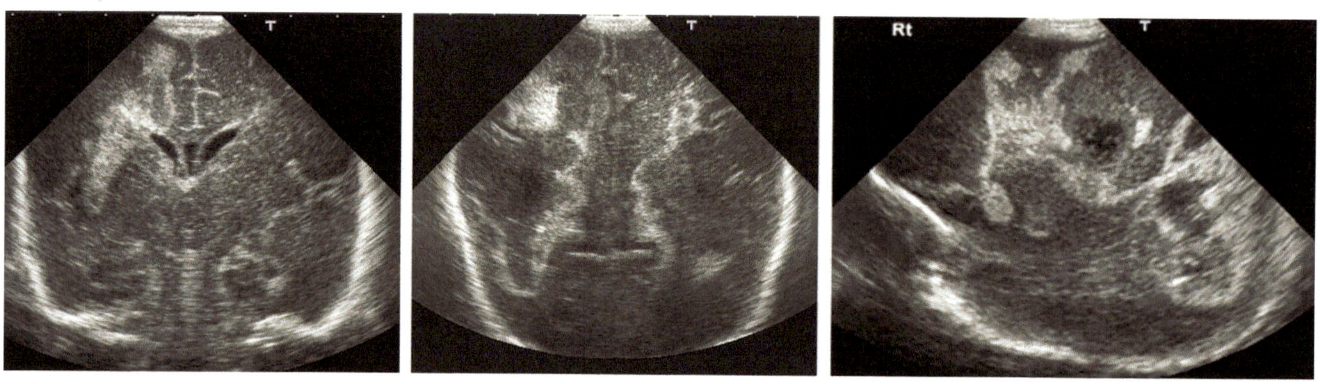

FIGURE 7.6E—A, B AND C

8 OTHER EEG TRENDS AND COMPUTATIONAL MEASURES

Sampsa Vanhatalo

Trends in the patient monitors are used for visualizing long-term changes in physiological parameters, such as heart rate (ECG), temperature, blood pressure or cortical activity (EEG). The trends facilitate clinical assessment and patient monitoring by offering a time-compressed display of clinically useful information that would be difficult to discern by visual review of the raw signals. The rationale of generating (computing) the aEEG trend is presented with visual examples in Chapter 2 (Figure 2.1), highlighting the way how aEEG supports clinically meaningful discrimination of the five key cortical states: inactive, burst-suppression, discontinuous, continuous and seizures.

The rationale of trends for newborn brain monitoring can be broadly categorized into two approaches: First, the conventional trends use simple computational measures, akin to aEEG, and they don't provide clinical interpretation. Their use needs a human expert for interpretation (hence, the need for this aEEG atlas!). Second, the more modern trends can display detections (e.g. seizures or sleep states) or other measures (e.g. background activity) using algorithms that were specifically trained for a physiologically and/or clinically meaningful interpretation. They can hence directly support the clinical decision-making.

8.1 Feature-Based Trends

Many computational trends have been introduced for a time-compressed display of EEG signals, and some of them have been already implemented for decades in the conventional EEG devices. They are typically visualizing one computational feature of the EEG signal, such as the total signal amplitude, power spectral density, symmetry of alpha power or interburst interval (Figure 8.1). They are mathematically very clear, but they lack a solid physiological or clinical interpretation. Apart from the aEEG, these features have not seen a wider clinical uptake in the neonatal EEG monitoring.

Some common examples of these trends include:

Power Spectral Density (*PSD*) shows the distribution of different frequency components (i.e. power spectrum) as a function of time, and it is sensitive to relative changes between different oscillatory frequencies.

Spectral Edge Frequency (*SEF*) shows the frequency under which a given proportion of EEG power is located. For instance, the SEF90 value shows that 90% of EEG power is below this frequency. The SEF measures reflect shape of the spectrum in a clean EEG signal, but they can be significantly confounded by both artefacts and the amplifier characteristics.

Total power, in turn, indicates the full signal power within a specified frequency.

Notably, all these are measuring EEG activity both inside and outside of the aEEG frequency (see Figure 2.1), so they are analytically complementary to the aEEG, though with a less clear clinical bedside value.

Some middle-ground solutions between simple and more elaborated measures have been introduced during the last two decades: They focus on measuring a clinically or physiologically recognized characteristic, such as *EEG bursts and burst shapes*, or visually assessed EEG characteristics like *interhemispheric synchrony* or *sleep-wake cycling*. These metrics are only used in clinical research so far, and they do not fully correspond to the visual review using the same EEG terminology. Several studies using these measures have clearly highlighted the ambiguity in the visual aEEG/EEG review of many EEG characteristics, such as "burst", "interburst", interhemispheric synchrony or cycling. Future studies and clinical trials are needed to establish the clinical potential of these novel measures as trend paradigms.

8.2 Interpreting Trends

Introduction of machine learning (ML)–based methods in the early 2000s made it possible to train algorithms for making clinically meaningful EEG interpretations. These algorithms were trained using input ("benchmark", reference) from the expert's EEG review rather than by developing heuristic mathematical measures. For instance, it became possible to train the algorithms to detect seizures by learning from the seizure annotations by the human experts. Automated algorithmic detectors have been now developed for many other types of complex EEG interpretations, such as sleep states, EEG background states and many types of artefacts (see Figures 8.2–8.4). While their clinical validation and implementation are still ongoing, it seems clear that such algorithms may perform at the level of human expert. It has become apparent that the most valid measure of the algorithm's performance is how it compares with the interrater agreement across human experts, i.e. whether a human expert could be replaced by the algorithm without compromising the agreement.

The next generation of EEG trends will likely provide users with clinically meaningful, transparent and intuitive interpretations. Such EEG classifiers employ modern machine learning methods, either based on combining heuristic signal features (e.g. the classic features earlier) or using data-driven, deep learning–based methods. Most importantly, the new algorithms are going beyond simple mimicking of conventional reviews or verbal rules of the EEG classifications. Instead, the modern algorithms are "trained" and "validated" with principled methodological pipelines using multicenter EEG data and large expert groups as benchmarks.

8.3 Visualization of Trends Other Than aEEG

There are multiple ways to display the outputs of ML-based algorithms as trends in the patient monitors.

A *direct trend* shows the actual output of the algorithm, such as the following:

- occurrence of seizures (seizure detector),
- presence of quiet sleep state (sleep state detector), or
- the type of cortical background activity (background classifier).

DOI: 10.1201/b22858-8

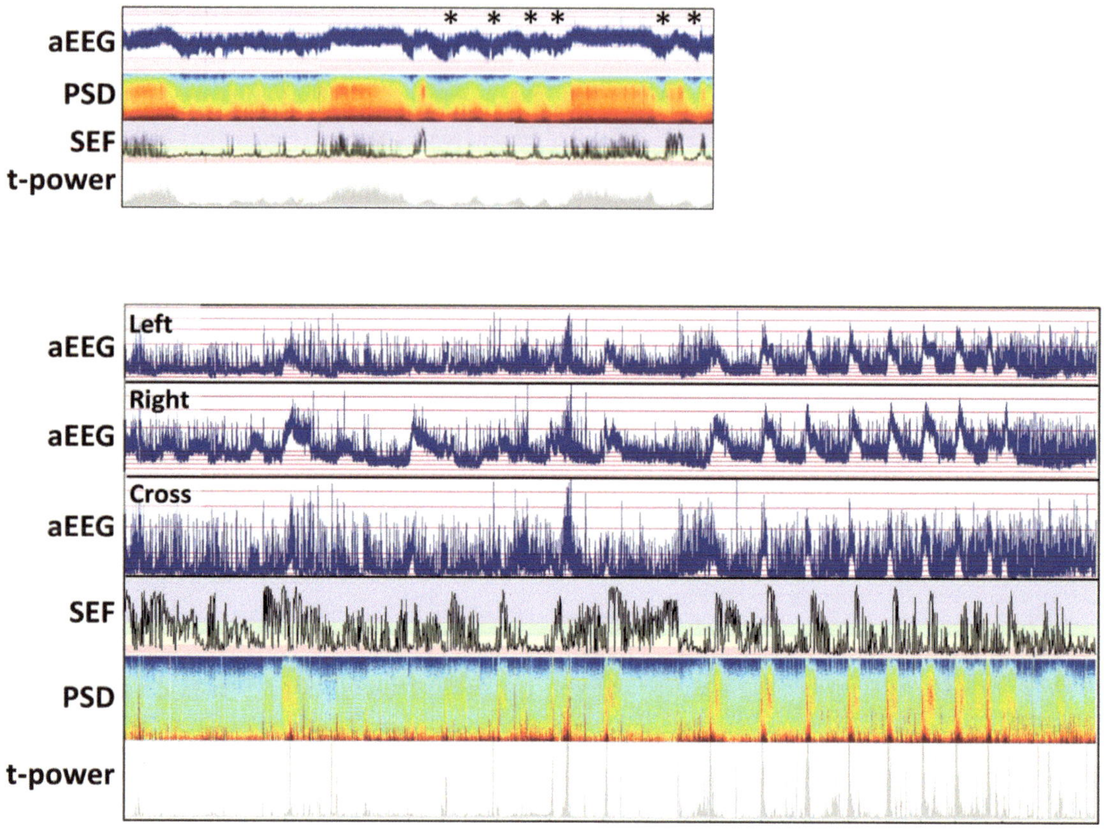

FIGURE 8.1 Comparison of simple feature-based trends that are commonly available in the EEG monitors.

Upper figure: Twelve hours of monitoring with some changes in the overall aEEG level and clear periods with SWC (quiet sleep epochs are indicated with asterisks). In this particular example, note how the PSD, SEF and total power fluctuate together with the aEEG trend, reflecting their common origins in the EEG signal content. However, this correlation is not always clear (see Figure 8.2), and clinician's interpretation is required separately for each of these trends.
Lower figure: Trend comparison during 8 hours of recovery from birth asphyxia, with initial burst-suppression activity with frequent seizures. Note the artefactual rise in the aEEG lower border in the left and right hemisphere aEEG trends, which is not seen in the cross-cerebral aEEG (because the artefact is apparently seen in the frontal EEG signals). All the other trends (SEF, PSD, total power) show clear changes during seizures (spiky appearance) and a loose correlation to the other aEEG changes.

More recently, algorithms like background classifier have been trained to show the output on a continuous scale rather than discrete categories (e.g. *BSN, Brain State of the Newborn;* Figures 8.2–8.3, 8.5). A continuous value output avoids ambiguities related to discrete categories, and it could also give the clinician an intuitively clearer interpretation. In addition, trends based on modern ML-algorithms can visualize the confidence (or uncertainty) of the displayed interpretation, akin to the uncertainty that is inherent to all clinical assessments. For example, it is more transparent and perhaps clinically more useful to display the likelihood (i.e. (un)certainty) of seizure detections rather than only showing dichotomic detections. Algorithms have been also developed to identify artefacts that would provide quality surveillance of the EEG data as a real-time feedback to the bedside staff for maintaining a good signal quality or to improve performance of the other algorithms by automatically removing the artefacts from the analyses.

An *indirect trend* shows a further elaboration of the algorithmic output, similar to the common heart rate trend that is based on R peak detections from the ECG signal. For example, the seizure detections can be visualized as a seizure burden (SB; Figure 8.4) trend showing minutes of seizures per hour, which may be more informative for treatment decisions. An indirect trend of the EEG background, in turn, may visualize the average of cortical activity background over longer time periods (e.g. every hour or multiple hours) together with the confidence of the finding, which may facilitate bedside assessment of cortical recovery over multiple days. Likewise, detections of quiet sleep state can be used for visualizing sleep state/depth trends (SST or SDT, respectively) that directly reflects sleep-wake cycling (SWC) and supports even SWC quantification (see Figures 8.2 and 8.5).

Taken together, the new EEG trends offer tailored interpretations to assist the bedside clinicians and clinical researcher. It is important that the treating clinician understands the nature of information shown in each trend, as well as their clinical implications for the patient care. The new trends are parts of the modern clinical decision support systems (CDSS) that should not make autonomic decisions. Understanding their role is crucial before the new trends can be widely implemented in the routine bedside monitors. Thereafter, much more collective clinical experience needs to be gathered to support evidence-based guidelines about the use of new trends in the routine care.

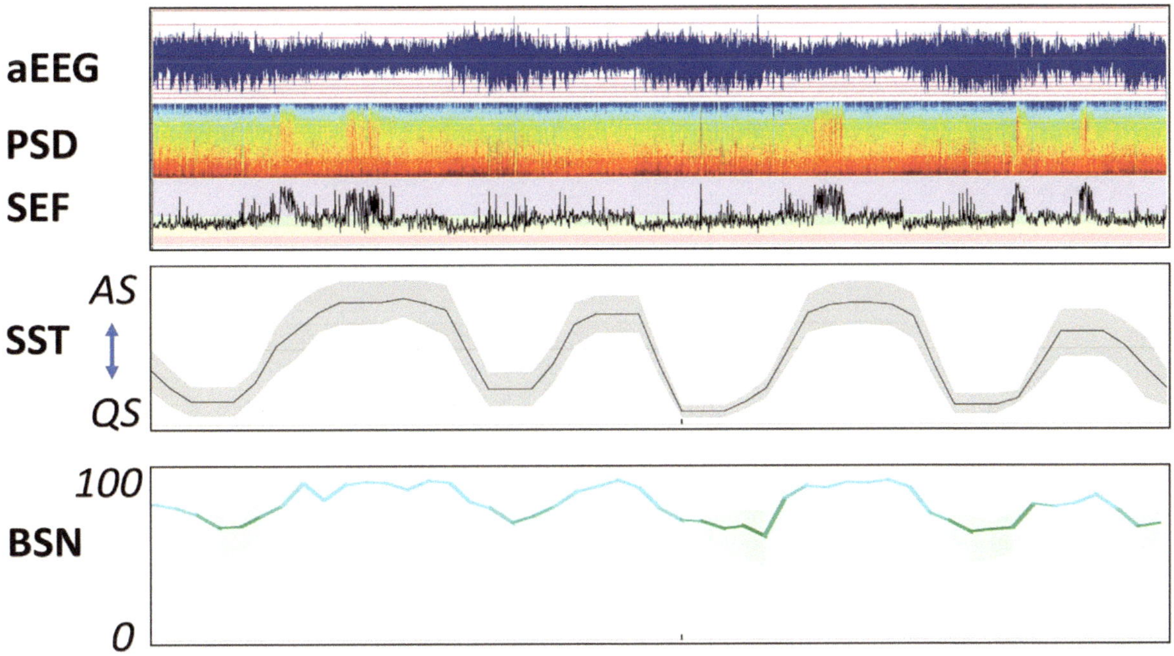

FIGURE 8.2 Comparison of the simple trends (aEEG, PSD, SEF) and novel interpreting trends (SST, BSN) in 8 hours of normal brain activity with a clear sleep-wake cycling (8 hours). The alteration between states, SWC, is apparent in the aEEG trend but hardly visible in the PSD and SEF trends. In contrast, the Sleep State Trend (SST; also called sleep depth trend, SDT) shows the likelihood of quiet sleep (QS) in a very robust way. This same SWC-related fluctuation is also visible in the more holistic trend, Brain State of the Newborn (BSN). The dark line indicates algorithms' output with shades indicating confidence of the output at each time point; colors indicate the level of BSN that may assist its visual review. (Courtesy of Saeed Montazeri.)

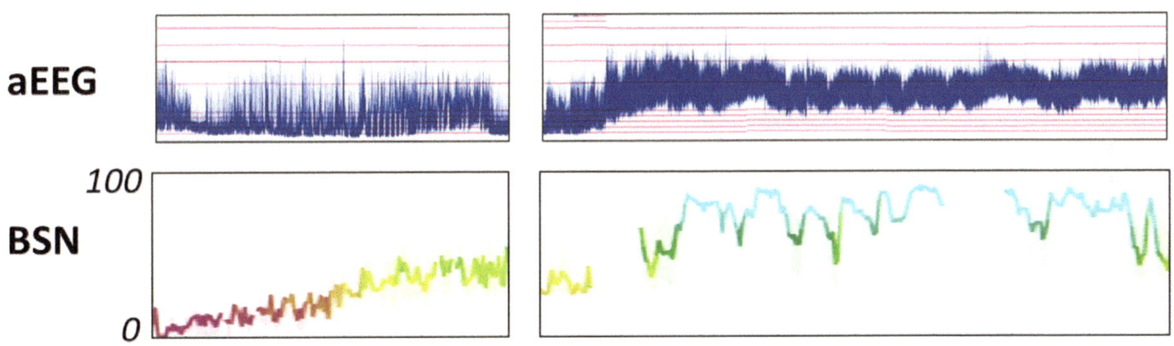

FIGURE 8.3 Comparison of aEEG and BSN trends during 3 days of the infant's recovery from birth asphyxia (gap, 16 hours). The aEEG trend shows an initial low activity typical of burst-suppression, then a relatively rapid recovery in the aEEG trend towards more normal levels and irregular fluctuations reminiscent of sleep-wake cycling. The corresponding BSN trend shows very low values (red) with gradual increase to higher yet abnormal levels (yellow) and a later rise to higher (green and blue) levels. The BSN trend also shows the fluctuations in brain state that resemble SWC in the aEEG. However, the state fluctuations are long-lasting and abnormal, being compatible with a delayed recovery from asphyxia. (Courtesy of Saeed Montazeri.)

8.4 Other Computational Measures

In addition to the trends that visualize changes in the cortical activity (EEG) over time, it is also possible to compute EEG measures from limited time epochs, such as minutes or hours. These measures can be either directly comparable to the conventional visual EEG assessments (e.g. maturation), or they may assess characteristics of the (a)EEG recording that go beyond visual perceptions.

8.4.1 Measures with Correlates in Visual Review

Visual recognition of "bursts", their shape in the EEG signal or their frequency are key characteristics in the newborn EEG review. The bursts are most prominent during early preterm development (tracé discontinu; see Chapter 7) or in the pathological state of burst-suppression. Several computational "*burst detectors*" have been developed during past decades. They use very different computational approaches, and they show varying correlation to the visual burst detection by human experts. It is also important to note that visual detection of bursts, especially their exact onsets or durations, is far more ambiguous than commonly considered. Burst detectors can be used further to assess *interburst intervals* (*IBI*), which is commonly assessed in the visual EEG review of both preterm and pathologic recordings. While IBI can be broadly useful, its accuracy is limited due to the ambiguity in burst detections in the first

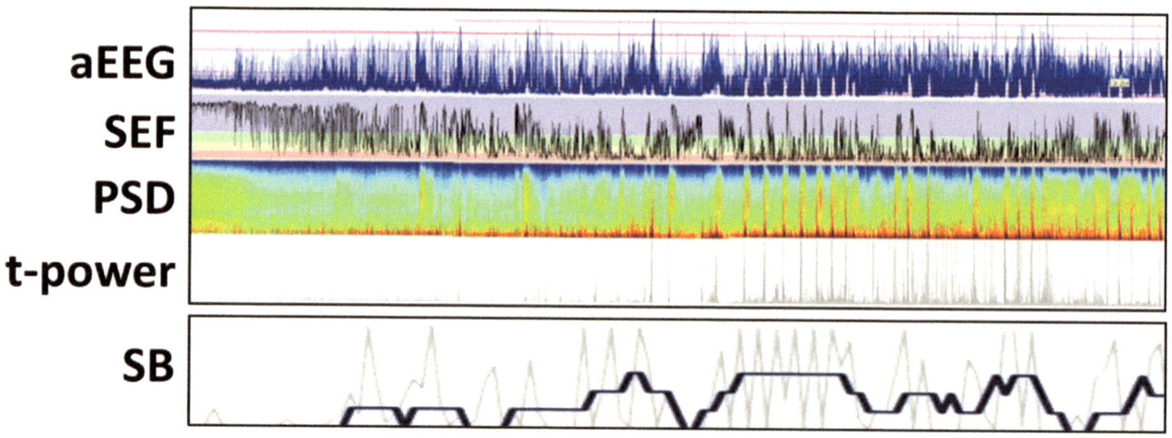

FIGURE 8.4 Comparison of conventional trends (aEEG, SEF, PSD, total power) and a seizure burden trend (SB) based on seizure detection algorithm. The conventional trends show typical seizure-related changes (see also Figure 8.1), whereas SB trend depicts the hourly cumulative amount of seizures (scale 0–6 min/h). Note how it is difficult to visually quantify hourly SB from the conventional trends, although they show the individual seizure occurrences clearly in this example. The grey line behind the SB trend depicts seizure likelihood over time. (SB trend courtesy of Saeed Montazeri and Nathan Stevenson.)

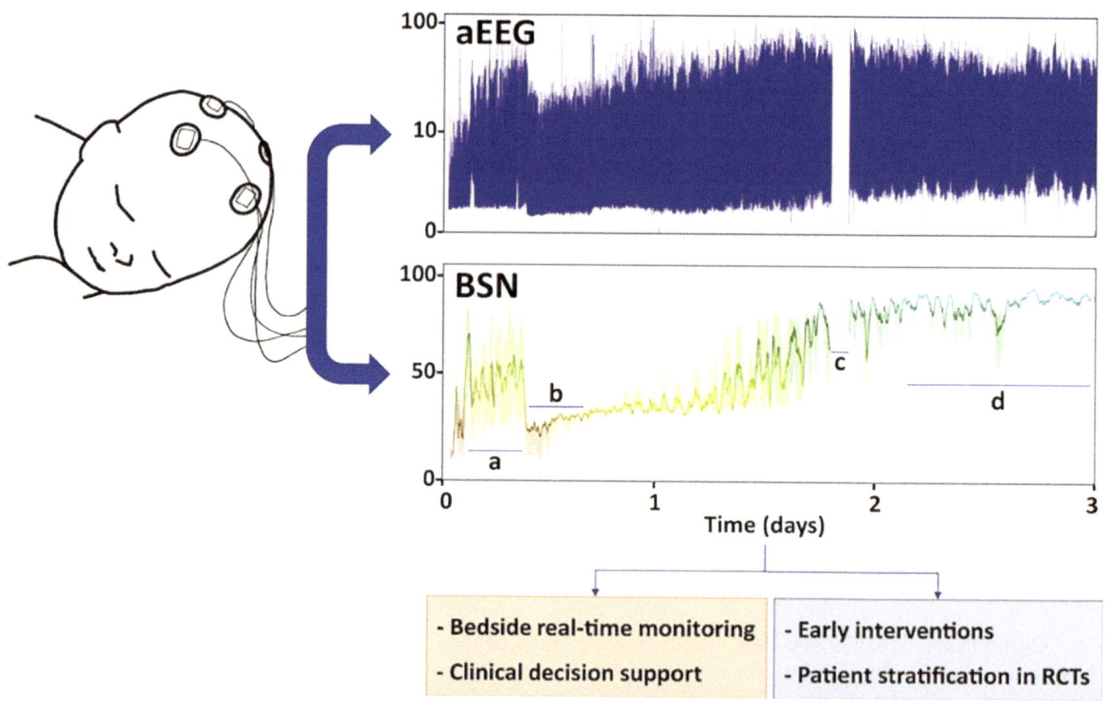

FIGURE 8.5 Comparison of the aEEG and the BSN trends in an example of 3-day brain monitoring in an infant recovering from perinatal asphyxia. The automated EEG background classifier BSN can provide substantial added information to several periods of clinical interest: a, initial brain recovery; b, transient suppression; c, care procedure; and d, emergence of an apparent sleep-wake cyclicity. (Modified from *Baud et al.*)

place. An indirect alternative to IBI is *suppression curve (SC)*, which aims to quantify the relative proportion of EEG signal in the "suppressed state".

Interhemispheric synchrony is another key aspect in the visual review of neonatal EEG recordings. High interhemispheric synchrony means that the bursting activity appears to be mostly co-incident between two hemispheres during quiet sleep (background categories *tracé discontinu* or *tracé alternant*); however, there are no clear or physiologically sound criteria for its visual quantitation. Recently, a computational measure *Activation Synchrony Index* (*ASI*) was developed to provide an objective and quantitative metric, a mimic of visual assessment.

Sleep-wake cycling (*SWC*) is a key characteristic in the visual EEG or aEEG review, and it refers to an alternation between successive sleep states (see SST in Figures 8.2, 8.3, 8.5). Identifying SWC requires detecting at least one sleep state, followed by observing their alternation over hours. However, the visual assessment is always qualitative and usually dichotomic, with high interrater variability and without established objective definitions. Some clinicians note SWC when they identify a single quiet sleep epoch during the reviewed time (range from tens of minutes to multiple hours), whereas other clinicians may apply stricter criteria and consider SWC only when they see rhythmic recurrence of quiet sleep epochs over multiple hours. To reduce variability and ambiguity, a novel measure *Brain Activity Cycling* (*BAC*) was recently developed as an objective and quantitative measure of SWC from multiple hours of brain monitoring signal.

8.4.2 Computational Measures beyond the Visually Reviewed EEG Properties

The raw EEG signal contains (patho)physiologically meaningful information that can be measured computationally from very long-time epochs (tens of minutes to hours). Such signal properties cannot be assessed visually, so these computational measures cannot be directly compared to visual aEEG/EEG review. For instance, EEG signal at one moment can statistically correlate to EEG signal many minutes away from it, and such correlation can be effectively measured with *Detrended Fluctuation Analysis* (*DFA*) *or its multifractal component* (*MFDFA*). These measures are sensitive to discontinuity in the EEG background, so they are also indirect measures of IBI without an actual burst detection. Alternatively, it is possible to measure statistical properties of the EEG bursts from very large (hundreds or thousands) collections of bursts using fully automated burst detections. This analysis can measure "burst shapes" or "burst scaling", which are strongly related to early cerebral hemorrhage, cortical maturation and long-term outcome in the preterm infants, as well as to early outcomes in the asphyxiated infants. All these fully methods can be fully automated; however, they are still waiting for prospective clinical validations and testing of bedside utility.

Maturation of cortical activity is routinely assessed in the visual review (Chapter 7); however, it can be done even more accurately with machine learning–based algorithms that provide a fully automated measure of *Functional Brain Age* (*FBA*). The FBA measures may track maturation of EEG activity longitudinally or detect developmental delays (Predicted Age Difference, PAD), which may link to abnormal long-term neurodevelopment.

8.4.3 Future Directions in the Computational Analyses of the Newborn EEG

Recent advances in computational methods have shown that it is possible to develop a fully automated EEG assessment for the newborn recordings, with a clinical meaning and accuracy that even compares with the expert's visual EEG review. It is important to note, however, that computational measures are supporting but not replacing clinical decision-making. The computational measures are designed, trained and validated for their respective roles, which may vary widely between use contexts. For instance, automated seizure detection can be used for assessing drug efficacy objectively in real time or post hoc, or it can be used for supporting clinician treatment decisions in individual infants. Likewise, an automated EEG background assessment could be used as a surrogate measure for stratification or as early endpoint in treatment trials, as well as for assessing recovery in individual patients. The technical and practical requirements for the novel computational tools vary widely, and they depend on the exact use cases. Therefore, it will be important to form international networks where novel tools can be assessed and validated specifically for each use case without immediate commercial interests. Such communal efforts created the success of the aEEG monitoring paradigm, and it will be needed again for building global experience and trust, with the ultimate aim at informing the next generation of guidelines.

References

Baud O, Arzounian D, Bourel-Ponchel E. Continuous monitoring of neonatal cortical activity: A major step forward. *Cell Rep Med.* 2022;3:100864.

Dereymaeker A, Koolen N, Jansen K, et al. The suppression curve as a quantitative approach for measuring brain maturation in preterm infants. *Clin Neurophysiol.* 2016;127:2760–2765.

Iyer KK, Roberts JA, Hellström-Westas L, et al. Cortical burst dynamics predict clinical outcome early in extremely preterm infants. *Brain.* 2015a;138:2206–2218.

Iyer KK, Roberts JA, Hellström-Westas L, et al. Early detection of preterm intraventricular hemorrhage from clinical electroencephalography. *Crit Care Med.* 2015b;43:2219–2227.

Kidokoro H, Inder T, Okumura A, et al. What does cyclicity on amplitude-integrated EEG mean? *J Perinatol.* 2012;32:565–569.

Koolen N, Dereymaeker A, Räsänen O, et al. Interhemispheric synchrony in the neonatal EEG revisited: Activation synchrony index as a promising classifier. *Front Hum Neurosci.* 2014;8:1030.

Montazeri S, Airaksinen M, Nevalainen P, et al. An automated bedside measure for monitoring neonatal cortical activity: A supervised deep learning-based electroencephalogram classifier with external cohort validation. *Lancet Digit Health.* 2022a;4:e884–e892.

Montazeri S, Nevalainen P, Metsäranta M, et al. Clinical outcome prediction using an automatically computed EEG background trend, Brain state of the newborn (BSN), after perinatal asphyxia. *Clin Neurophysiol.* 2024;162:68–76.

Montazeri S, Nevalainen P, Stevenson NJ, et al. Sleep state trend (SST), a bedside measure of neonatal sleep state fluctuations based on single EEG channels. *Clin Neurophysiol.* 2022b;143:75–83.

Navakatikyan MA, O'Reilly D, Van Marter LJ. Automatic measurement of interburst interval in premature neonates using range EEG. *Clin Neurophysiol.* 2016;127:1233–1246.

O'Toole JM, Boylan GB, Lloyd RO, et al. Detecting bursts in the EEG of very and extremely premature infants using a multi-feature approach. *Med Eng Phys.* 2017;45:42–50.

Palmu K, Wikström S, Hippeläinen E, et al. Detection of 'EEG bursts' in the early preterm EEG: Visual vs. automated detection. *Clin Neurophysiol.* 2010;121:1015–1022.

Pavel AM, Rennie JM, de Vries LS, et al. A machine-learning algorithm for neonatal seizure recognition: A multicentre, randomised, controlled trial. *Lancet Child Adolesc Health.* 2020;4:740–749.

Pillay K, Dereymaeker A, Jansen K, et al. Applying a data-driven approach to quantify EEG maturational deviations in preterms with normal and abnormal neurodevelopmental outcomes. *Sci Rep.* 2020;10:7288.

Plomgaard AM, Stevenson N, Roberts JA, et al. Early EEG-burst sharpness and 2-year disability in extremely preterm infants. *Pediatr Res.* 2023;95(1):193–199.

Räsänen O, Metsäranta M, Vanhatalo S. Development of a novel robust measure for interhemispheric synchrony in the neonatal EEG: Activation synchrony Index (ASI). *NeuroImage.* 2013;69:256–266.

Stevenson N, Oberdorfer L, Tataranno M-L, et al. Automated cot-side tracking of functional brain age in preterm infants. *Ann Clin Transl Neurol.* 2020a;7:891–902.

Stevenson N, Palmu K, Wikström S, et al. Measuring brain activity cycling (BAC) in long term EEG monitoring of preterm babies. *Physiol Meas.* 2014;35:1493–1508.

Stevenson N, Tataranno M-L, Kaminska A, et al. Reliability and accuracy of EEG-based age estimates in the preterm infant: Comparison of conventional EEG, amplitude-integrated EEG and an age prediction algorithm. *Ann Clin Transl Neurol.* 2020b;7:1564–1573.

Tapani K, Nevalainen P, Vanhatalo S, et al. Validating an SVM-based neonatal seizure detection algorithm for generalizability, non-inferiority and clinical efficacy. *Comput Biol Med.* 2022;145:105399.

9 ADVANCING NEONATAL NEUROCRITICAL CARE WITH BRAIN MONITORING

Sonia L Bonifacio

9.1 Introduction

Over the past 30 years, the availability and use of bedside neurological monitoring in the neonatal intensive care unit has increased substantially. What was previously employed in research studies to better understand the impact of illness and neonatal care on the immature newborn brain has translated to daily clinical practice with the goals of providing individualized and precise care. As our ability to resuscitate and support life in small and critically ill newborns continues to improve, brain monitoring is critical to monitor and support the developing brain with a goal of assuring the best possible neurologic outcome. Advances in monitoring technology (digitization and internet-based streaming) allow for broad implementation even in historically disadvantaged settings. Implementation of monitoring improves our identification and management of seizures and allows us to respond in real time, a substantial improvement of prior practice that was fraught with poor accuracy and/or delays in treatment leading to over and under treatment with antiseizure medications. Multimodal monitoring also allows for real-time adjustments in care practices such as ventilation and hemodynamic support with a goal of maintaining homeostasis in brain perfusion and potentially reducing harm.

9.2 Neurocritical Care for Neonates

The first formally dedicated Neuro-Intensive Care Nursery Program was developed in 2007 in San Francisco. However, the concept of specialized neurocritical care units and the practice of neurocritical care for neonates began to emerge in Europe and in the US already in the late 1990s and was based on results from observational studies of acute brain injury investigated with aEEG, EEG, ultrasound/Doppler, MRI, and NIRS in high-risk neonates (e.g. very preterm infants, asphyxiated infants and newborns with seizures). The increased scientific knowledge and awareness that these studies created were further amplified by the trials of therapeutic hypothermia for the treatment of moderate to severe encephalopathy due to perinatal hypoxia-ischemia. Therapeutic hypothermia is the first treatment with demonstrated efficacy for infants with hypoxic-ischemic encephalopathy (HIE), a diagnosis that carries high morbidity and mortality. Prior to this, neuroprotection in the neonatal care units was focused on prevention of intraventricular hemorrhage and in the provision of developmentally supportive care for preterm infants. In parallel, there was increased recognition and use of aEEG as a bedside brain monitoring device for high-risk infants. Advances in technology, such as the digitization of aEEG and conventional EEG, facilitated the uptake of use of aEEG in neonatal intensive care units, and aEEG was rapidly adopted in many centers worldwide. With use of bedside brain monitoring and neonatal neurocritical care services, the possibility to identify patients with seizures increased, and also improved the diagnostic accuracy of individual seizures, which prevents over-treatment of abnormal movements that are not seizures and improves treatment of electrographic seizures. So far, there have been no randomized controlled studies evaluating effects of the concept of neurocritical care. However, several observational studies have demonstrated that the neurocritical care concept is associated with less administration (around 30%) of antiseizure medication, reduced duration of exposure to antiseizure medications, and decreased hospital length of stay likely due to increased precision in the identification and treatment of seizures. New patient groups, such as infants with surgical problems, have also been increasingly recognized.

The fundamental aspects of the neonatal neurocritical care (NNC) model are the co-management of care between neonatologists and child neurologists and the use of care protocols and guidelines focused on the protection of the newborn brain. Patients include those with acute, emergent neurological diagnoses as well as those with more subacute and chronic neurological conditions that may present in term newborns or in those preterm newborns with neurologic morbidity. While the impetus for starting this program was the need to develop a therapeutic hypothermia program, it also opened the door for more deliberate collaboration between multiple groups, including neonatology, neurology/neurophysiology, nursing, neuroradiology, occupational and physical therapy, specialized neurodevelopmental care, and long-term follow-up. The creation of such a program provided a mechanism to develop focused neuroprotective strategies in the NICU.

Neuroprotective strategies from adult NCC, which is heavily focused on maintaining homeostasis and continuous monitoring, were translated into the NICU program with increased focus on regulation of temperature, glucose, ventilation and oxygenation, nutrition, and neuro-supportive care. Adult NCC is also highly focused on the use of care practice guidelines or protocols to standardize care and reduce variation which has resulted in reduced morbidity, mortality, and length of stay in the hospital. Specialized nursing care and nursing leadership support are another important element of both adult and neonatal NCC. Nurses are the team members that are present at the bedside 24 hours a day. They require advanced education and knowledge about neurological conditions and must be able to recognize abnormal neurologic findings in their patients. Trained nurses can apply brain monitoring quickly, learn to identify changes in brain activity by reviewing aEEG with regular frequency, and notify physicians to these changes. See Table 9.1A.

Recognizing that access to pediatric or neonatal neurology may be limited, a framework to prioritize which conditions could benefit from early co-management in the acute phase should be developed at each individual center. Table 9.1B provides an example of how different conditions can be prioritized based on acuity and the most prevalent neurological conditions that are cared for by the neonatal NCC team. The table shows the suggested time frame by which neurologists should be involved, anticipated duration of co-management between neonatology and neurology, and the type of neuromonitoring that should be performed.

DOI: 10.1201/b22858-9

TABLE 9.1A: Key Elements Necessary to Develop a Neonatal Neurocritical Care Programme

Key elements	Rationale
Self-identified physician and nursing leaders	This model of care requires consistent presence and culture change which can only be accomplished with dedicated leaders.
Training of all nursing staff	Nurses need training to recognize neurological conditions, identify seizures, develop competence in aEEG application and interpretation, implement TH, and facilitate neurodevelopmental care.
Protocols and guidelines • Brain monitoring • Seizure management • Stroke evaluation • Therapeutic hypothermia • Neuroimaging • Neuroprotective care	Use of protocols and guidelines are an effective means of providing evidence-based care and reducing variation in care. They should be updated with regular frequency. Using brain monitoring as an example, a guideline should contain information on who should be monitored, in what clinical circumstance, why it is important, and how long monitoring should be continued.
Daily collaboration between neonatology and neurology	Multi-specialty collaboration is important to ensure we broadly evaluate each patient and formulate a plan of care that addresses both the complex physiology present in NICU patients as well as the more nuanced neurological evaluation that may be required. It is critical for families to familiarize themselves with the teams that will provide care once discharged from the hospital. Collaboration between teams also assures consistent messaging to families, especially important for conversations about outcome and goals of care.

TABLE 9.1B: Suggested Framework for Co-Management between Neonatology and Neurology and Recommended Neuromonitoring by Neurological Condition

Neurological condition	Type of brain monitoring	Timing of notification of neurologist	Anticipated duration of co-management between neonatology and neurology
Acute/Emergent			
• Neonatal encephalopathy (due to hypoxia-ischemia or other causes)	aEEG/EEG, NIRS	As soon as patient is admitted to the NICU	Five to six days (cover period of TH, seizures and early imaging)
• Diagnosed or suspected seizures	aEEG/EEG	As soon as patient is being evaluated for possible seizures	Two to four days (cover acute treatment and investigations, planning follow-up)
• Known or suspected stroke	aEEG/EEG	As soon as patient is being evaluated for stroke	Same as those with seizures
• Acute intracranial hemorrhage	aEEG/EEG	At time intracranial hemorrhage is identified	Two to four days to cover period of active brain monitoring and imaging, then as needed to manage post hemorrhagic complications
• Acute CNS infection—meningitis/encephalitis	aEEG/EEG	At time CNS infection is identified	Two to four days to cover period of active brain monitoring and imaging, then at least once prior to discharge
Subacute/Chronic			
• Preterm infant with large IVH (grade III/IV)	aEEG/EEG	At time of recognition of hemorrhage	Two to four days, then 1/week to monitor for PVHD
• CNS malformation	Consider aEEG/EEG if clinical concern for seizures	At time of recognition	Two to four days then establish outpatient f/u plan
• Critical illness (sepsis, ECMO, cardiac malformation, post-major surgery)	aEEG/EEG, NIRS	At time of recognition of neurologic compromise	Two to four days, then consider risk of ongoing neurological injury

The concept of neurocritical care needs to adapt to local conditions. For example, in Brazil, remote evaluation of neuromonitoring with aEEG and consultation with neonatologists with expertise in neonatal neurology have resulted in significant uptake of brain monitoring (Figure 9.1). This is a successful model of care that may be applied to many other countries to provide neuroprotective care in an equitable fashion.

9.3 All Care Is Brain Care—Applying Principles of NeuroNICU Care to Every Baby in Every Unit

Attention to the impact of neonatal care on the developing brain is needed to optimize the neurodevelopmental outcomes of all NICU patients. Common practices and

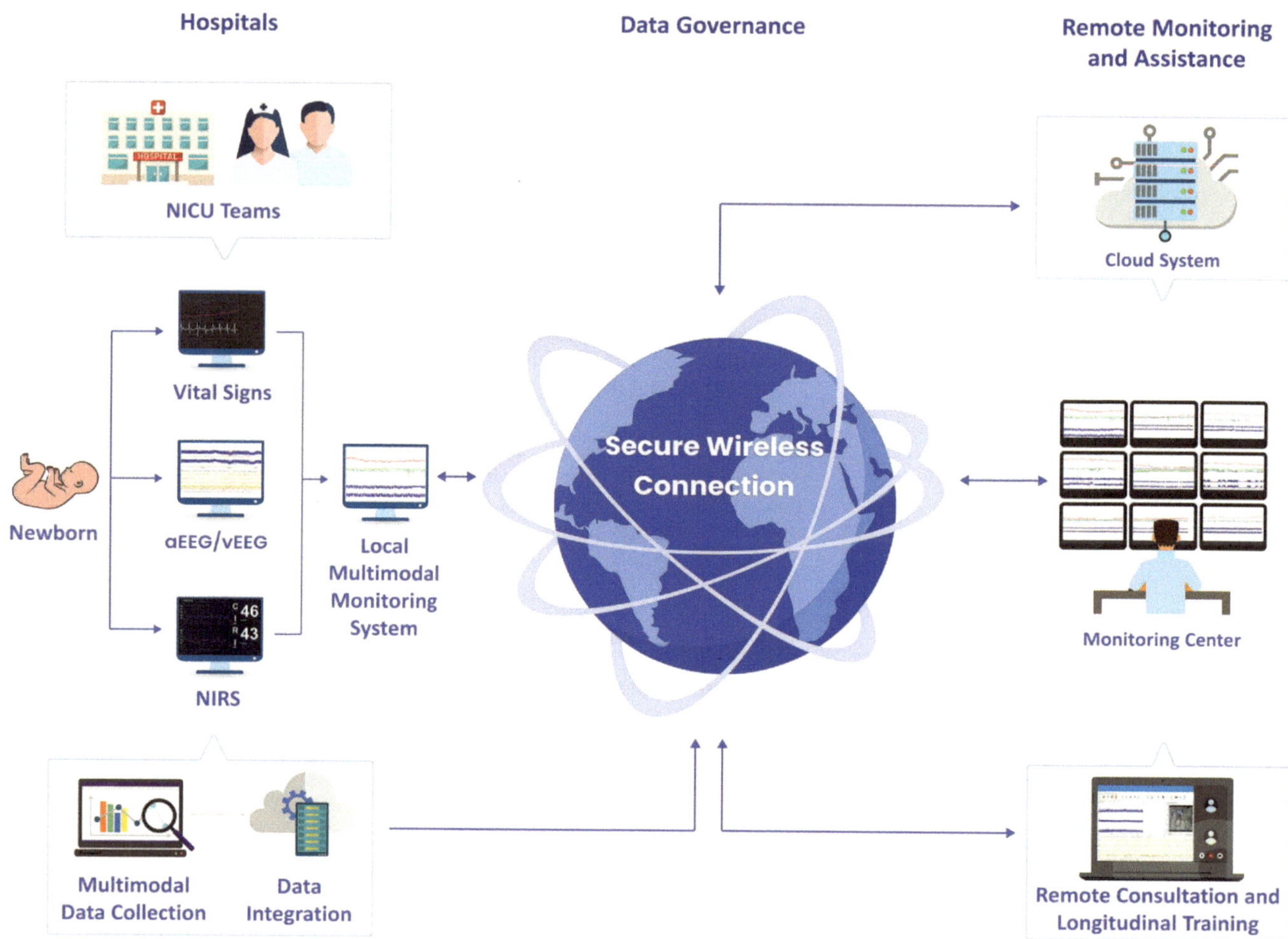

FIGURE 9.1 The organization of neonatal brain monitoring and neurology consultation within a large network of NICUs in Brazil: multimodality monitoring is supported by machine learning and AI; remote consultation and training is assisted by immersive reality tools. (Courtesy of Gabriel Variane.)

comorbid conditions such as mechanical ventilation, supplemental oxygen, use of inotropes, numerous painful and stressful procedures, inadequate nutrition/poor growth, bloodstream infections, and necrotizing enterocolitis all have the ability to negatively impact the developing brain. Consequently, both preterm and term infants can benefit from a neuro-protective, -supportive, -preventative approach to care. To reduce variations in care, care guidelines and care bundles should be developed that represent evidence-based care or local adaptations to current evidence.

Neuromonitoring with aEEG plays a key role in this framework. Extremely preterm infants and those with extremely low birthweight carry a significant risk of developing intraventricular hemorrhage, white matter injury and maldevelopment/dysmaturation of the cerebral white matter. Those who suffer high-grade intraventricular hemorrhage or parenchymal hemorrhagic infarctions are also at significant risk of seizures. aEEG monitoring in this population has identified that 30–40% of these infants have seizures diagnosed on monitoring. Seizures in the first week of life in preterm infants are associated with impaired neurodevelopment. Infants who are critically ill, sedated and/or paralyzed will also benefit from brain monitoring since they are at increased risk of neurological complications, including seizures. This includes infants on extracorporeal membrane oxygenation (ECMO) who are anticoagulated with an increased risk of intracranial/intraparenchymal hemorrhages that may necessitate the need for urgent imaging and a possible change in care. Newborns with congenital heart disease may also benefit from neuromonitoring, particularly in the immediate postoperative period as they, too, are at risk for cerebral hypoxia-ischemia and developing seizures.

9.4 Multimodal Monitoring

Multimodal monitoring in the form of combining aEEG with near-infrared spectroscopy (NIRS) is now common in neonatal care. NIRS monitoring can be used as a proxy of cerebral perfusion. NIRS is used primarily as a trending device and can assist with titration of mechanical ventilation settings, may inform providers about possible anemia and guide red blood cell transfusion, and may identify newborns who require inotropic support in the setting of hypotension in order to maintain adequate cerebral perfusion. There is no evidence that cerebral oximetry in ELBW infants during the first day of life would reduce the incidence of neonatal death or severe brain injury. However, in infants with HIE, the combination of regional oxygen saturation monitoring with NIRS and aEEG background pattern during the first days of life provides complementary information for outcome assessment. High cerebral saturations and lack of cerebral saturation variability are NIRS findings that are concerning.

Another clinically useful multimodal paradigm is the combination of cerebral activity monitoring (aEEG) to measuring subcortical functions with somatosensory evoked potentials (SEP). They can be performed at the same time by stimulating median nerve at wrists, followed by computing the SEP responses from the raw EEG signal available in the current aEEG monitors. Presence of cortical SEP responses indicates functional somatosensory pathways, and in particular the thalamus and thalamocortical pathways. Such finding provides a strong prediction of poor vs good outcomes over and beyond the prediction available from the aEEG/EEG review or neuroimaging. However, measuring SEP responses during the (a)EEG monitoring requires special training.

9.5 Suggested Clinical Practice Guidelines for Review of aEEG/vEEG

Table 9.1C shows an example of written recommendations for clinical review of aEEG once monitoring is initiated. The systematic approach to reviewing the recording as described in Chapter 2 should be used. In the neonatal intensive care unit, it is important to have clear delineation of roles and responsibilities amongst the staff for review of the aEEG to maximize the benefit of monitoring. Neonates with suspected seizures may need more frequent review of the aEEG trace and marking of the trace at the time of suspicious clinical events. Marking the aEEG is important to facilitate the review of the raw EEG that corresponds to such events. All physicians and advanced practice providers who work in the neonatal intensive care unit should have working knowledge of aEEG with the ability to place the device on patients, interpret the background, and identify common artefacts and seizures. The nursing staff who care for patients on aEEG monitoring should have the same knowledge as well as the ability to troubleshoot the monitoring device and identify changes in the aEEG background and seizures to notify providers in a timely fashion. It is vital that nurses understand how to annotate the monitor in real time so that the aEEG can be appropriately evaluated. When a patient is on monitoring, nurses can document the background pattern and presence of seizures in the electronic medical record with a prescribed frequency.

References

Bonifacio SL, Glass HC, Peloquin S, Ferriero DM. A new neurological focus in neonatal intensive care. *Nat Rev Neurol.* 2011;7(9):485–494.

Chock VY, Rao A, Van Meurs KP. Optimal neuromonitoring techniques in neonates with hypoxic ischemic encephalopathy. *Front Pediatr.* 2023;11:1138062.

Chock VY, Vesoulis ZA, El-Dib M, et al. The future of neonatal cerebral oxygenation monitoring: Directions after the SafeBoosC-III trial. *J Pediatr.* 2024;270:114016.

Das Y, Leon RL, Liu H, et al. Wavelet-based neurovascular coupling can predict brain abnormalities in neonatal encephalopathy. *Neuroimage Clin.* 2021;32:102856.

Duerden EG, Grunau RE, Chau V, et al. Association of early skin breaks and neonatal thalamic maturation: A modifiable risk? *Neurology.* 2020;95(24):e3420–e3427.

Glass HC, Bonifacio SL, Peloquin S, et al. Neurocritical care for neonates. *Neurocrit Care.* 2010;12(3):421–429.

Hansen ML, Pellicer A, Hyttel-Sørensen S, et al. Cerebral oximetry monitoring in extremely preterm infants. *N Engl J Med.* 2023;388(16):1501–1511.

Lemmers PM, Zwanenburg RJ, Benders MJ, et al. Cerebral oxygenation and brain activity after perinatal asphyxia: Does hypothermia change their prognostic value? *Pediatr Res.* 2013;74(2):180–185.

Murthy P, Zein H, Thomas S, et al. Neuroprotection care bundle implementation to decrease acute brain injury in preterm infants. *Pediatr Neurol.* 2020;110:42–48.

TABLE 9.1C: Example of aEEG/EEG Review Recommendations in a NNC Unit

Initiate monitoring as soon as possible § The goal is to start monitoring as soon as possible in a high-risk infant or infant with suspected seizures. § In these infants, the unit should establish an expected time limit for starting monitoring, for example, within 30 minutes of arrival of symptoms.
Frequent aEEG review during the first hour after recording initiated § Review the aEEG background pattern. § Look for suspected seizures on the aEEG trend and review the raw EEG for marked episodes corresponding to suspicious clinical seizures. § Be aware of common artefacts that may be confused with seizures. § The frequency of subsequent aEEG review is adjusted to the clinical situation, such as seizure occurrence or other adverse events. § In high-risk patients, for example, those with HIE and an abnormal electrocortical aEEG background activity, review should be performed every 1 to 2 hours in the first 12 hours, then every 2 hours for next 12–18 hours.
If seizures are identified § Treat according to your institutional guidelines. § Review aEEG closely and frequently after antiseizure medication (ASM) are administered. Note that electrographic seizures (aEEG/EEG) may continue even after stopping of clinical seizures. § If seizures continue 30 minutes after ASM, consider further medication. § If seizures stop after ASM, develop a plan to review the aEEG/EEG to identify seizure recurrence. § Make a plan for future aEEG/EEG review during the highest risk period.
If uncertain, ask for help § Call the physician in charge. § If suspicion is high on aEEG and raw EEG, consider administering phenobarbital.

Nevalainen P, Metsäranta M, Marchi V, et al. Towards multimodal brain monitoring in asphyxiated newborns with amplitude-integrated EEG and simultaneous somatosensory evoked potentials. *Early Hum Dev.* 2021;153:105287.

Shah DK, Zempel J, Barton T, et al. Electrographic seizures in preterm infants during the first week of life are associated with cerebral injury. *Pediatr Res.* 2010;67(1):102–106.

Smith GC, Gutovich J, Smyser C, et al. Neonatal intensive care unit stress is associated with brain development in preterm infants. *Ann Neurol.* 2011;70(4):541–549.

Variane GFT, Dahlen A, Pietrobom RFR, et al. Remote monitoring for seizures during therapeutic hypothermia in neonates with hypoxic-ischemic encephalopathy. *JAMA Netw Open.* 2023;6(11):e2343429

Wietstock SO, Bonifacio SL, McCulloch CE, et al. Neonatal neurocritical care service is associated with decreased administration of seizure medication. *J Child Neurol.* 2015;30(9):1135–1141.

Wietstock SO, Bonifacio SL, Sullivan J, et al. Continuous video electroencephalographic (EEG) monitoring for electrographic seizure diagnosis in neonates: A single-center study. *J Child Neurol.* 2016;31(3):328–332.

Case 9.1 Term Infant with Congenital Heart Defect

This is a term infant with a prenatal diagnosis of Tetralogy of Fallot with Pulmonary Atresia with Multiple Aorto-Pulmonary Collaterals (TOF/PA/MAPCAs) and left-sided congenital diaphragmatic hernia (CDH). At birth, the infant was intubated due to known CDH. An umbilical arterial line and a peripherally inserted central venous line were placed. After birth, the infant was somewhat pale with poor perfusion but showed improvement. First blood gas demonstrated mild acidosis with a pH of 7.1 and a base deficit of 5 mmol/L. The following morning, about 12 hours after birth, there was an acute drop in hematocrit and a mild coagulopathy.

Cranial ultrasound demonstrated an intraparenchymal left temporal occipital hemorrhage.

Brain monitoring in the form of *aEEG*/cEEG was initiated, and multiple seizures were identified. The initial three-channel aEEG shows left, right and cross-cerebral channels and corresponding raw EEG trace (Figure 9.1A). "The initial activity shows a slightly discontinuous pattern with suspected seizures." As more time passes, between 10:55 and 12:00, there are seven discrete areas of elevation of the lower and upper margin that should be investigated for seizure and were confirmed on review of the raw trace. Two doses of phenobarbital, 20 mg/kg/dose, were administered at the following times: 11:36–11:56; 14:00–14:29. At about 12:20, we can see the emergence of a more appropriate background pattern for a term infant who has received phenobarbital. The background appears discontinuous. The raw trace below the aEEG trace demonstrates seizure occurring at a time later than what is shown on the compressed trace.

The next day, another seizure was detected, best seen on the cross-cerebral recording (P3-P4) (Figure 9.1B). The background pattern has recovered to a CNV with imminent SWC. In Figure 9.1C, the full EEG is shown, with seizures best seen in C3-Fp and T3-O1.

Cranial *ultrasound* (Figure 9.1D) (a) shows a midline shift and a left-sided irregular area of increased echogenicity suggestive of a hemorrhage. The *MRI*-T2 (b) and DWI (c) demonstrate a subpial hemorrhage with adjacent ischemia of the cortex and white matter as well as parenchymal hemorrhage.

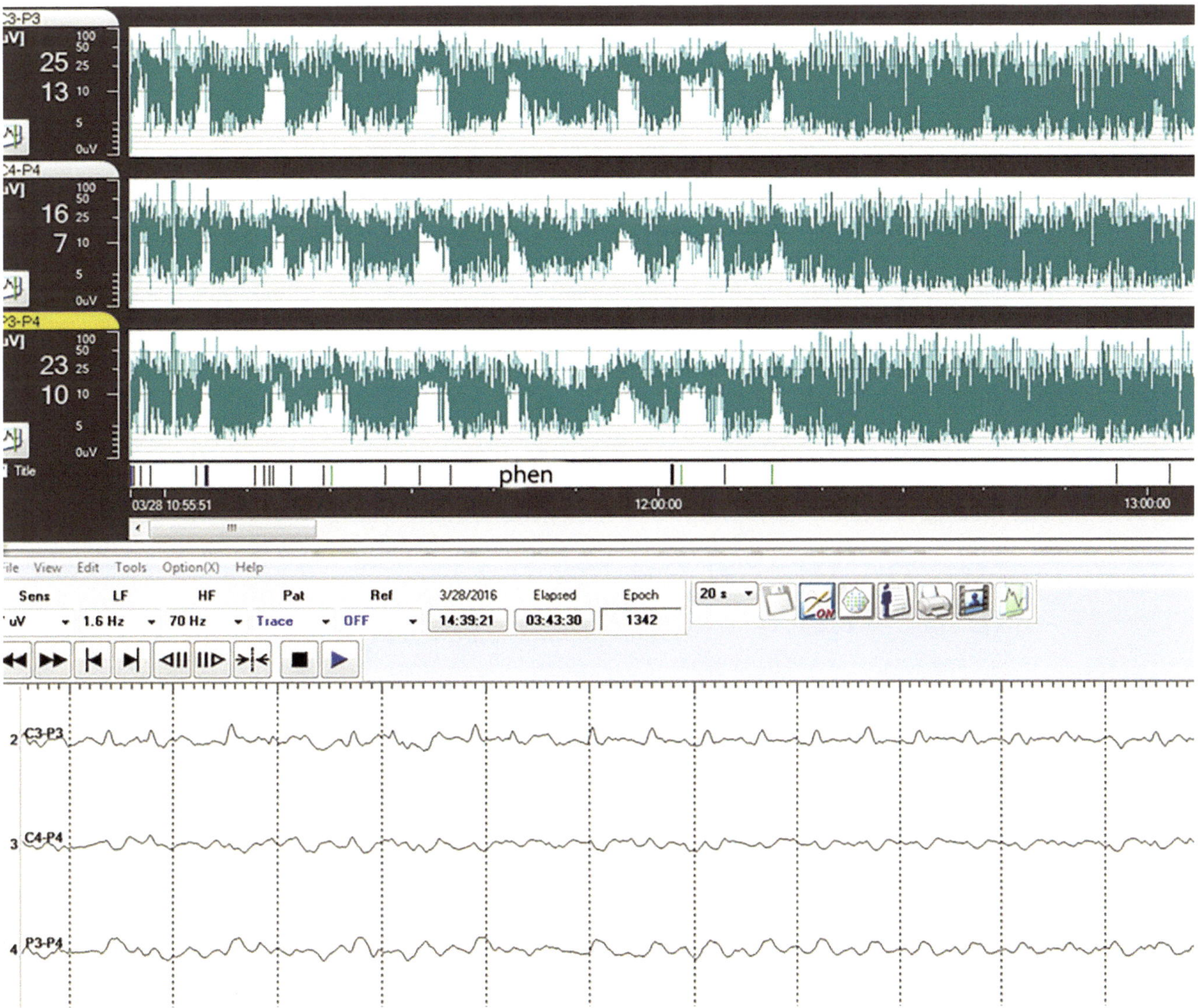

FIGURE 9.1A

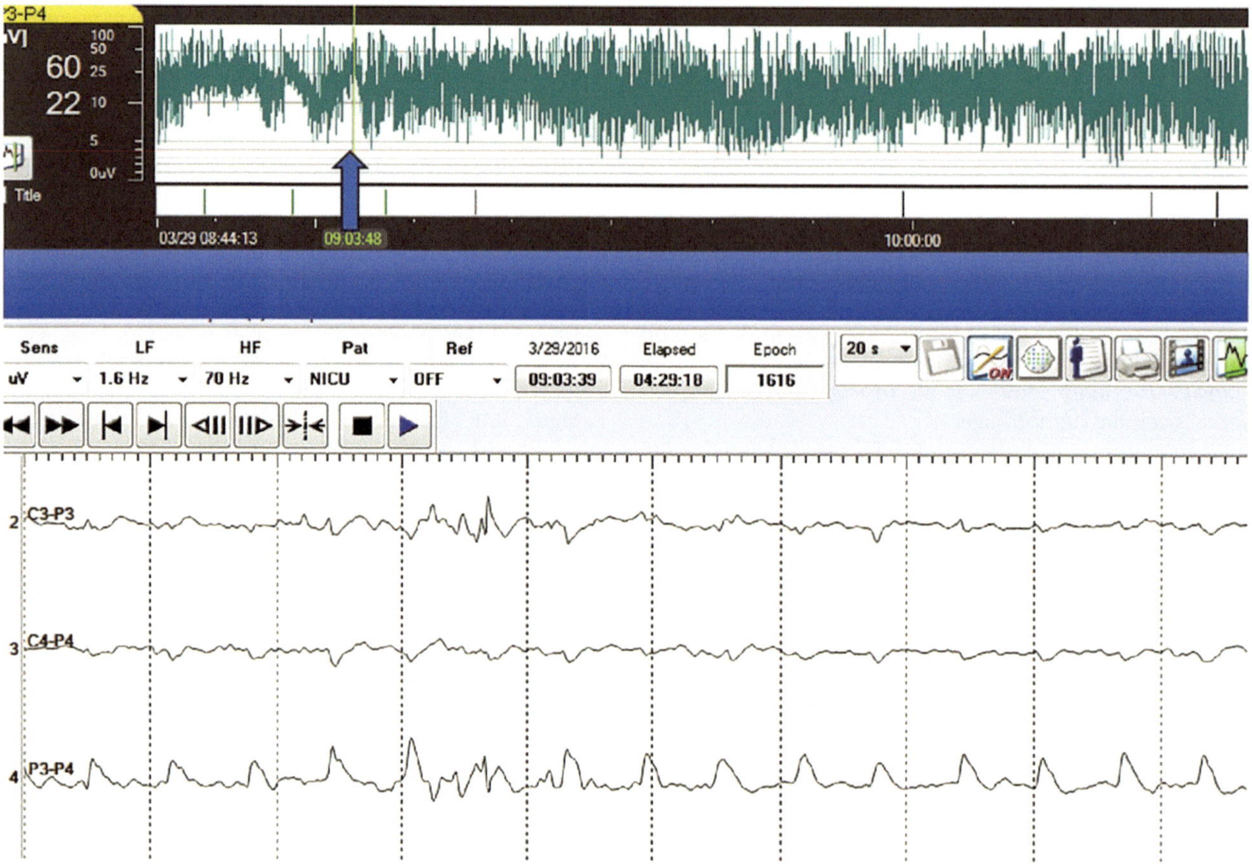

FIGURE 9.1B

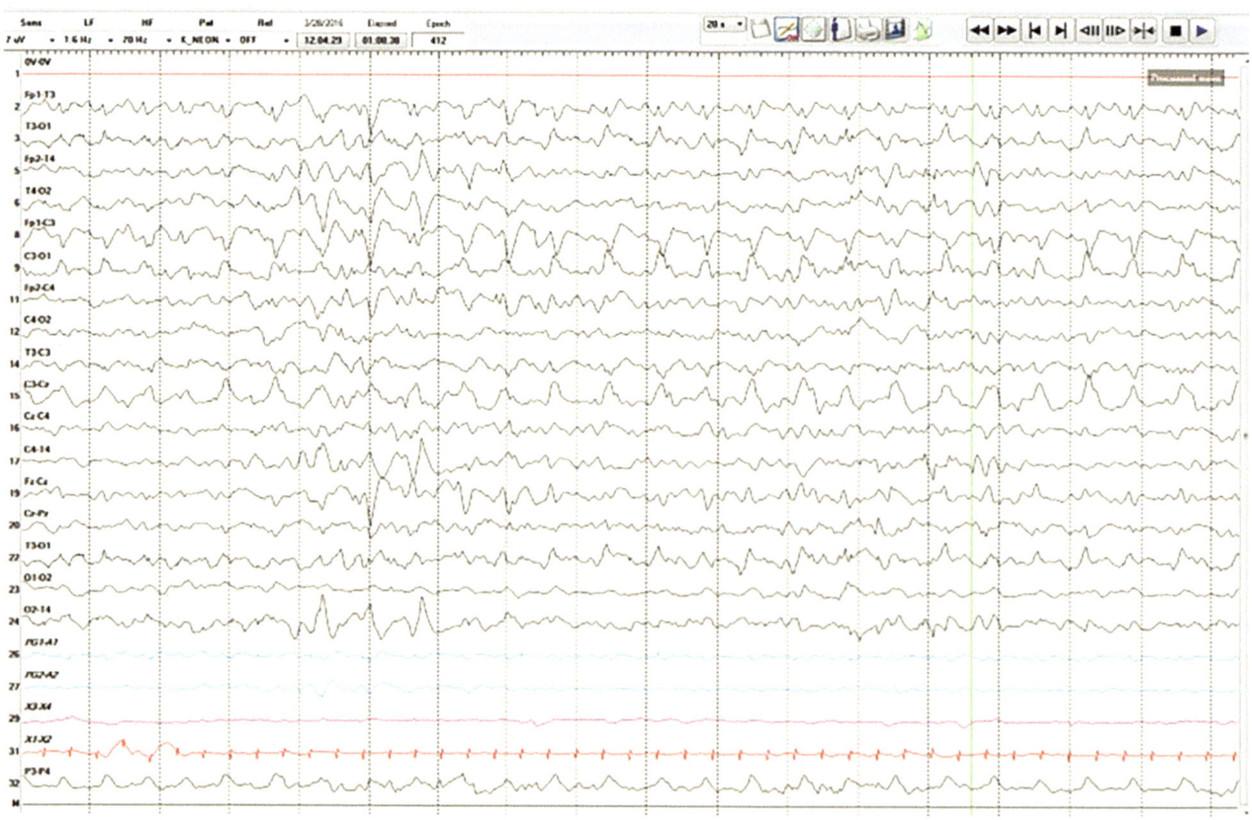

FIGURE 9.1C

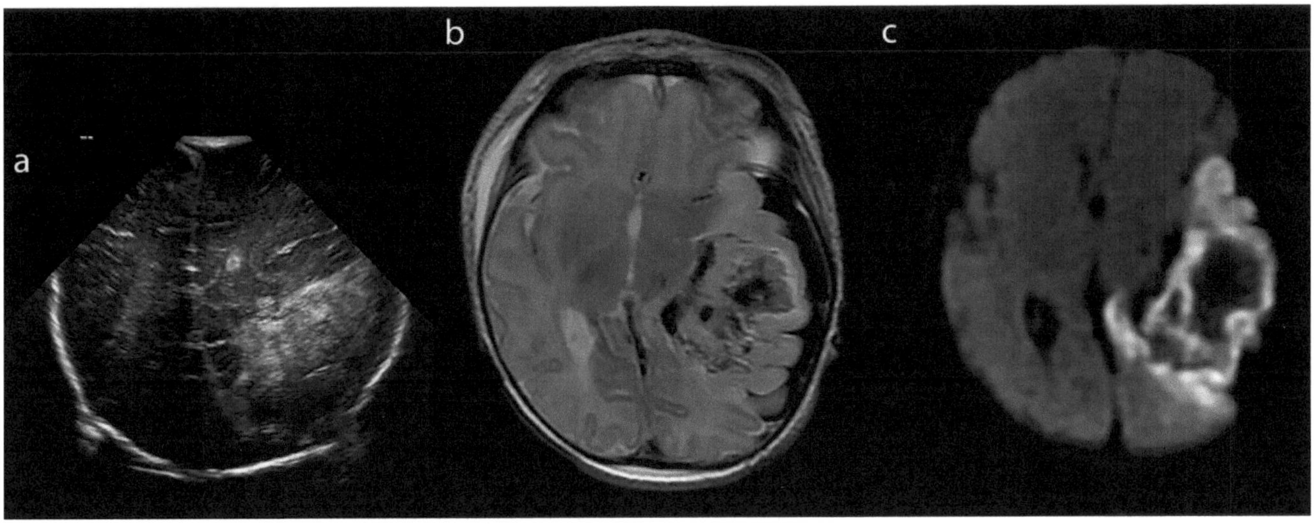

FIGURE 9.1D

Case 9.2 Preterm Infant with Pericardial Effusion, Severe Metabolic Acidosis, and Brain Injury

This is a 32-week preterm infant with acute onset of profound metabolic acidosis at 24 hours after birth. At the time of delivery, the infant was intubated, surfactant administered, umbilical lines placed, and then extubated to CPAP. Infant was found mottled with poor perfusion, low blood pressure, and low oxygen saturation. A blood gas was obtained and revealed a pH of 6.7, a base deficit of −30, and a lactate of 17 mmol/L. The infant was transferred to a tertiary hospital, and follow-up blood gas had persistent metabolic acidosis. An emergent echocardiogram was performed and revealed pericardial tamponade. The fluid was drained and found to have a glucose of >1200 mg / dL and was consistent with extravasated parenteral nutrition. The infant had ongoing profound metabolic acidosis for greater than 12 hours with anuria, coagulopathy, liver dysfunction and brain injury.

The *aEEG* at the time of admission to the tertiary center shows the left, right, and cross-cerebral channels. The background pattern is most consistent with burst-suppression (Figure 9.2A). In Figure 9.2B, you can see there are elevations of the lower margin, starting around 7:00, that are concerning for seizures. On this aEEG device, we can see the red line/arrow that correlates the aEEG trace with the raw EEG trace. We see rhythmic ictal activity in the raw EEG trace. Figure 9.2C demonstrates recurrent repetitive seizures predominantly on the right and identified by elevation of the lower and upper margin.

Cranial *ultrasound* was obtained (Figure 9.2D) and demonstrated a right-sided germinal matrix hemorrhage, diffuse increased echogenicity of the white matter and loss of grey-white differentiation.

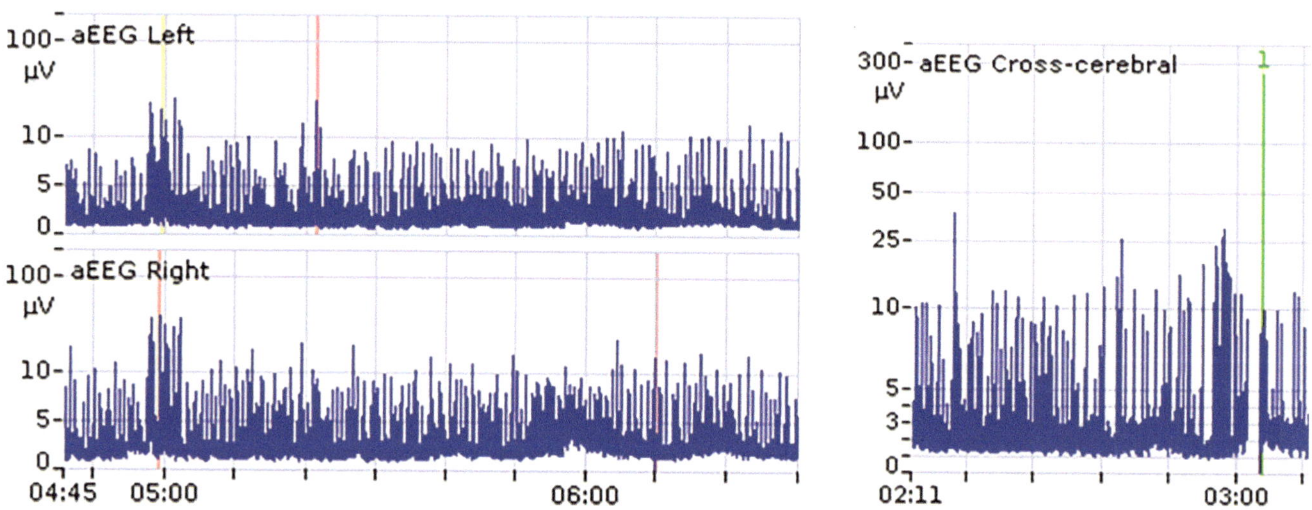

FIGURE 9.2A

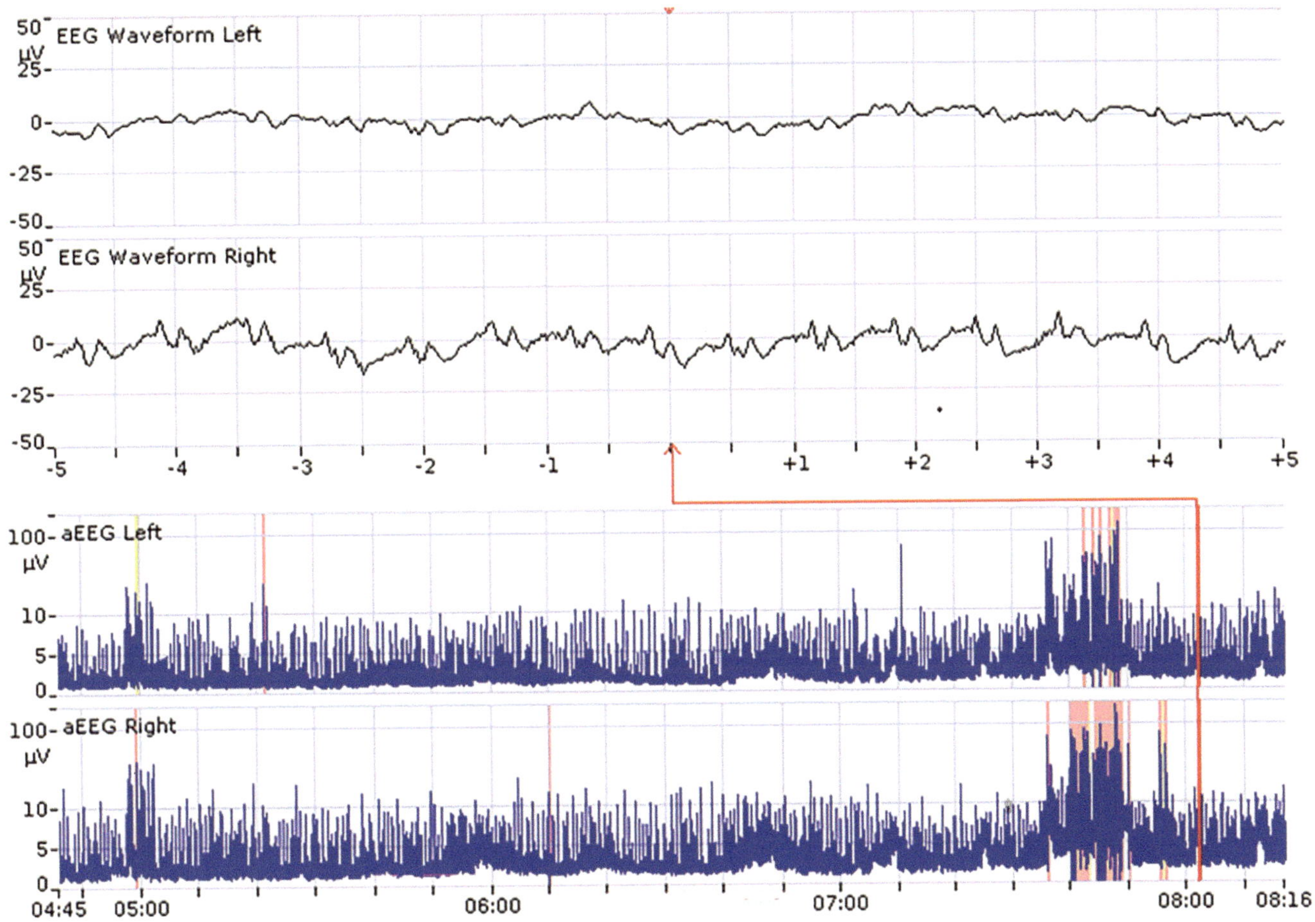
EEG Waveform Left
EEG Waveform Right
aEEG Left
aEEG Right
µV
04:45
05:00
06:00
07:00
08:00
08:16

FIGURE 9.2B

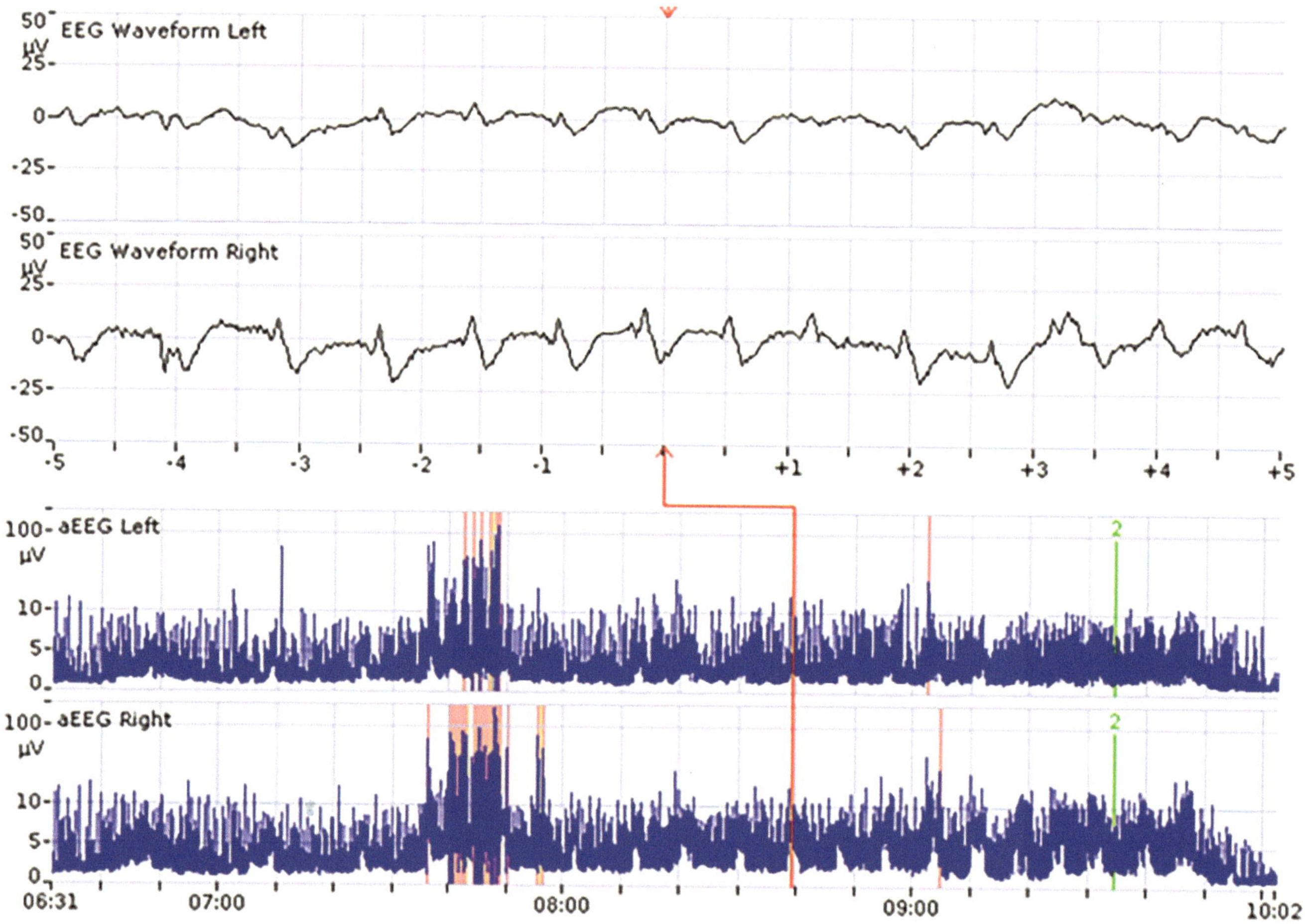

FIGURE 9.2C

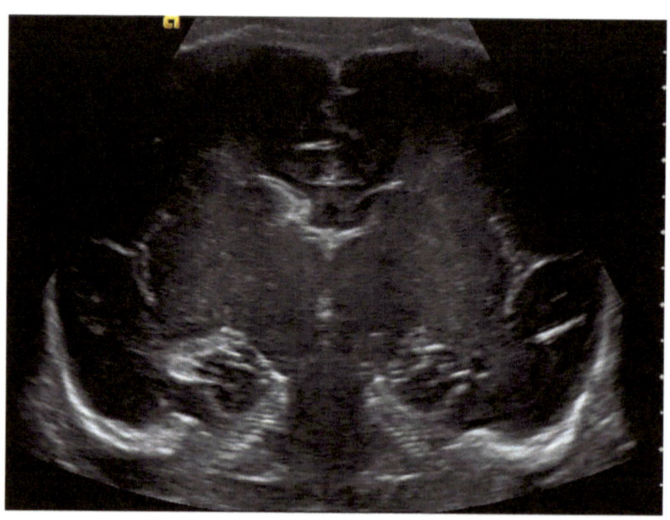

FIGURE 9.2D

Case 9.3 Multimodal Monitoring in a Preterm Infant (couresy of Gabriel Variane)

A preterm infant of 29 weeks and birthweight of 970 g was admitted to the neonatal intensive care unit with respiratory distress and was stable on CPAP. During the fourth day after birth, oxygen saturation dropped to 20%, and HR decreased from ~160 bpm to ~100 bpm associated with a depression on aEEG background activity, evolving from a discontinuous to continuous low-voltage pattern. The $rScO_2$ and $rSrO_2$ were noted to trend downward 2 and 8 hours, respectively, earlier than other vital signs abnormalities. The infant was diagnosed with a pericardial effusion by cardiac echo. After pericardiocentesis, a recovery of SpO_2, HR, $rScO_2$, $rSrO_2$ and aEEG background activity was immediately seen (Figure 9.3).

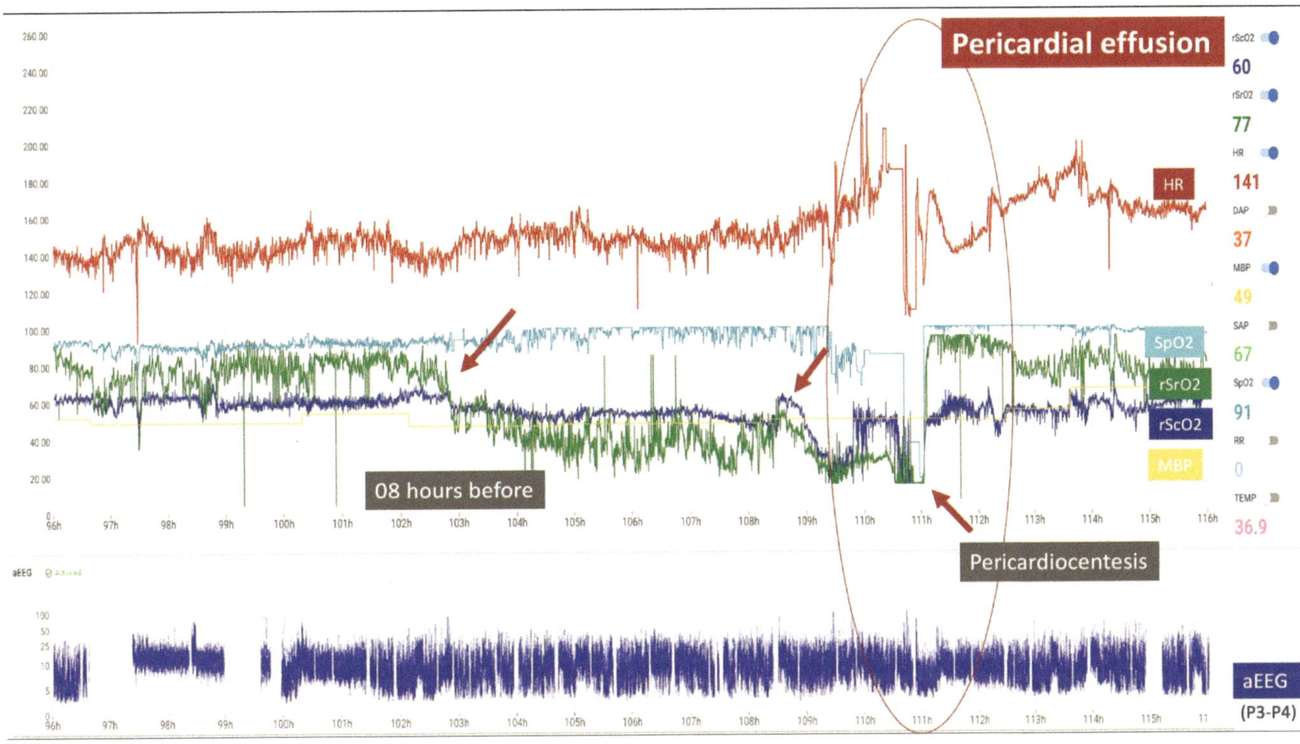

FIGURE 9.3 HR, heart rate; $rScO_2$, regional cerebral saturation; $rSrO_2$, regional renal saturation; SpO_2, pulse oximetry.

Case 9.4 Full-Term Infant with Progressing Mild to Moderate Encephalopathy with Seizures (courtesy of Lina Chalak)

This male infant was born at 41 weeks' gestation with a birthweight of 4360 grams by caesarean section. The membranes ruptured 16 hrs prior to delivery, and there was meconium-stained liquor. Apgar scores were 3 and 9 at 1 and 5 minutes, respectively, with an arterial umbilical pH of 7.26 and a base deficit of 16 mmol/L. He needed CPAP for a few days for respiratory distress.

Cranial *ultrasound* on admission showed no abnormalities. The initial Sarnat exam showed evidence of mild HIE at 3 and 6 hours after birth (incomplete weak Moro reflex and mild increase in tone).

cEEG was started at 6 hrs of age (Figure 9.4A). Repetitive right-sided seizures were confirmed on the aEEG at 22 hrs on a DNV background pattern, and phenobarbital and diazepam were required to control these seizures (Figure 9.4B). Hypothermia was started following the onset of seizures.

NIRS values remained in the normal range (75–85). Combining both NIRS and EEG in real time to evaluate very low frequencies signals revealed changes in neurovascular coupling as encephalopathy progressed from mild to moderate. Figure 9.4C shows in (a) wavelet-based MAP → $S_{ct}O_2$ coherence; the x-axis represents time, the y-axis represents scale (which has been converted to equivalent Fourier period), and the color scale represents the magnitude of R^2. The cone of influence (COI), where edge effects should be considered, is shown as a lighter shade. The black line contours designate areas of significant coherence ($p < 0.05$). The arrows designate the relative phase between MAP and $S_{ct}O_2$: a rightward-pointing arrow indicates in-phase coherence between the two signals ($\Delta\phi = 0$); a leftward-pointing arrow indicates anti-phase coherence ($\Delta\phi = \pi$). (a) First segment of the real-time MAP and $S_{ct}O_2$ data. Time zero indicates start of the EEG recording at 6 hours. In this squared cross-wavelet coherence, $R_{MAP \rightarrow SctO2}{}^2(n, s)$, red indicates normal neurovascular coupling at low frequency. The two signals fluctuate synchronously in a clear in-phase relationship indicating cerebral blood perfusion is matching the neuronal oscillations at the very low frequencies (0.0001–0.001).

Figure 9.4D: Impaired neurovascular coupling from the neonate after he progressed to have seizures and was treated with hypothermia for moderate encephalopathy. The two signals fluctuate in a clear anti-phase relationship with a periodicity of around 2 hours in very low frequencies of oscillations indicating mismatch at the very low frequencies (0.0001–0.001).

An MRI diffusion-weighted imaging (Figure 9.4E) showed diffusion restriction in the right frontal lobe.

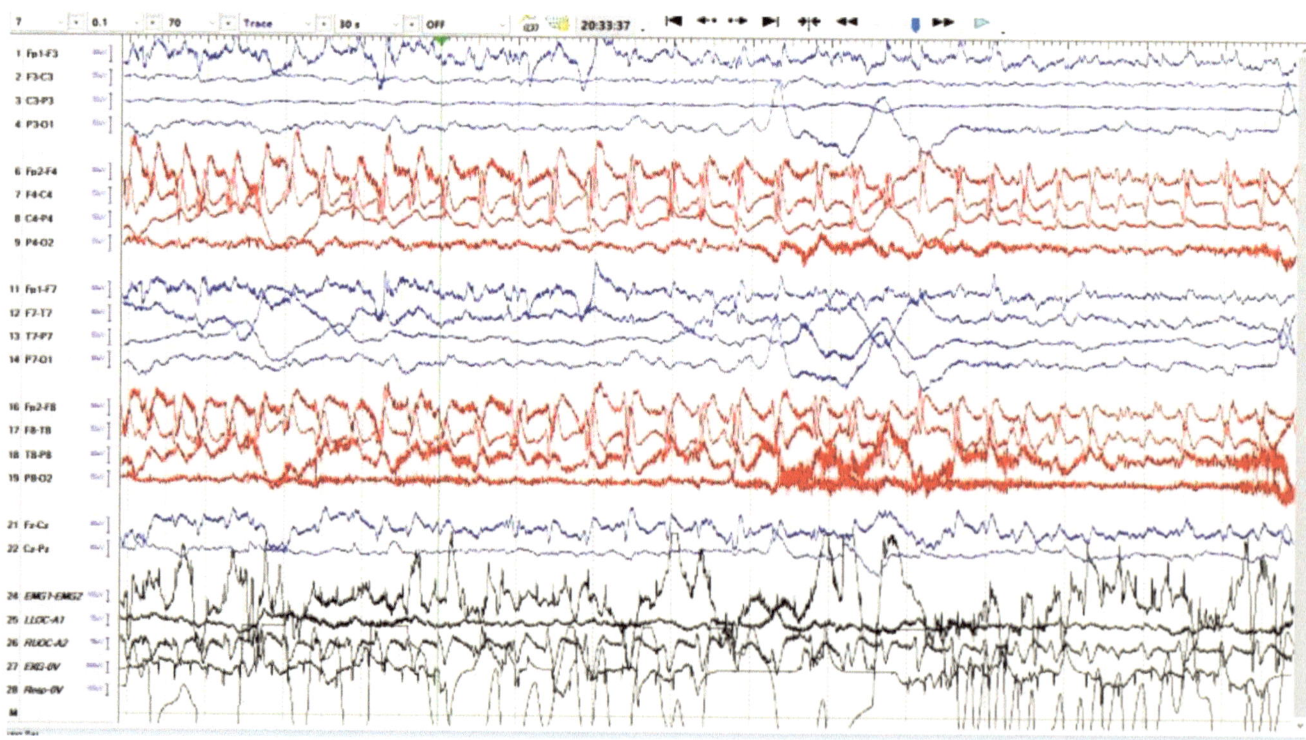

FIGURE 9.4A

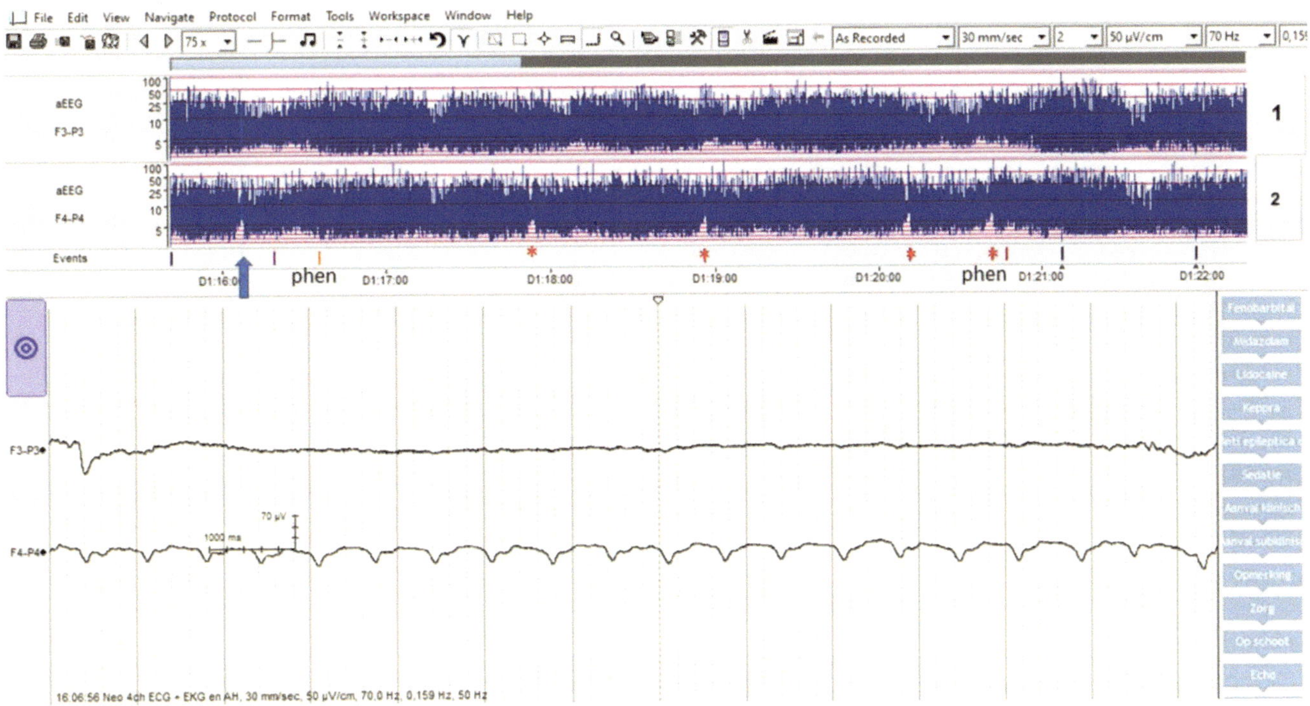

FIGURE 9.4B

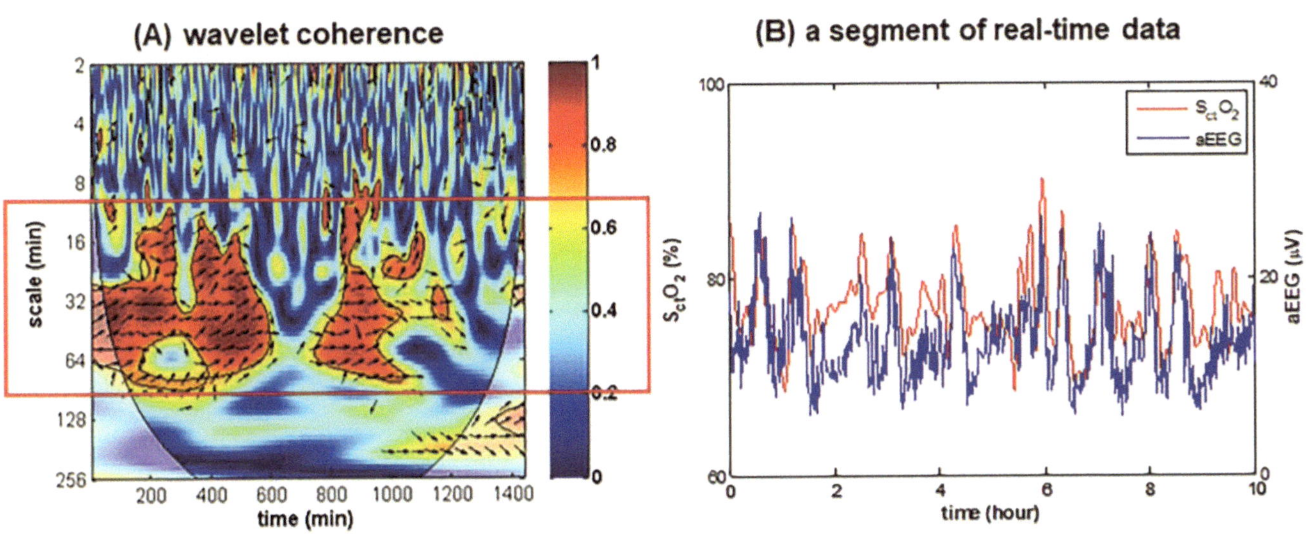

FIGURE 9.4C

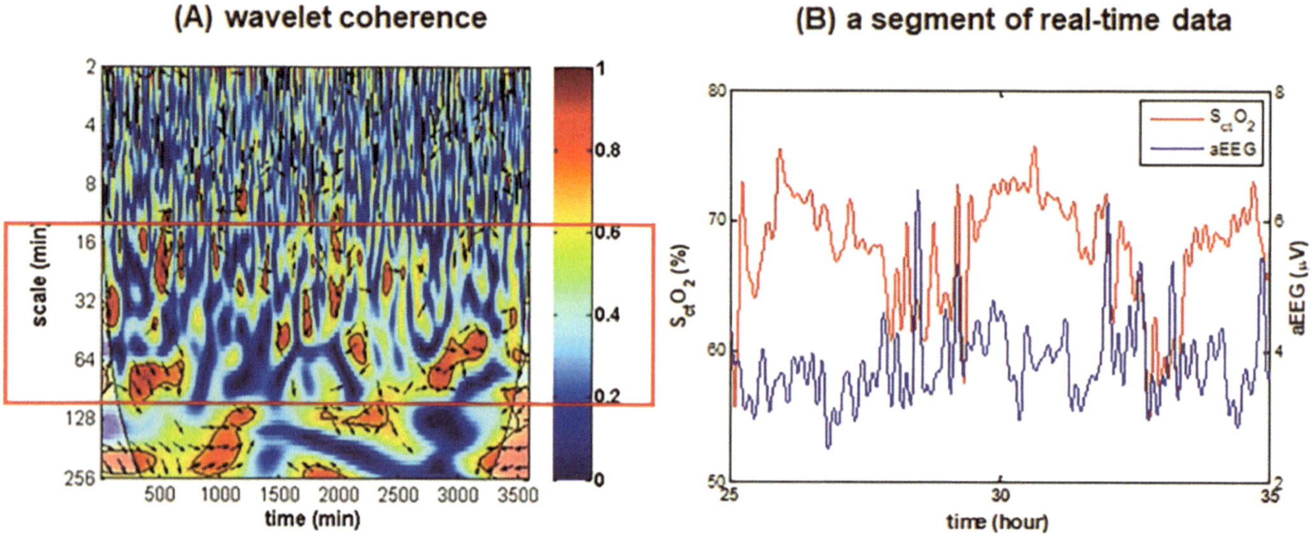

FIGURE 9.4D

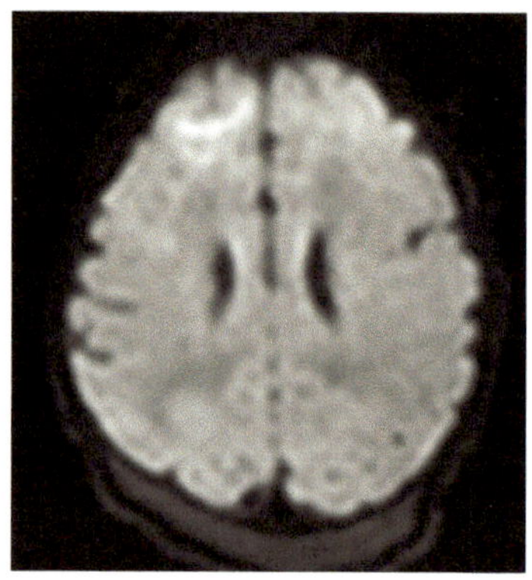

FIGURE 9.4E